SPECIALTY IMAGING™

GYNECOLOGIC ONCOLOGY

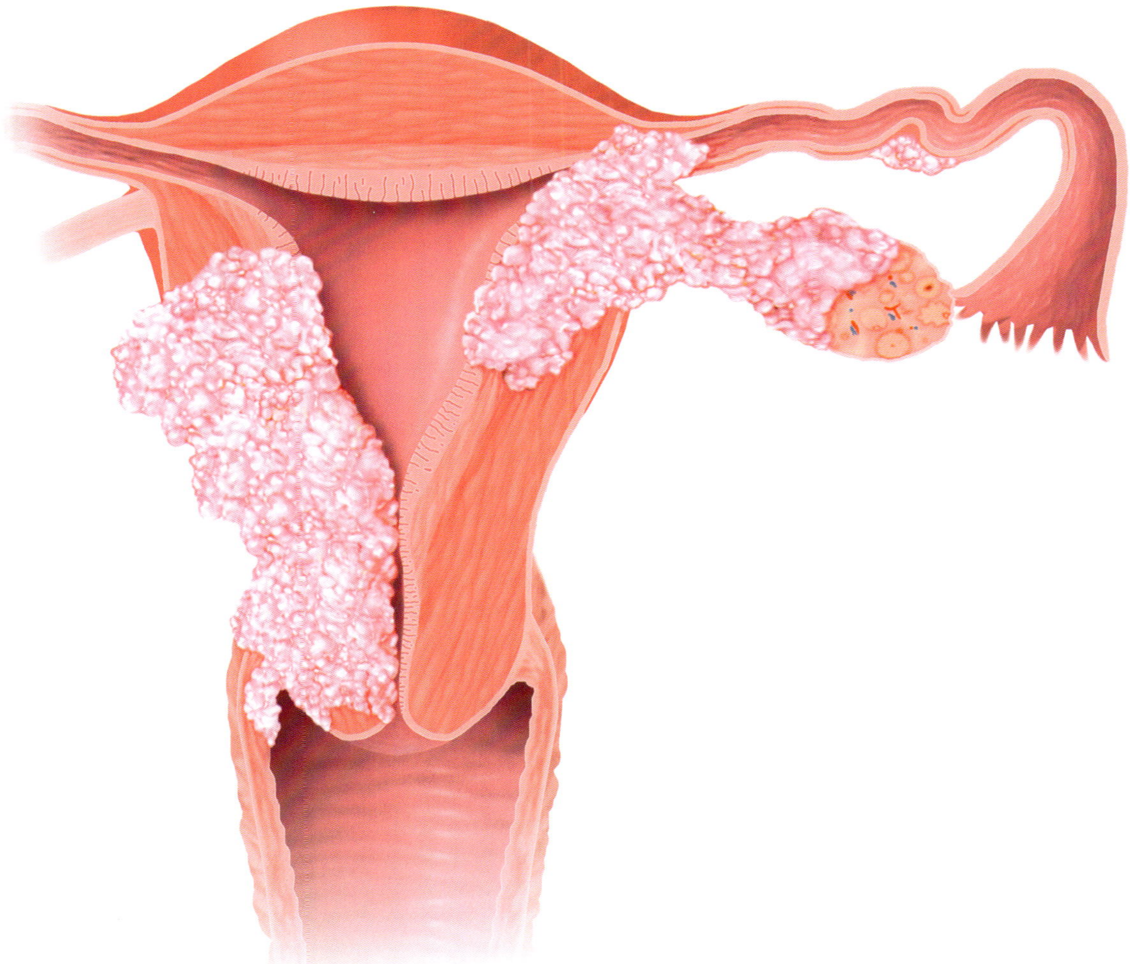

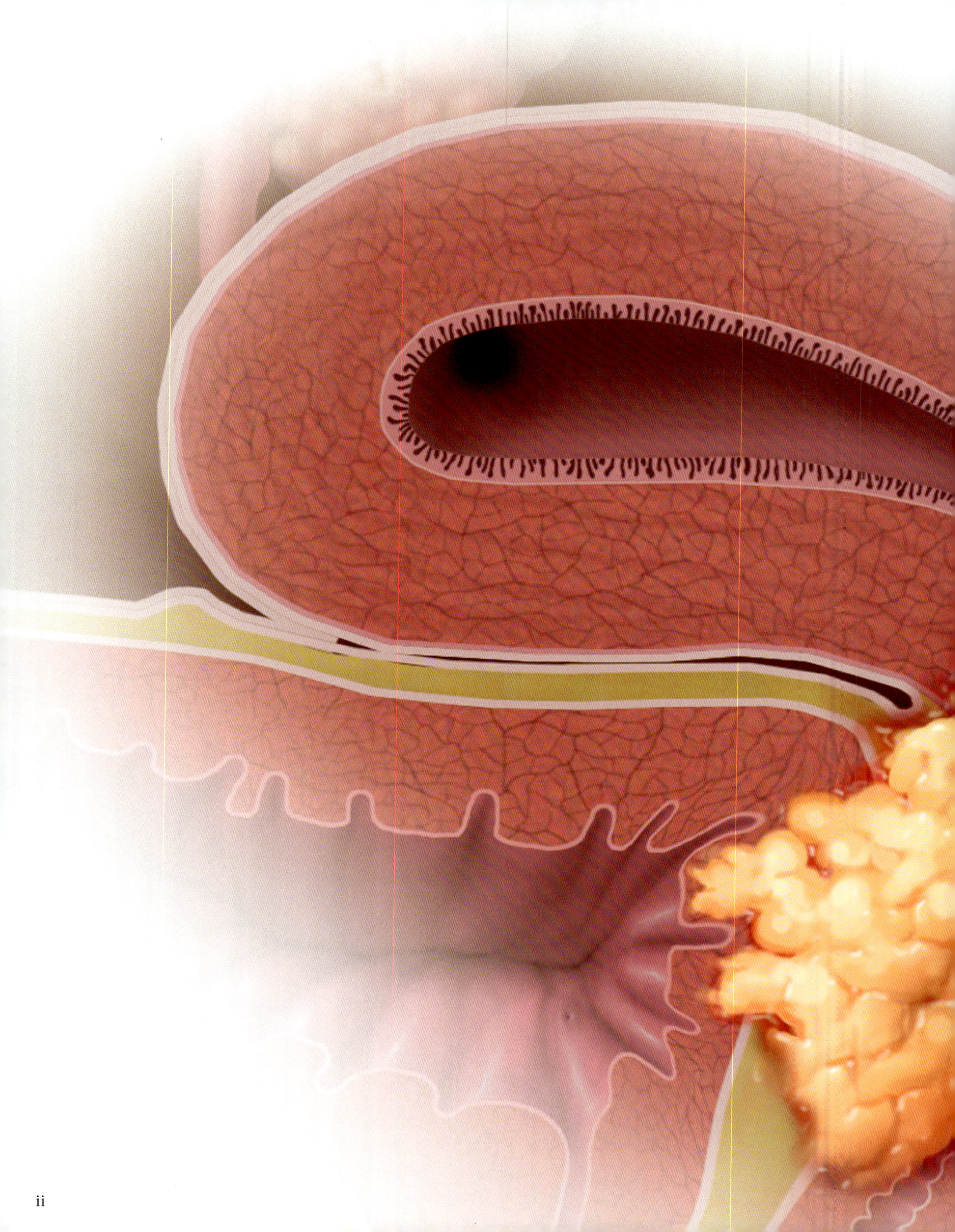

SPECIALTY IMAGING™

GYNECOLOGIC ONCOLOGY

Akram M. Shaaban, MBBCh

Associate Professor of Radiology

University of Utah School of Medicine

Salt Lake City, UT

Maryam Rezvani, MD

Assistant Professor of Radiology

University of Utah School of Medicine

Salt Lake City, UT

Todd M. Blodgett, MD

Adjunct Assistant Professor

University of Pittsburgh Medical Center

President, FRG Molecular Imaging

Foundation Radiology Group

Pittsburgh, PA

AMIRSYS®
Names you know. Content you trust.®

Printed in Canada by Friesens, Altona, Manitoba, Canada

ISBN: 978-1-931884-22-8

Notice and Disclaimer

Library of Congress Cataloging-in-Publication Data

Shaaban, Akram M.
Specialty imaging. Gynecologic oncology / Akram M. Shaaban, Maryam Rezvani, Todd M. Blodgett. -- 1st ed.
p. ; cm.
Other title: Gynecologic oncology
Includes index.
ISBN 978-1-931884-22-8
1. Generative organs, Female--Cancer--Imaging--Handbooks, manuals, etc. I. Rezvani, Maryam. II. Blodgett, Todd M. III. Title. IV. Title: Gynecologic oncology.
[DNLM: 1. Genital Neoplasms, Female--diagnosis. 2. Magnetic Resonance Imaging--methods. WP 145 S524s 2010]
RC280.G5S43 2010
616.99'465--dc22

2010014986

To my parents, I truly owe you everything.
To my wife Inji, son Karim and daughter May, the jewels of my life, thanks for your understanding and tremendous support.
AMS

To Mary Lou Magee, a great friend, confidant, and mother,
who developed a malignant brain tumor during the creation of this book.
I love you!
TMB

To my parents, Houshmand and Shahla, I dedicate not just this work
but all my efforts in life and faith.
To my sister, Sara, for believing in me and everything I humbly attempt.
MR

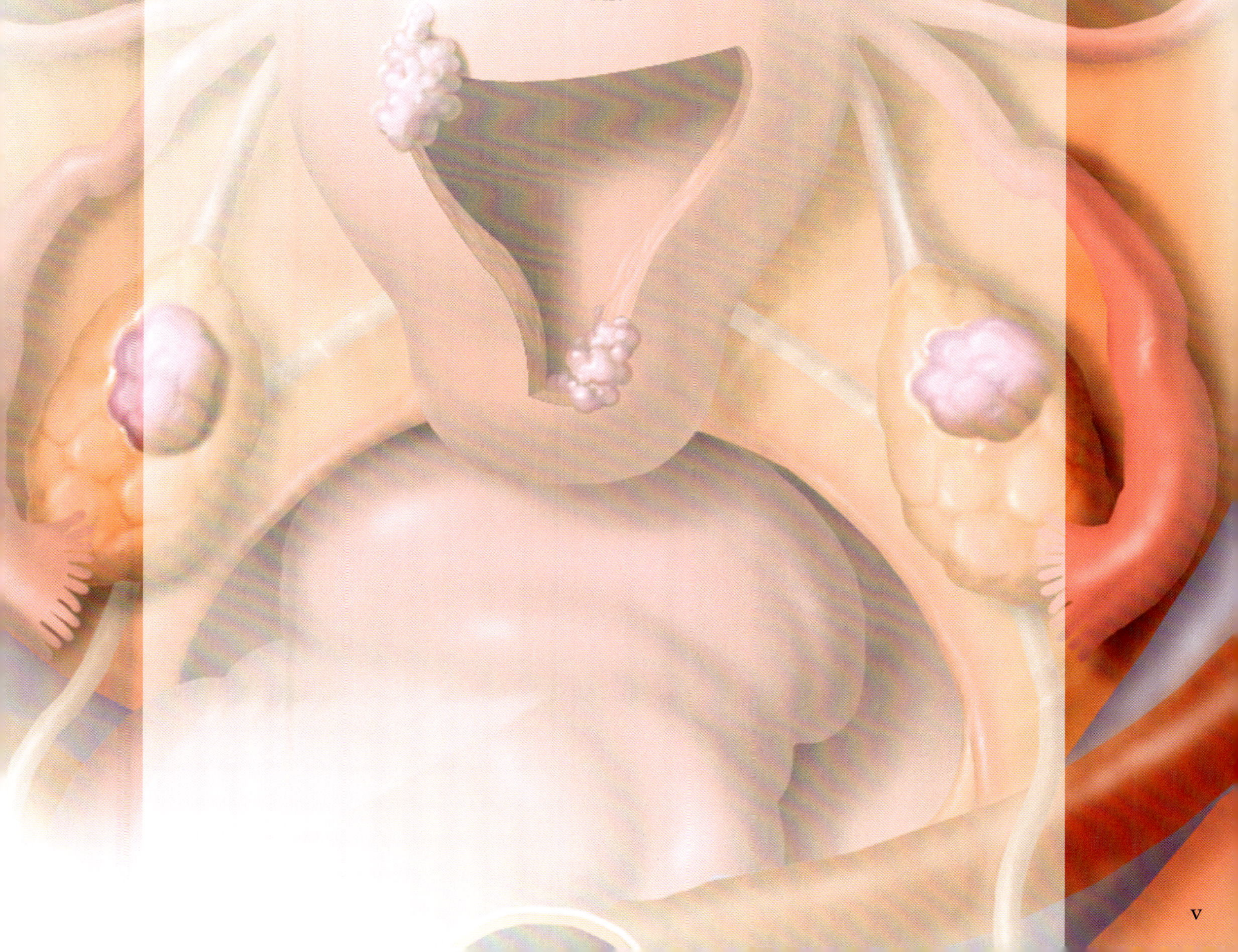

PREFACE

In *Specialty Imaging: Gynecologic Oncology*, Amirsys proudly presents the most up-to-date staging and imaging for gynecologic cancers—less than one year after the introduction of the 7th edition of the AJCC Cancer Staging Manual. This includes the redefined TNM and prognostic stage grouping for cancers of the vulva, cervix uteri, and corpus uteri, along with thorough discussion of gestational trophoblastic disease and cancers of the vagina, ovary, and fallopian tube.

Each lavishly illustrated chapter offers multiple ways to make sense of a particular gynecologic cancer. Quick reference tables provide the definitions for TNM, FIGO stages, and AJCC prognostic groups. Rich drawings illuminate these stages. High-quality images of practically every stage of every tumor demonstrate clinical appearances. All of these vivid images—more than 400 in the volume—are fully annotated to maximize their illustrative potential. Bulleted text distills the pertinent information to the essentials. Whether you are looking for routes of spread, imaging techniques for local staging, or treatment options, you will find it quickly in this easy-to-use yet comprehensive reference.

Like other Amirsys books, *Specialty Imaging: Gynecologic Oncology* was designed with you, the reader, in mind. We think you'll find this new volume a handy and wonderfully rich resource that will significantly enhance your practice—and find a welcome place on your bookshelf.

Paula J. Woodward, MD
David G. Bragg, MD and Marcia R. Bragg Presidential Endowed
Chair in Oncologic Imaging
Professor of Radiology
University of Utah School of Medicine
Salt Lake City, UT

ACKNOWLEDGEMENTS

Contributing Author

Mohamed E. Salama, MD
Assistant Professor
Department of Pathology
University of Utah and ARUP Reference Laboratory
Salt Lake City, UT

Text Editing

Kellie J. Heap
Arthur G. Gelsinger, MA
Katherine Riser, MA
Dave L. Chance, MA

Image Editing

Jeffrey J. Marmorstone
Danny C. La

Medical Editing

Jonathan Shakespear, MD

Illustrations

Lane R. Bennion, MS
Richard Coombs, MS
Laura C. Sesto, MA

Art Direction and Design

Laura C. Sesto, MA

Associate Editor

Ashley R. Renlund, MA

Production Lead

Melissa A. Hoopes

AMIRSYS®
Names you know. Content you trust.®

TABLE OF CONTENTS

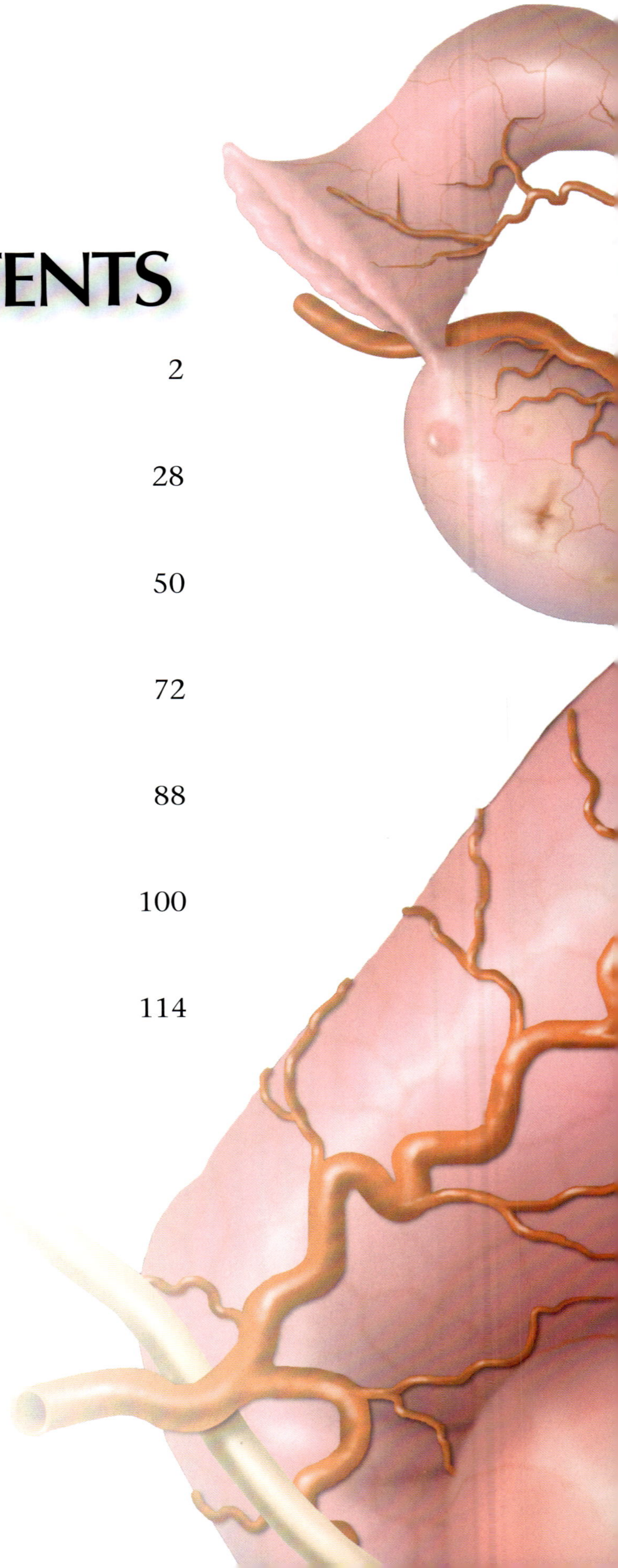

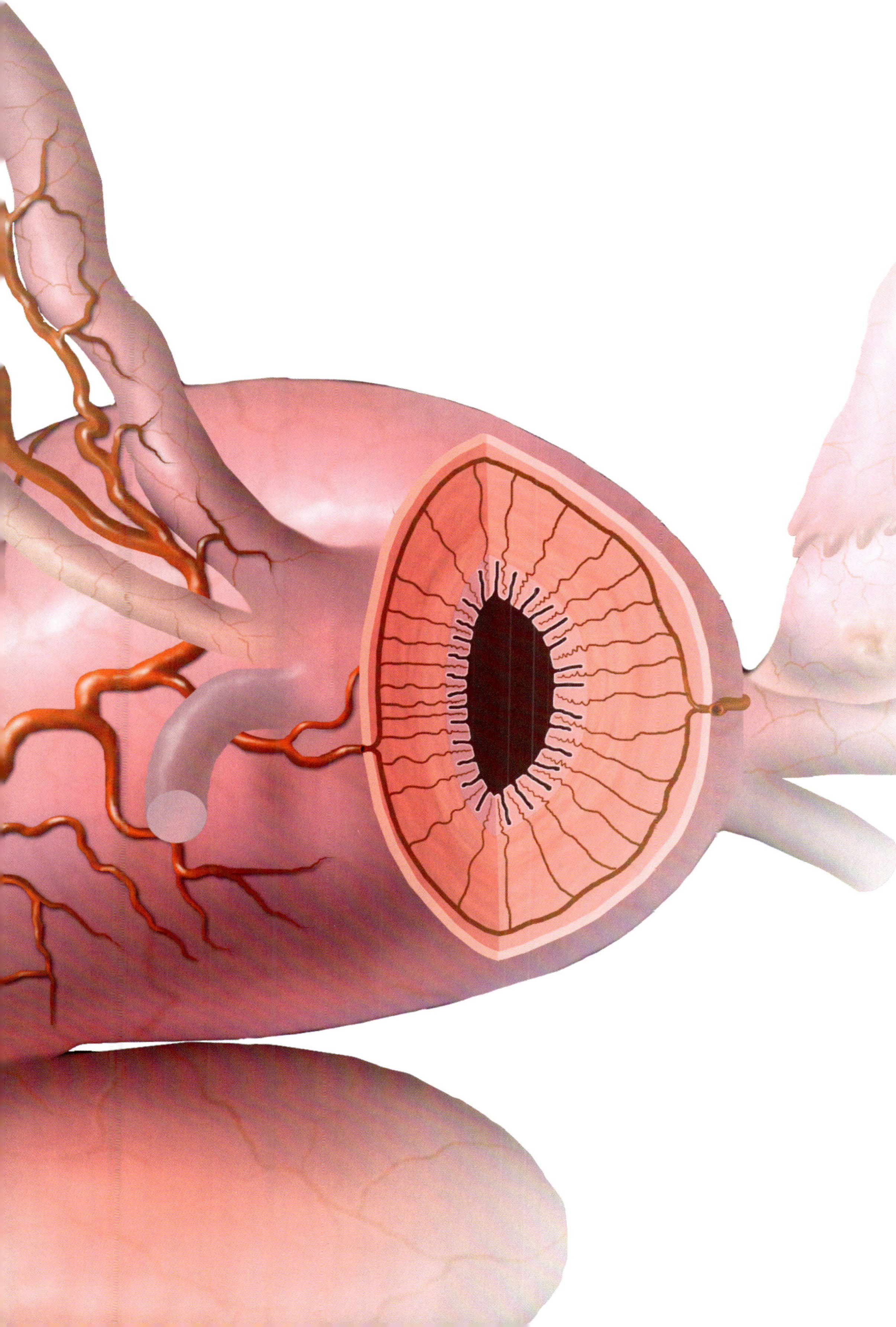

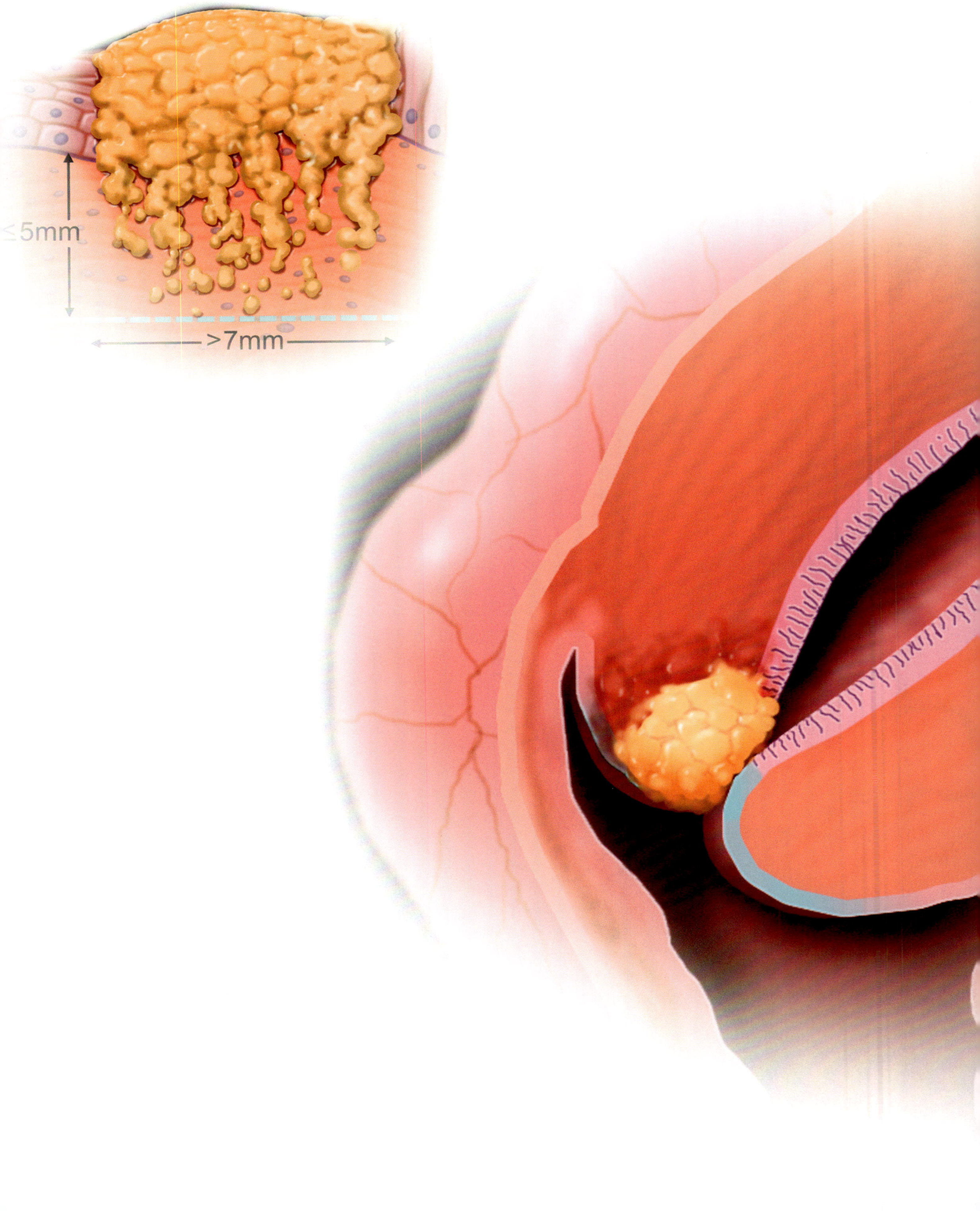
≤5mm
>7mm

Cervix Uteri Carcinoma

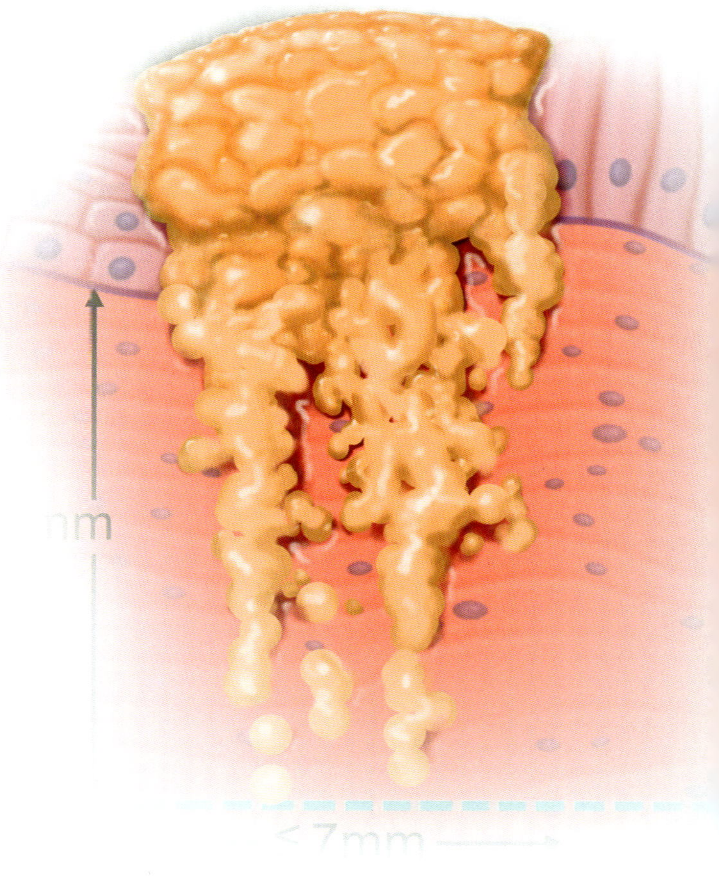

CERVIX UTERI CARCINOMA

(T) Primary Tumor

Adapted from 7th edition AJCC Staging Forms.

TNM	*FIGO*	*Definitions*
TX		Primary tumor cannot be assessed
T0		No evidence of primary tumor
Tis[1]		Carcinoma in situ (preinvasive carcinoma)
T1	I	Cervical carcinoma confined to uterus (extension to corpus should be disregarded)
T1a[2]	IA	Invasive carcinoma diagnosed only by microscopy; stromal invasion with a maximum depth of 5.0 mm measured from the base of the epithelium and a horizontal spread of ≤ 7.0 mm; vascular space involvement, venous or lymphatic, does not affect classification
T1a1	IA1	Measured stromal invasion ≤ 3.0 mm in depth and ≤ 7.0 mm in horizontal spread
T1a2	IA2	Measured stromal invasion > 3.0 mm and ≤ 5.0 mm with a horizontal spread ≤ 7.0 mm
T1b	IB	Clinically visible lesion confined to the cervix or microscopic lesions greater than T1a/IA2
T1b1	IB1	Clinically visible lesion ≤ 4.0 cm in greatest dimension
T1b2	IB2	Clinically visible lesion > 4.0 cm in greatest dimension
T2	II	Cervical carcinoma invades beyond uterus but not to pelvic wall or to lower 1/3 of vagina
T2a	IIA	Tumor without parametrial invasion
T2a1	IIA1	Clinically visible lesion ≤ 4.0 cm in greatest dimension
T2a2	IIA2	Clinically visible lesion > 4.0 cm in greatest dimension
T2b	IIB	Tumor with parametrial invasion
T3	III	Tumor extends to pelvic wall &/or involves lower 1/3 of vagina, &/or causes hydronephrosis or nonfunctioning kidney
T3a	IIIA	Tumor involves lower 1/3 of vagina, no extension to pelvic wall
T3b	IIIB	Tumor extends to pelvic wall &/or causes hydronephrosis or nonfunctioning kidney
T4	IVA	Tumor invades mucosa of bladder or rectum, &/or extends beyond true pelvis (bullous edema is not sufficient to classify a tumor as T4)

(N) Regional Lymph Nodes

NX		Regional lymph nodes cannot be assessed
N0		No regional lymph node metastasis
N1	IIIB	Regional lymph node metastasis

(M) Distant Metastasis

M0		No distant metastasis
M1	IVB	Distant metastasis (including peritoneal spread, involvement of supraclavicular, mediastinal, or paraaortic lymph nodes, lung, liver, or bone)

[1]*FIGO no longer includes stage 0 (Tis).* [2]*All macroscopically visible lesions, even with superficial invasion, are T1b/IB.*

CERVIX UTERI CARCINOMA

AJCC Stages/Prognostic Groups

Adapted from 7th edition AJCC Staging Forms.

Stage	*T*	*N*	*M*
0	Tis	N0	M0
I	T1	N0	M0
IA	T1a	N0	M0
IA1	T1a1	N0	M0
IA2	T1a2	N0	M0
IB	T1b	N0	M0
IB1	T1b1	N0	M0
IB2	T1b2	N0	M0
II	T2	N0	M0
IIA	T2a	N0	M0
IIA1	T2a1	N0	M0
IIA2	T2a2	N0	M0
IIB	T2b	N0	M0
III	T3	N0	M0
IIIA	T3a	N0	M0
IIIB	T3b	Any N	M0
	T1-3	N1	M0
IVA	T4	Any N	M0
IVB	Any T	Any N	M1

CERVIX UTERI CARCINOMA

Tis

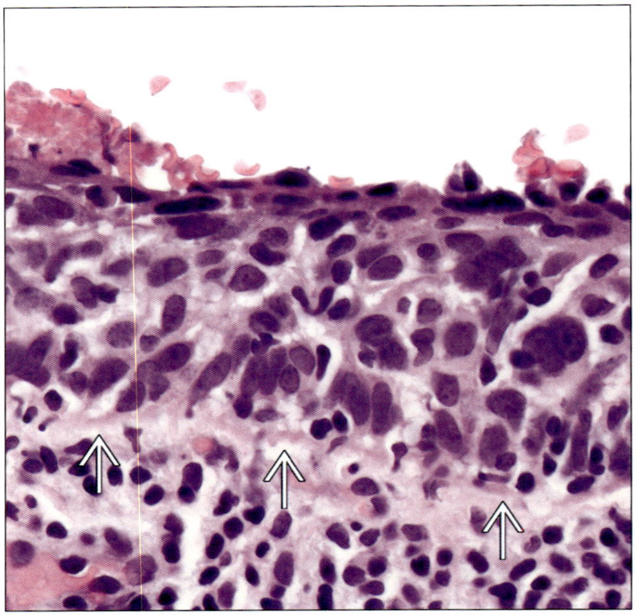

H&E stain shows high-grade squamous intraepithelial lesion. Cells have hyperchromatic nuclei, lack maturation, lack normal organization, and show indistinct cell membranes. Neoplastic cells are limited by the intact eosinophilic basement membrane, leading to the term "preinvasive carcinoma."

Methods for Microscopic Measurement of Depth of Invasion

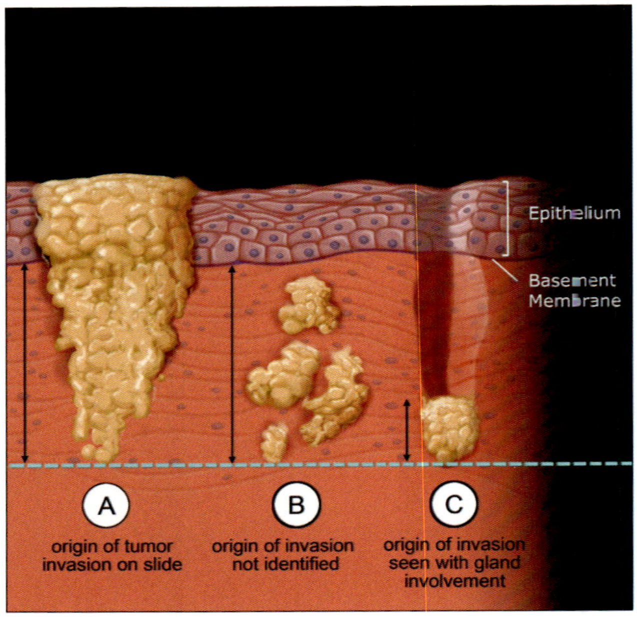

A. The depth of invasion is measured from the origin of invasion to the last cell of the invasion focus. B. Invasion is measured from the basement membrane to the last cell of the invasion focus. C. Invasion is measured from the site of origin to the last cell of the invasion focus.

T1a1

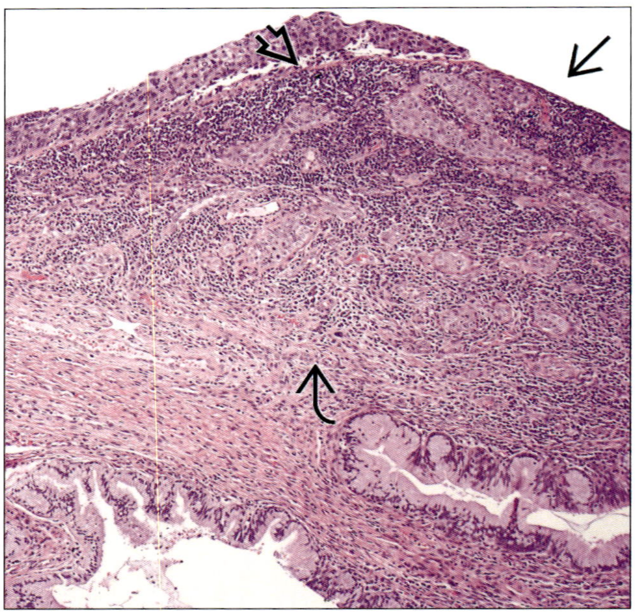

Low-power magnification H&E of cervix shows there is loss of squamous epithelium on the right with underlying moderately differentiated carcinoma characterized by irregular nests of squamous cells invading the stroma. Nests extend to a depth of 1.5 mm from basement membrane.

T1a1

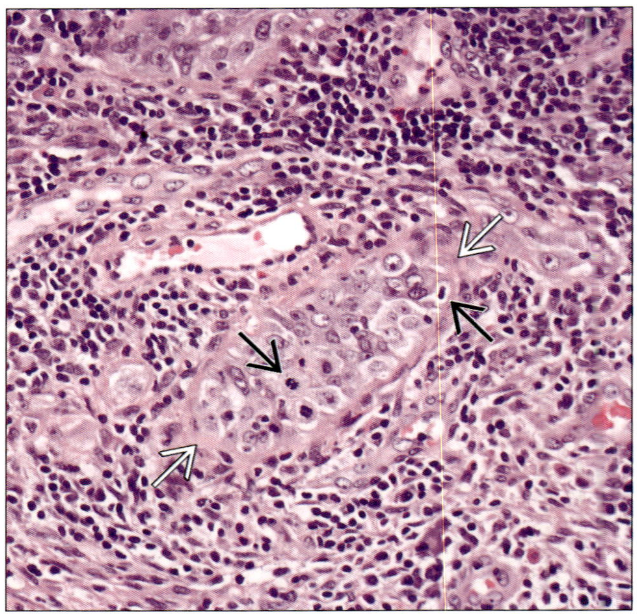

Higher power magnification shows the invasive squamous nests with mitotic figures and prominent surrounding inflammatory infiltrate. (Original magnification 400x.)

CERVIX UTERI CARCINOMA

T1a2

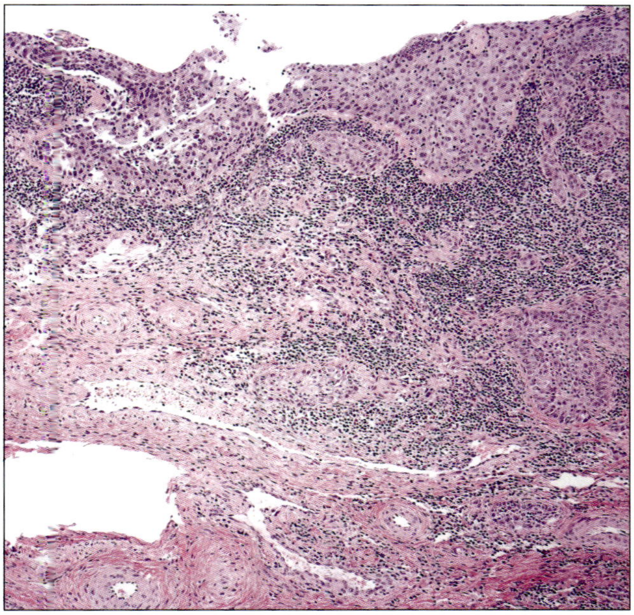

H&E section of the cervix with stromal depth of invasion of 3.5 mm is characteristic of tumor stage T1a2. (Original magnification 40x.)

T1b1

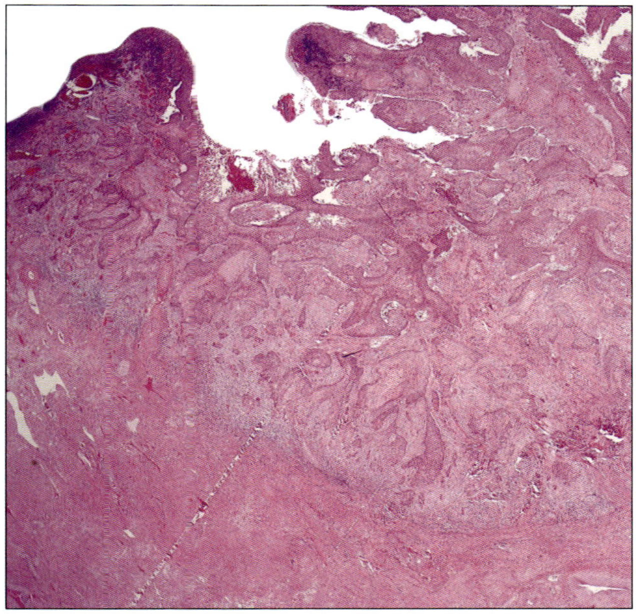

H&E stain shows invasive squamous cell carcinoma with a microscopic depth of invasion of 6 mm. Clinically, this lesion was visible; however, it was confined to the cervix and less than 4 cm in greatest dimension. (Original magnification 20x.)

T3

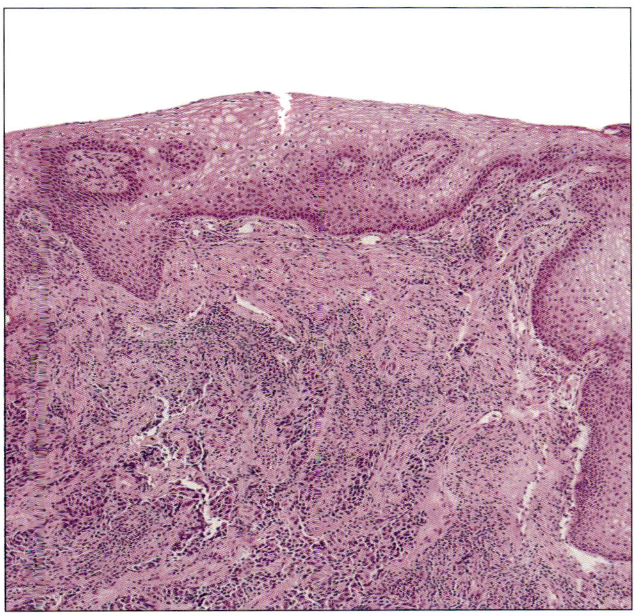

Low-power magnification of H&E stained slide shows cervical squamous cell carcinoma involving the lower 1/3 of the vagina. (Original magnification 40x.)

T3

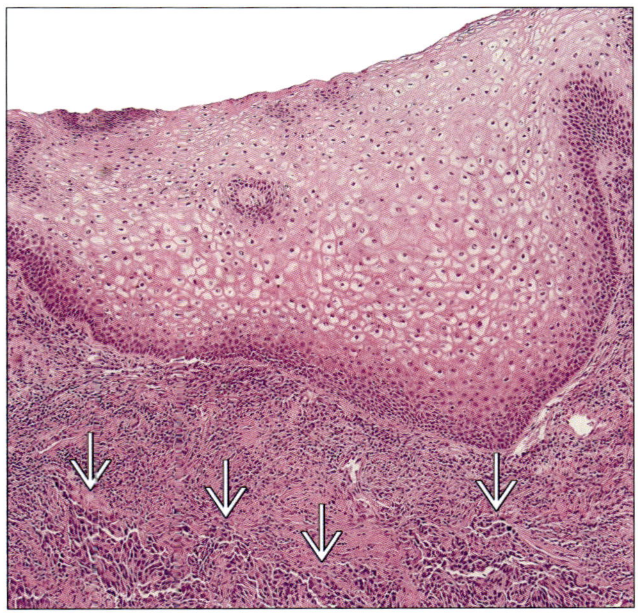

Higher power magnification shows uninvolved nonkeratinized vaginal surface epithelium with the subepithelial cords and nests of neoplastic cells ➔. (Original magnification 100x.)

CERVIX UTERI CARCINOMA

T1a1

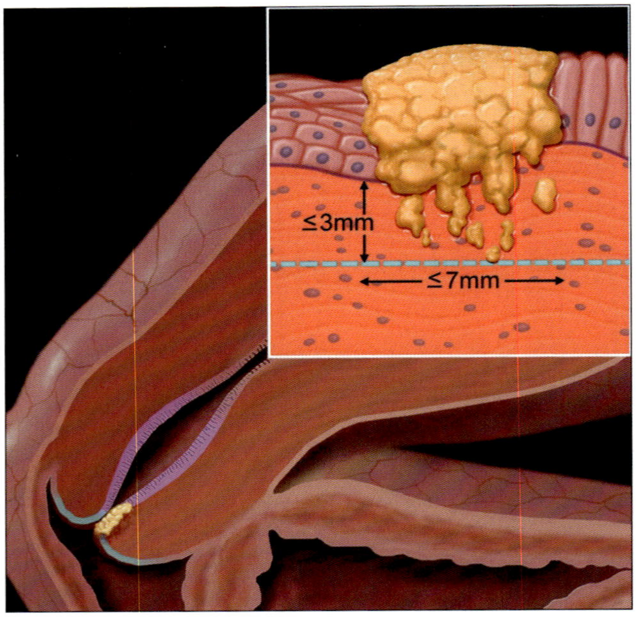

Stage T1a1 cervical carcinoma is defined as microscopic tumor with stromal invasion of ≤ 3 mm in depth and ≤ 7 mm in horizontal spread.

T1a2

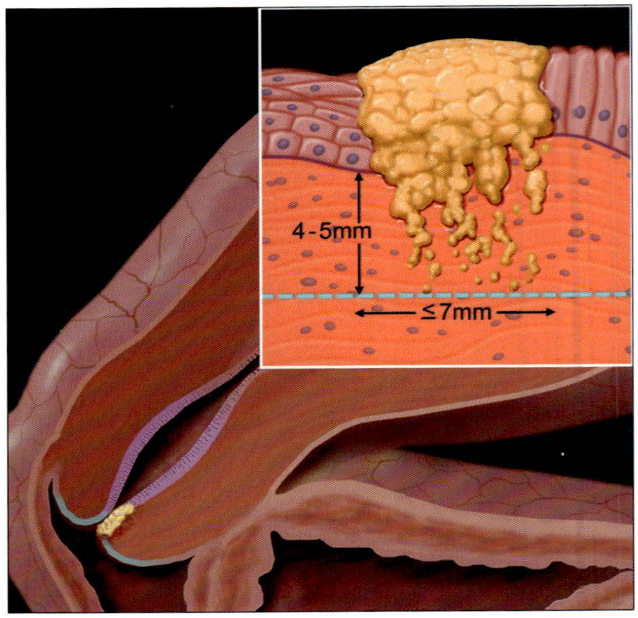

Stage T1a2 cervical carcinoma is microscopic tumor with stromal invasion of 4-5 mm in depth and ≤ 7 mm in horizontal spread.

T1b1

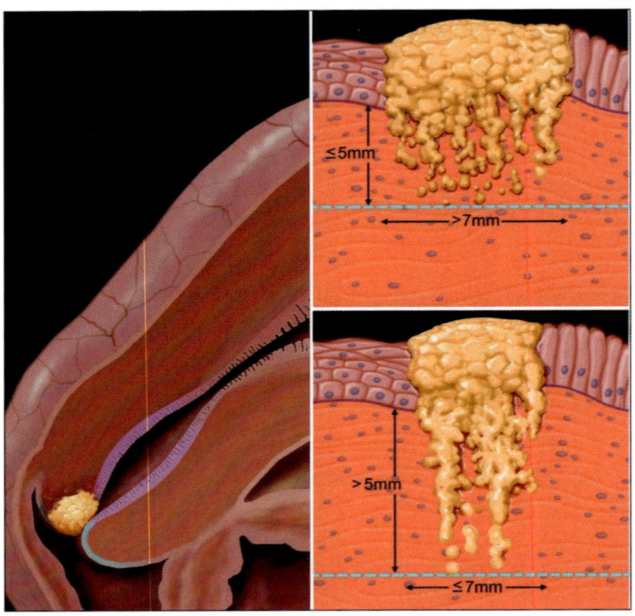

Stage T1b1 cervical carcinoma is a microscopic or clinically visible lesion. Microscopic tumors have stromal invasion > 5 mm in depth or > 7 mm in horizontal spread. Clinically visible tumors are ≤ 4 cm in size. All lesions at this stage are confined to the cervix.

T1b2

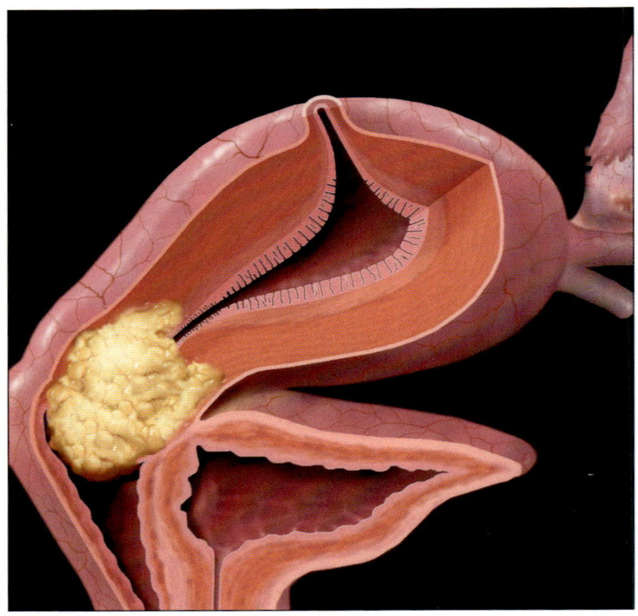

Stage T1b2 cervical carcinoma is a clinically visible lesion > 4 cm in size. Tumors at this stage are confined to the cervix. Tumor may be exophytic extending into the vaginal vault; however, there is no invasion of adjacent structures.

CERVIX UTERI CARCINOMA

T2a1 and T2a2

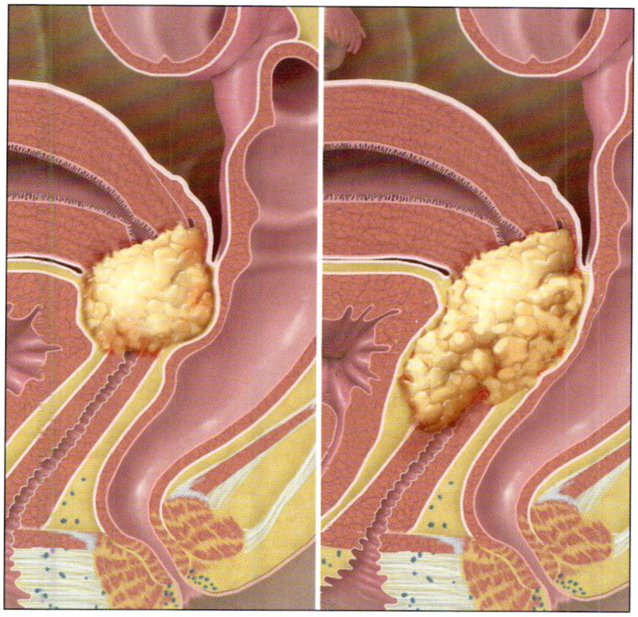

Stage T2a tumor extends beyond the cervix to invade the upper 2/3 of the vagina. Graphics are sagittal views of the pelvis showing tumor invading the upper vagina. Left graphic depicts stage T2a1 with tumor ≤ 4 cm in size. Right graphic depicts stage T2a2 with tumor > 4 cm in size.

T2b

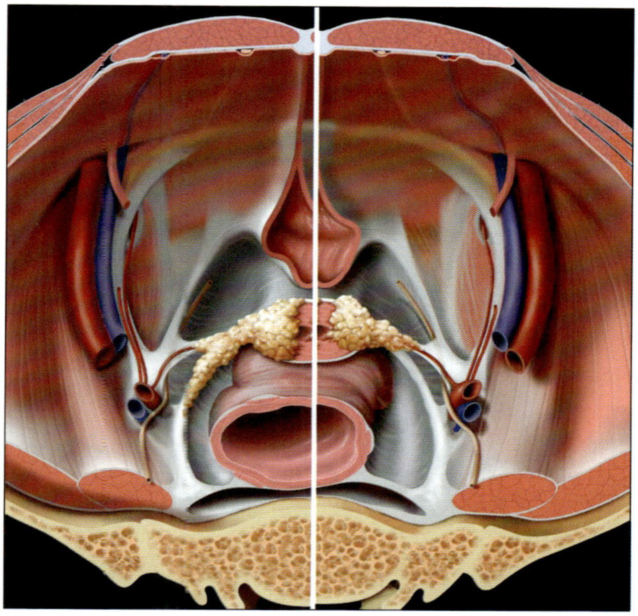

Stage T2b tumor extends beyond the cervix to invade the parametrium. Graphic looks into the pelvic bowl and depicts tumors invading the parametrium including fat, uterine ligaments, and paracervical vessels.

T2b

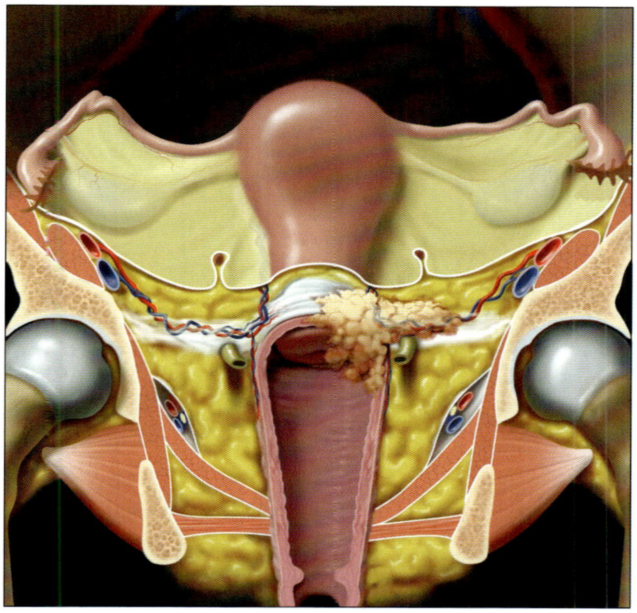

Stage T2b tumor extends beyond the cervix to invade the parametrium. Graphic is a view in the coronal plane depicting tumor invading the parametrium including fat, uterine ligaments, and paracervical vessels. There is encasement of the ureter; however, no hydronephrosis is present.

T3a

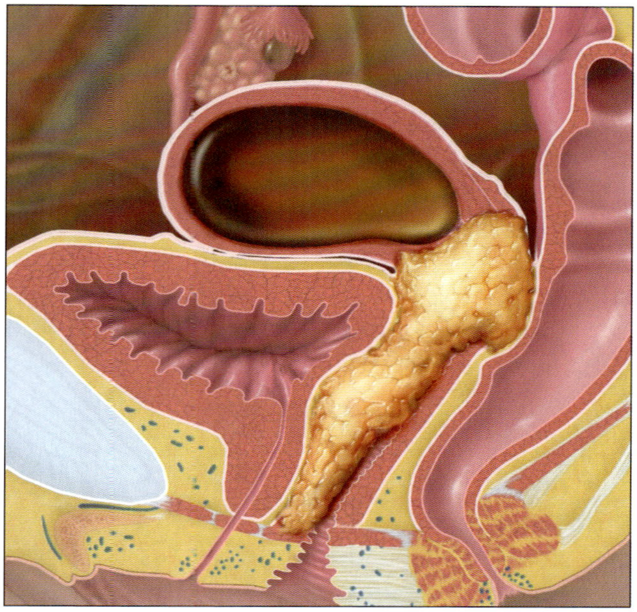

Stage T3a tumor invades the lower 1/3 of the vagina. Graphic is a sagittal view of the pelvis showing tumor invading the lower vagina.

CERVIX UTERI CARCINOMA

T3b

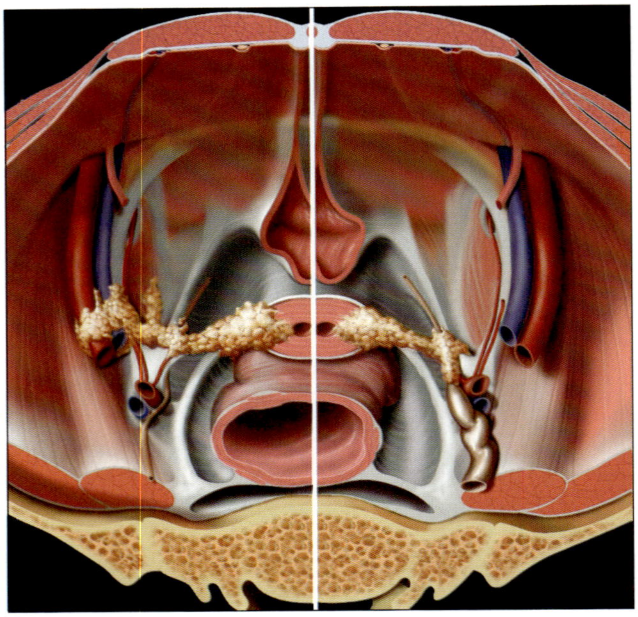

Stage T3b tumor extends to the pelvic sidewall or causes hydronephrosis. Graphics are views looking into the pelvic bowl. Left graphic depicts tumor extending to the pelvic sidewall to encase the iliac vessels and invade the musculature. Right graphic depicts tumor invading the ureter, resulting in hydronephrosis.

T3b

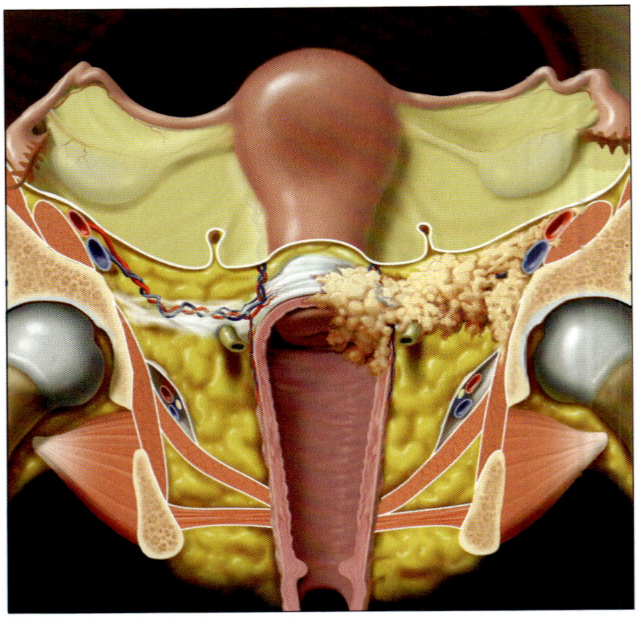

Stage T3b tumor extends to the pelvic sidewall or causes hydronephrosis. Graphic is a view in the coronal plane showing tumor extending to the pelvic sidewall to encase the external iliac vessels and invade the musculature. Tumor invades the ureter, causing hydronephrosis (not shown).

T4

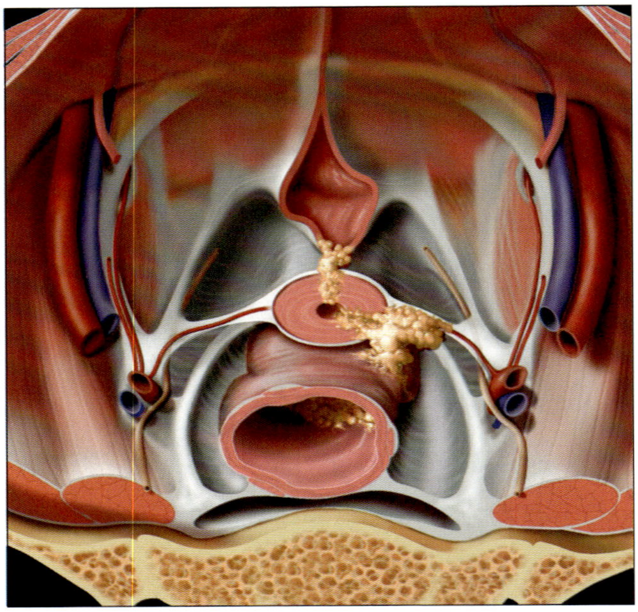

Stage T4 tumor invades the urinary bladder or rectal mucosa. Graphic looks into the pelvic bowl and shows tumors invading the urinary bladder mucosa anteriorly and the rectal mucosa posteriorly.

T4

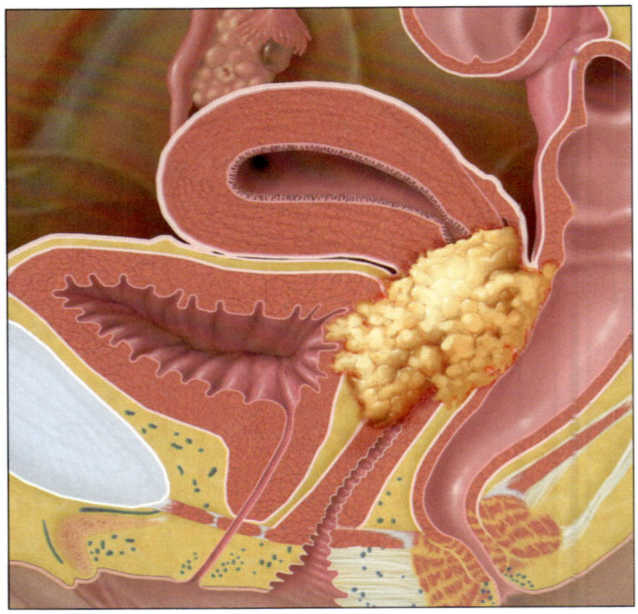

Stage T4 tumor invades the urinary bladder or rectal mucosa. Graphic is a sagittal view of the pelvis showing tumor invading the urinary bladder mucosa anteriorly and the rectal mucosa posteriorly.

CERVIX UTERI CARCINOMA

N1

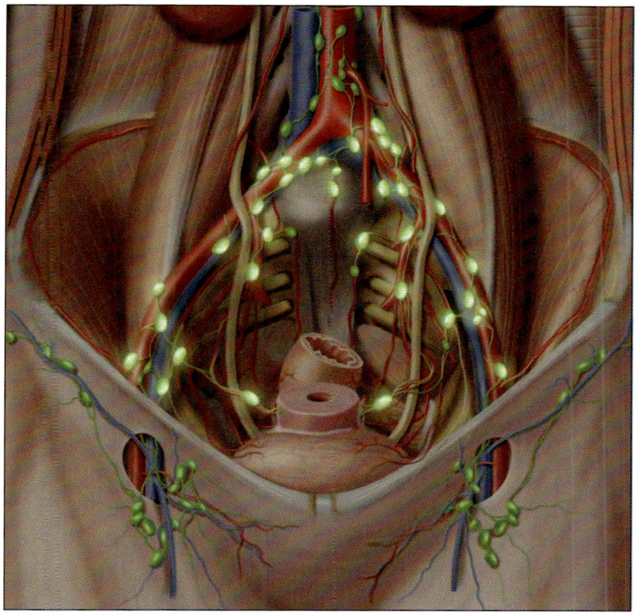

Frontal view of the female pelvis depicts lymph node chains. Regional lymph nodes in cervical carcinoma are highlighted and include parametrial, obturator, internal iliac, external iliac, common iliac, sacral, and presacral lymph nodes.

N1

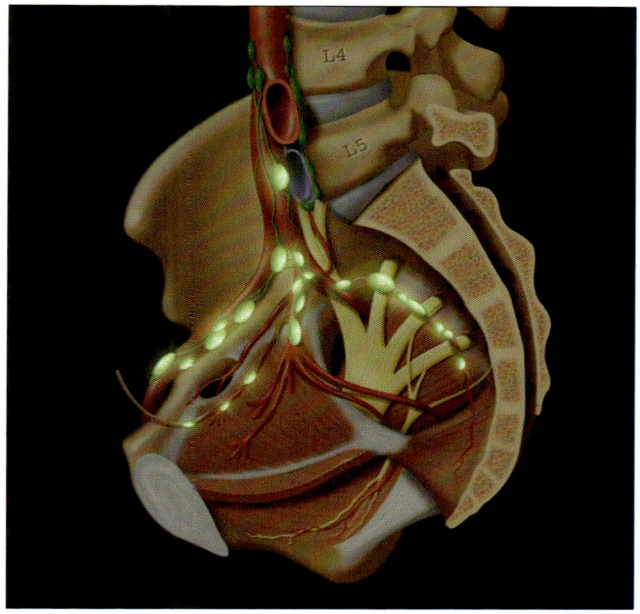

Lateral view of the pelvis shows the presacral and hypogastric routes of lymphatic drainage more clearly. The obturator lymph node, often the sentinel node in cervical carcinoma, is also shown.

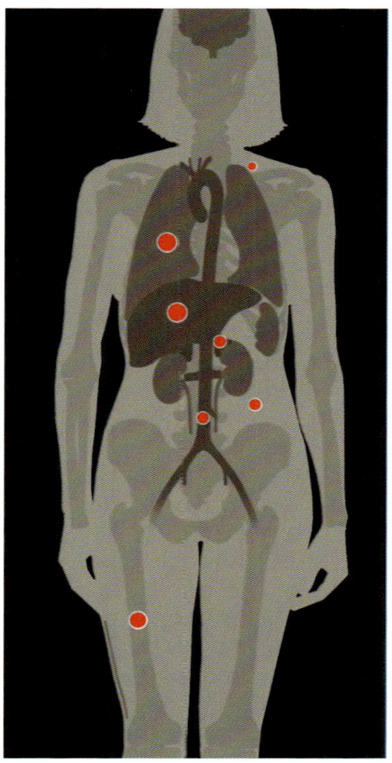

METASTASES, ORGAN FREQUENCY

Liver	33%
Pulmonary	33-38%
Bone	15-29%
Adrenal gland	15%
Paraaortic lymph nodes	15%
Supraclavicular nodes	7%
Abdominal cavity	5-27%

Reported organ frequency of metastatic disease is based on findings at autopsy in patients with recurrent cervical cancer.

CERVIX UTERI CARCINOMA

OVERVIEW

General Comments

- 3rd most common gynecologic malignancy
- 80% are squamous cell carcinoma

Classification

- Histopathologic types
  - Cervical intraepithelial neoplasia, grade III
  - Squamous cell carcinoma in situ
  - Squamous cell carcinoma
    - Invasive
    - Keratinizing
    - Nonkeratinizing
    - Verrucous
  - Adenocarcinoma in situ
  - Invasive adenocarcinoma
  - Endometrioid adenocarcinoma
  - Clear cell adenocarcinoma
  - Adenosquamous carcinoma
  - Adenoid cystic carcinoma
  - Adenoid basal cell carcinoma
  - Small cell carcinoma
  - Neuroendocrine
  - Undifferentiated carcinoma

PATHOLOGY

Routes of Spread

- **Contiguous spread**
  - Most common mode of spread
  - Caudally to invade
    - Vagina
  - Anteriorly to invade
    - Vesicouterine ligament
    - Urinary bladder
  - Laterally to invade
    - Cardinal ligaments
    - Paracervical tissues
      - Fat, vessels, ureters, lymphatics
    - Pelvic sidewall in advanced disease
      - Iliac vessels, pelvic musculature
  - Posteriorly to invade
    - Uterosacral ligaments
    - Rectum
- **Lymphatic spread**
  - Significant prognostic indicator
  - ↑ incidence with advancing stage of disease
  - Correlates with ↓ disease-free survival
  - ↑ incidence of recurrence at each stage with lymphatic invasion
  - Lymphatic drainage of cervix
    - Parametrial → obturator → internal/external iliac
  - 3 pathways of lymphatic drainage of cervix
    - Lateral route
      - Parallels external iliac vessels
      - Tumor drains 1st to medial external iliac chain, then to middle and lateral chains
      - Deep inguinal lymph nodes drain via lateral route
    - Hypogastric route
      - Parallels internal iliac vessels
      - Lymph nodes along internal iliac branches drain to junctional lymph nodes
      - Junctional lymph nodes lie between internal and external iliac vessels
    - Presacral route
      - Along uterosacral ligament
      - Uterosacral ligament → lymphatic plexus anterior to sacrum
  - All 3 routes of lymphatic drainage of cervix drain to common iliac chains
  - Common iliac chains drain to paraaortic lymph nodes
  - Depth of invasion of cervix and adjacent structures may affect nodal involvement
    - Parametrial and pelvic sidewall invasion
      - Drainage by external iliac lymph nodes
    - Invasion of lower 1/3 of vagina
      - Inguinal lymph node metastases
    - Rectal wall invasion
      - Drainage by inferior mesenteric lymph nodes
- **Peritoneal seeding**
  - Peritoneal metastasis varies from 5-27% in autopsy series
  - Mesenteric or omental metastases are uncommon
  - "Sister Joseph" nodule
    - Umbilical metastasis
    - Direct extension of tumor from anterior peritoneal surface
- **Hematogenous spread**
  - Liver is most common abdominal organ with metastases
  - Adrenal gland is 2nd most common metastatic site in abdomen
  - Pulmonary metastases are relatively common in autopsy series (33-38%)
    - May be present for significant period of time; however, may remain asymptomatic
    - 1/3 will have mediastinal or hilar adenopathy
    - Lymphangitic carcinomatosis occurs in < 5%

General Features

- Comments
  - Cervical cancer originates at squamocolumnar junction (SCJ)
    - SCJ is originally located in ectocervix (intravaginal)
    - SCJ moves to endocervix with advancing age
    - Cancer arises in transformation zone between old and new SCJ
  - Migration of SCJ accounts for age-related change in tumor growth pattern
    - Young women: Exophytic growth
    - Older women: Endophytic growth
  - Adenocarcinoma and small cell cervical cancer
    - Aggressive histologic subtypes
    - More often advanced at presentation
  - Adenoma malignum
    - Subtype of adenocarcinoma (3%)
    - Arises from columnar epithelium of endocervical canal
    - Composed of well-differentiated endocervical glands
    - History of copious watery discharge
    - Prognosis is poor
      - Early peritoneal metastases

- Poor response to chemoradiation therapy
  - Associated with Peutz-Jeghers syndrome
- Clear cell adenocarcinoma
  - Rare histologic subtype of adenocarcinoma
  - Associated with in utero diethylstilbestrol (DES) exposure
  - Case reports suggest possible association with cervical endometriosis

- Etiology
  - Risk factors for cervical cancer
    - High-risk strains of human papilloma virus (HPV)
    - Sexual activity at early age
    - Multiple sexual partners
    - Sexually transmitted disease
    - Multiparity
    - Low socioeconomic status
    - Cigarette smoking
    - Immunosuppression
    - Long-term use of oral contraceptives
    - In utero DES exposure
      - Clear cell adenocarcinoma
  - 70% of cervical cancer is caused by HPV 16 and 18
  - 27% of women in USA age 14-59 years are positive for at least 1 strain of HPV
    - 15.2% are positive for 1 of high-risk strains
  - Women with HIV/AIDS have poor prognosis, often rapidly progressive cancer
- Epidemiology & cancer incidence
  - 3rd most common gynecologic malignancy following endometrial and ovarian cancer
  - Decreased incidence since introduction and widespread use of Papanicolaou smear
  - Estimated 11,270 women diagnosed in 2009 in the USA
  - Estimated 4,070 cervical cancer-related deaths in 2009 in the USA

Gross Pathology & Surgical Features

- Gross appearance
  - Poorly circumscribed granular or eroded appearance
  - Nodular, ulcerated lesion or exophytic mass
  - Diffuse enlargement and hardening of cervix
    - Endophytic infiltrative lesion in cervical canal
  - Barrel-shaped cervix
    - Diffusely enlarged, bulky, and > 6 cm
    - Most common with adenocarcinoma

Microscopic Pathology

- H&E
  - Large-cell keratinizing squamous cell carcinoma
    - Sheets & nests of malignant squamous cells invade stroma
    - Abundant cytoplasm
    - Large pleomorphic nuclei & inconspicuous nucleoli
    - Keratin pearls & intercellular bridges
    - Occasional mitotic figures
    - Infiltrative growth pattern
  - Large-cell nonkeratinizing squamous cell carcinoma
    - Large cells of similar size and shape
    - Moderate cytoplasm
    - May have individual cell keratinization
    - Keratin pearls are absent
    - Prominent nucleoli
    - Mitotic figures are common
    - Invasive edge is smooth
  - Histologic grade
    - Degree of differentiation of tumor cells
    - Based on amount of keratin, degree of nuclear atypia, mitotic activity
    - Correlates with frequency of pelvic nodal metastasis
    - Grade 1: Well differentiated
      - Abundant intercellular bridging
      - Cytoplasmic keratinization
      - Keratin pearls
      - Cells are uniform with minimal nuclear pleomorphism
      - Mitotic rate is < 2 mitotic figures per high-power field
    - Grade 2: Moderately differentiated
      - Individual cell keratinization
      - Moderate nuclear pleomorphism
      - Mitotic rate is ≤ 4 mitotic figures per high-power field
    - Grade 3: Poorly differentiated
      - Minimal evidence of squamous differentiation
      - Cells are immature with marked nuclear pleomorphism and scant cytoplasm
      - Mitotic rate is > 4 mitotic figures per high-power field

IMAGING FINDINGS

Detection

- **Ultrasound**
  - Inadequate for diagnosis, staging, and surveillance for recurrence
  - Technically limited by body habitus, low signal-to-noise ratio, and lack of tissue characterization
- **CT**
  - 92% accuracy for assessment of stage IIIB-IVB disease
  - CT can demonstrate
    - Pelvic sidewall extension
    - Ureteral obstruction
    - Advanced bladder and rectal invasion
    - Adenopathy
    - Extrapelvic spread of disease
  - May see distention of uterine cavity with fluid/blood if tumor obstructs endocervical canal
  - CT can guide lymph node biopsy and radiation planning
  - CT has high sensitivity and specificity for detection of recurrent tumor
    - Soft tissue mass with variable degrees of necrosis
    - Cystic mass with minimal soft tissue
  - Limitations of CT
    - Limited visualization of primary tumor
      - Hypodense or isodense to normal cervical stroma
      - Tumor detection and depth of invasion difficult
    - Inaccurate for detection of parametrial invasion
      - Only 30-58% accuracy
      - Parametrial inflammation can mimic parametrial tumor infiltration
      - Paracervical ligaments and vessels may be mistaken for soft tissue strands

CERVIX UTERI CARCINOMA

- **MR**
  - Ideal for local cervical cancer staging
    - Superior soft tissue contrast
    - Multiplanar capability
  - Superior to clinical evaluation and other imaging modalities with regard to tumor characteristics that determine prognosis and stage
    - Tumor size
    - Parametrial invasion
    - Vaginal wall invasion
    - Pelvic sidewall extension
  - Accuracy of MR is 94% in selecting operative candidates
    - Compared with 76% for CT
  - Including MR in pre-treatment work-up significantly decreases number of procedures and invasive studies
  - Typical MR findings of cervical cancer
    - T2 hyperintense mass disrupting normal hypointense cervical stroma
    - Endophytic: Arises from endocervical canal
    - Exophytic: Arises from ectocervix and extends into vaginal vault
  - MR technique
    - T2WI best for visualization of tumor and local staging
      - FSE, small field of view (FOV), high resolution
    - Coronal oblique T2WI: Long & short (donut view) axis of cervix
      - Evaluation of depth of cervical stromal invasion
      - Evaluation of parametrial invasion
    - Sagittal T2WI
      - Depth of cervical stromal invasion
      - Visualization of invasion of vagina and urinary bladder
      - Helpful to distend vagina with gel
    - Axial T2WI
      - Parametrial invasion
      - Pelvic sidewall invasion
      - Rectal invasion
    - T2WI with fat saturation
      - Helpful if prominent paracervical venous plexus
    - IV contrast reportedly not helpful for depth of stromal invasion or parametrial involvement
      - Loss of soft tissue contrast due to enhancement of normal cervical stroma and variable tumor enhancement
      - May result in overestimation of tumor size
    - IV contrast is useful in advanced disease to evaluate
      - Rectal, urinary bladder, pelvic sidewall invasion
      - Pelvic fistulas
      - Recurrent/residual disease post radiation or surgery
  - Characteristic features of adenoma malignum
    - Multicystic mass extending from superficial to deep cervical wall
    - Mass may be nodular or annular
    - Mass invades deep into cervical stroma
    - Cystic components are hyperintense on T2WI with intervening low signal septations
    - Solid enhancing components help differentiate adenoma malignum from benign entities
  - Limitations of MR
    - Differentiating tumor recurrence from early radiation change and infection
    - May overestimate parametrial invasion with large tumors
      - Due to surrounding stromal edema from tumor compression or inflammation
- **PET/CT**
  - Excellent for detection of lymphadenopathy and distant metastatic disease
    - 100% sensitivity and 99.6% specificity for lymph nodes > 5 mm in short axis
    - 100% sensitivity and 94% specificity for distant metastatic disease
  - PET is superior to MR and CT for depiction of adenopathy
    - Metabolic changes may precede morphologic changes
    - Moderate to marked increase FDG uptake relative to normal structures
    - SUV is not helpful when characterizing lymph node lesions
  - Limitations
    - Lower spatial resolution compared to CT and MR
    - Cannot differentiate malignant from reactive adenopathy
    - Cannot differentiate malignant, infectious, or inflammatory processes
  - Poor anatomic resolution of PET is overcome by fusion with CT

Staging

- **General comments**
  - Accurate staging is critical for guiding management
  - Important to avoid upstaging at time of surgery
    - Significant increase in morbidity when surgery and radiotherapy are combined
  - International Federation of Gynecology and Obstetrics (FIGO)
    - Clinical staging of cervical cancer
    - Preferred staging system in order to provide uniformity
    - Results of imaging technologies (CT, MR, PET) should **not** be used to determine clinical stage
      - Not universally available
      - Can be used for prognostic information and treatment planning
    - Surgical and pathologic findings should not change clinical stage
      - Can be used in TNM staging
    - Clinical stage must not be changed for subsequent findings once treatment started
    - If there is doubt regarding stage, the lesser stage should be used
  - FIGO staging system is based on
    - Clinical examination (under anesthesia)
    - Chest x-ray
    - Intravenous pyelogram
    - Barium enema
    - Cystoscopy and proctoscopy
    - Aforementioned radiologic and endoscopic studies are often not used in clinical practice
  - MR is more accurate for staging compared to clinical FIGO staging
    - Particularly in patients with ≥ stage IIA disease
- **Stage IA**

CERVIX UTERI CARCINOMA

- Microinvasive disease
- Traditionally not visible on MR
- Some reports describe area of enhancement in arterial phase on dynamic post-contrast imaging

- **Stage IB**
  - Clinically visible (> 5 mm); however tumor remains confined to cervix
  - Hyperintense mass disrupting low signal cervical stroma on T2WI
  - Partial stromal invasion
    - Preservation of outer rim of normal low signal cervical stroma on T2WI
    - Parametrial invasion can reliably be excluded if rim of normal stroma is ≥ 3 mm
  - Full thickness stromal invasion
    - No outer rim of normal cervical stroma
    - Parametrial tissue is symmetric and normal in signal intensity
    - Preservation of sharp, distinct parametrial fat planes
    - Excluding parametrial invasion is more difficult with full thickness invasion
    - If vaginal fornices are not invaded, tumor is likely confined to cervix
  - Exophytic cervical mass can fill and expand vaginal fornices
    - If low signal vaginal wall is preserved (no invasion), this remains stage IB tumor
- **Stage IIA**
  - Invasion of upper 2/3 of vagina
  - Disruption of normal low signal vaginal wall by hyperintense cervical mass on T2WI
- **Stage IIB**
  - Invasion of parametrial tissues
    - Vessels, fat, and lymphatics between leaves of broad ligament
  - Probability of parametrial invasion is 28% for tumors > 2 cm
  - Specific signs of parametrial invasion
    - Frank extension of mass into parametrial tissues
    - Encasement of parametrial vessels
    - Encasement of ureter (no hydronephrosis)
    - Nodular thickening of uterine ligaments
  - Early parametrial invasion may manifest as
    - Full thickness cervical stromal invasion by tumor with irregularity of outer cervical contour
    - Stranding (> 3-4 mm in thickness) and nodularity of parametrial fat
    - These findings are nonspecific and can be secondary to parametrial inflammation
  - Coronal oblique and sagittal T2WI are best for identifying parametrial involvement
  - T2WI with fat saturation may be helpful in women with prominent paracervical venous plexus
- **Stage IIIA**
  - Invasion of lower 1/3 of vagina
  - Disruption of normal low signal vaginal wall by hyperintense cervical mass on T2WI
  - Best evaluated in axial and sagittal planes
- **Stage IIIB**
  - Hydronephrosis or pelvic sidewall invasion
    - Pelvic sidewall invasion manifests as
      - Tumor extension to within 3 mm of pelvic musculature
      - Invasion of obturator internus and piriformis muscles: Diffuse enlargement or mass
      - Encasement of iliac vessels by tumor
    - Ureteral invasion as manifested by hydronephrosis can be identified with US, CT, or MR
    - Enlarge FOV on coronal fluid-sensitive sequence to evaluate entire urinary tract
  - Any T stage with regional nodal metastases
    - Lymph node metastases are detected equally well with CT and MR
    - CT and MR are slightly better than lymphangiography
    - Anatomic imaging uses lymph node size and shape to predict presence of pathology
      - Spherical shape
      - Size > 1 cm in short axis: 75-88% accuracy
    - IV contrast aids in detection of lymph nodes
      - Lymph nodes avidly enhance
      - ↑ conspicuity in hypodense pelvic fat on CT or low signal pelvic fat on T1WI C+ FS MR
    - Central necrosis is highly predictive of metastasis
      - Lack of central enhancement
    - Metabolic imaging with PET utilizes presence of increased glucose metabolism to predict pathology
      - Relative increased FDG uptake compared to other lymph nodes is considered positive
    - Detection of micrometastases remains a challenge for both anatomic and metabolic imaging
    - Reactive adenopathy can be difficult to differentiate from malignant adenopathy
- **Stage IVA**
  - Invasion of urinary bladder or rectal mucosa
  - Disruption of normal low signal urinary bladder or rectal wall by high signal tumor on T2WI
  - Eccentric nodular wall thickening
  - Protrusion of tumor into lumen
  - Fistula formation: Tumor to urinary bladder or rectum
    - Enhancing tract on post-contrast sequences
    - Intraluminal air in urinary bladder
  - Bullous edema sign
    - High signal thickening of urinary bladder wall on T2WI
    - Reactive inflammation, not tumor invasion
    - Not stage IVA if occurring in isolation
  - Bladder and rectal mucosal involvement must be confirmed by biopsy and histology
- **Stage IVB**
  - Distant metastatic disease including extrapelvic lymph nodes
  - Metastatic disease is most commonly seen with recurrence or advanced disease
    - Overall incidence of 56%
    - 10% have metastatic disease at time of diagnosis
  - Factors influencing incidence of distant metastasis
    - Clinical stage at diagnosis
    - Endometrial extension as shown at pre-treatment dilation and curettage
    - Pelvic tumor control with treatment
  - Incidence of distant metastases increases with increasing stage of disease
    - Stage IA (3%) → stage IVA (75%)

CERVIX UTERI CARCINOMA

- Most common organs
  - Liver, lungs, abdominal cavity, and GI tract
- Most common lymph nodes
  - Periaortic, supraclavicular, and inguinal
- Most common bones
  - Thoracic and lumbar spine
  - Destructive lesions
  - Usually by contiguous extension from paraaortic lymph node mass
  - Pelvis, ribs, and extremities less frequently involved
- Liver is most common abdominal organ with metastases
  - Solid mass with variable enhancement on CECT or MR
  - Increased FDG activity compared with background liver on PET/CT
- Peritoneal carcinomatosis
  - Implants scalloping liver contour
  - Irregular and nodular peritoneal thickening
  - Mass or infiltrative soft tissue in mesentery or omentum
  - Soft tissue masses on serosal surface of bowel
  - Ascites is often present, though nonspecific
- Pleural involvement
  - Pleural thickening and nodularity
  - Hydrothorax (often seen with ascites)
  - More common with adenocarcinoma
- Pericardial metastasis is rare
  - Nodular pericardial thickening
  - Pericardial effusion
  - Spread via paraaortic lymph nodes
- Rare metastatic sites
  - Skin, brain, meninges, heart, and breast
  - Usually occur in recurrent cervical cancer

Restaging

- Recurrence is defined as development of tumor ≥ 6 months following disease regression
- Up to 20% of cases of cervical cancer recur
- Risk factors for recurrence include
  - Histologic grade
  - Tumor size
  - Depth of stromal invasion
  - Lymph node status at presentation
- Most common sites of local recurrence
  - Cervix
  - Vaginal cuff
  - Parametrial tissues
  - Pelvic sidewall
- Local recurrence in pelvis
  - Central
    - At remaining cervix or vaginal cuff
    - Can extend anteriorly to ureter or bladder
    - Posteriorly to invade rectum
      - ± rectovaginal fistula
    - Laterally to pelvic sidewall
  - Pelvic sidewall
    - Invasion precludes treatment with pelvic exenteration
- CT
  - Overall high sensitivity and specificity in detection of recurrent tumor
  - Limited ability to differentiate early radiation change/fibrosis from recurrence
  - Readily available
  - Short scan time eliminates bowel motion artifact
- MR
  - Contrast-enhanced MR: Accuracy of 82% for distinguishing recurrence from fibrosis
  - Can assess extent of vaginal and pelvic floor involvement
  - Disadvantages include cost and long scan time
- PET/CT
  - Able to differentiate metabolically active tumor from therapy-related fibrosis
  - Whole-body evaluation for distant metastases
  - Poor spatial resolution precludes evaluation of local tumor invasion of adjacent structures

CLINICAL ISSUES

Presentation

- Average age of presentation is 50 years
  - 2 peaks at age 38 and 62 years
- Most common symptoms are vaginal bleeding and discharge
- Precursor is cervical intraepithelial neoplasia (CIN)
  - CIN 1: Minor dysplasia
  - CIN 2: Moderate dysplasia
  - CIN 3: Severe dysplasia
    - 40% progress to invasive cancer if not treated
    - Average time to progression is 10-15 years

Cancer Natural History & Prognosis

- Major factors influencing prognosis
  - Histologic type and grade
  - Stage
  - Tumor volume
  - Depth of stromal invasion
  - Adjacent tissue extension
  - Lymphatic spread
  - Vascular invasion

Treatment Options

- Major treatment alternatives
  - Surgical resection
    - Trachelectomy
      - Maintains fertility
      - Depends on relationship of tumor to internal os
    - Wertheim-Meigs operation
      - Total abdominal hysterectomy
      - Resection of upper 1/3 of vagina
      - Excision of parametrial and uterosacral ligaments
      - Pelvic and periaortic lymph node dissection
  - Radiation therapy
    - External beam pelvic radiation and intracavitary brachytherapy
    - Can extend radiation field to include paraaortic lymph nodes
      - Long-term disease control if low volume (< 2 cm) nodal disease below L3
  - Chemotherapy
    - Survival advantage in stage IB2-IVA disease when concurrent with radiation therapy
    - Advantageous in stage I-IIA disease if found to have poor prognostic factors at surgery
    - Risk of death is decreased by 30-50%

CERVIX UTERI CARCINOMA

- **Stage 0**
  - Absence of invasion must be confirmed with colposcopic-directed biopsy or cone biopsy
  - Loop electrosurgical excision procedure (LEEP)
    - Outpatient, in-office procedure
    - Requires only local anesthesia
  - Laser or cold-knife conization
    - Preserves uterus
    - Avoids radiation therapy and surgery
    - Requires general anesthesia
    - Mandatory if
      - Extension of disease into endocervical canal
      - Lack of correlation between cytology and colposcopic-directed biopsy
      - Adenocarcinoma in situ
  - Most common cause of failure at this stage is unrecognized invasive disease treated with inadequate ablative therapy
- **Stage IA**
  - Total hysterectomy
    - Depth of tumor invasion < 3 mm (proven by cone biopsy)
    - Negative cone biopsy margins
    - No vascular or lymphatic channel invasion
  - Conization
    - Depth of tumor invasion < 3 mm (proven by cone biopsy)
    - Negative cone biopsy margins
    - No vascular or lymphatic channel invasion
    - Considered if desire to preserve fertility
  - Radical hysterectomy (including pelvic lymph node dissection)
    - Depth of tumor invasion 3-5 mm or unknown due to positive cone margins
    - Lymph node dissection done due to reported risk of lymph node metastasis of up to 10%
  - Intracavitary radiation therapy
    - Reserved for women who are not surgical candidates
    - Depth of tumor invasion < 3 mm
    - No lymphatic or vascular space invasion
- **Stage IB/IIA**
  - Identical overall and 5-year disease-free survival rates for radiation therapy and radical hysterectomy
    - Stage IB
      - 85-90% cure rate (small volume disease)
    - Stage IIA
      - 75-80% cure rate
  - Radiation therapy
    - External beam pelvic radiation combined with intracavitary brachytherapy
    - May also be beneficial in those with close vaginal margins (< 0.5 cm) at radical surgery
    - Extended field radiation
      - May be used to control small volume paraaortic nodal disease
      - Possible survival advantage with large tumors even without histologic evidence of paraaortic metastases
      - ↑ toxic effects if history of prior abdominopelvic surgery
  - Radical hysterectomy and bilateral pelvic lymph node dissection
    - Surgery indicated after radiation therapy if
      - Tumor is confined to cervix but responds incompletely to radiation therapy
      - Vaginal anatomy precludes optimal brachytherapy
  - Radical hysterectomy, lymph node dissection, radiation therapy, and chemotherapy
    - Considered if
      - Positive pelvic lymph nodes
      - Positive surgical margins
      - Residual parametrial disease
  - Radiation and chemotherapy
    - Considered for bulky tumors
    - Studies have shown overall survival advantage with concurrent chemoradiation therapy
- **Stage IIB/III/IVA**
  - Stage IIB
    - Survival and local control are better with unilateral parametrial involvement vs. bilateral
  - Stage III
    - Better survival outcome with unilateral pelvic sidewall involvement vs. bilateral
    - Lower 1/3 vaginal invasion has worse survival outcome than pelvic wall disease
  - Radiation and chemotherapy
    - External beam pelvic radiation combined with intracavitary brachytherapy
    - ↓ risk of death by 30-50% with use of concurrent chemotherapy
    - Resection of macroscopically involved pelvic nodes may improve rates of local control with postoperative radiation therapy
- **Stage IVB**
  - Radiation therapy may be used to palliate central disease or distant metastasis
  - No standard chemotherapy treatment is available
  - Clinical trials using single or multiple agents are ongoing

REPORTING CHECKLIST

T Staging

- Size
- Endophytic vs exophytic mass
- Obstruction of endocervical canal
  - Distention of uterine cavity
- Contiguous spread
  - Vagina
    - Upper 2/3
    - Lower 1/3
  - Parametrial invasion
    - Loss of outer rim of normal cervical stroma
    - Frank tumor extension
    - Encasement of pericervical vessels
    - Soft tissue nodules & strands (> 3 mm)
    - Uterosacral, cardinal, vesicouterine ligaments
      - Nodular thickening
  - Pelvic sidewall
    - Common, internal, & external iliac artery & vein
      - Vessel encasement
    - Pelvic musculature
      - Obturator internus, piriformis, psoas, iliacus
      - Tumor within 3 mm of muscle
      - Diffuse muscle enlargement or mass

- Ureteral invasion
  - Hydronephrosis
- Urinary bladder & rectal mucosa
  - Eccentric nodular wall thickening
  - Protrusion of tumor into lumen
  - Fistula from tumor to bladder or rectum
    - Enhancing tract
    - Intraluminal air in urinary bladder
  - Bullous edema sign
    - Reactive inflammation, not tumor invasion

N Staging

- Pelvic lymph nodes
  - Obturator
  - Internal, external, & common iliac
  - Presacral
- Anatomic imaging
  - Size > 1 cm in short axis
  - Spherical shape
  - Central necrosis
- Metabolic imaging
  - Relative increased FDG uptake

M Staging

- Hematogenous metastasis
  - Liver, adrenal gland, lung
- Extrapelvic lymph nodes
  - Paraaortic, inguinal, supraclavicular most common
- Peritoneal metastasis
  - Implants scalloping liver contour
  - Irregular & nodular peritoneal thickening
  - Soft tissue masses on serosal surface of bowel
  - Omental or mesenteric mass
  - Ascites
- Osseous metastasis
  - Thoracic & lumbar spine most common
    - Contiguous extension from paraaortic mass
  - Pelvis, ribs, extremities less common

SELECTED REFERENCES

1. American Joint Committee on Cancer: AJCC Cancer Staging Manual. 7th ed. New York: Springer, 2010
2. American Cancer Society. What are the key statistics about cervical cancer? http://www.cancer.org. Accessed May 30, 2009
3. National Institutes of Health. Cervical cancer treatment. http://www.cancer.gov/cancertopics/pdq/treatment/cervical/HealthProfessional. Accessed October 23, 2009
4. Rezvani M et al: Imaging of cervical pathology. Clin Obstet Gynecol. 52(1):94-111, 2009
5. Fu, Y: Pathology of cervical carcinoma. Glob. libr. women's med., (ISSN: 1756-2228); DOI 10.3843/GLOWM.10230, 2008
6. Akin O et al: Imaging of uterine cancer. Radiol Clin North Am. 45(1):167-82, 2007
7. Loft A et al: The diagnostic value of PET/CT scanning in patients with cervical cancer: a prospective study. Gynecol Oncol. 106(1):29-34, 2007
8. Sala E et al: MRI of malignant neoplasms of the uterine corpus and cervix. AJR Am J Roentgenol. 188(6):1577-87, 2007
9. Amit A et al: The role of hybrid PET/CT in the evaluation of patients with cervical cancer. Gynecol Oncol. 100(1):65-9, 2006
10. Unger JB et al: Detection of recurrent cervical cancer by whole-body FDG PET scan in asymptomatic and symptomatic women. Gynecol Oncol. 94(1):212-6, 2004
11. Jeong YY et al: Uterine cervical carcinoma after therapy: CT and MR imaging findings. Radiographics. 23(4):969-81; discussion 981, 2003
12. Kaur H et al: Diagnosis, staging, and surveillance of cervical carcinoma. AJR Am J Roentgenol. 180(6):1621-31, 2003
13. Metser U et al: MR imaging findings and patterns of spread in secondary tumor involvement of the uterine body and cervix. AJR Am J Roentgenol. 180(3):765-9, 2003
14. Okamoto Y et al: MR imaging of the uterine cervix: imaging-pathologic correlation. Radiographics. 23(2):425-45; quiz 534-5, 2003
15. Scheidler J et al: Imaging of cancer of the cervix. Radiol Clin North Am. 40(3):577-90, vii, 2002
16. Pannu HK et al: CT evaluation of cervical cancer: spectrum of disease. Radiographics. 21(5):1155-68, 2001
17. Nicolet V et al: MR imaging of cervical carcinoma: a practical staging approach. Radiographics. 20(6):1539-49, 2000
18. Yang WT et al: Comparison of dynamic helical CT and dynamic MR imaging in the evaluation of pelvic lymph nodes in cervical carcinoma. AJR Am J Roentgenol. 175(3):759-66, 2000
19. Fulcher AS et al: Recurrent cervical carcinoma: typical and atypical manifestations. Radiographics. 19 Spec No:S103-16; quiz S264-5, 1999
20. Yamashita Y et al: Adenoma malignum: MR appearances mimicking nabothian cysts. AJR Am J Roentgenol. 162(3):649-50, 1994
21. Hricak H et al: Invasive cervical carcinoma: comparison of MR imaging and surgical findings. Radiology. 166(3):623-31, 1988
22. LaPolla JP et al: The influence of surgical staging on the evaluation and treatment of patients with cervical carcinoma. Gynecol Oncol. 24(2):194-206, 1986
23. Van Nagell JR Jr et al: The staging of cervical cancer: inevitable discrepancies between clinical staging and pathologic findinges. Am J Obstet Gynecol. 110(7):973-8, 1971

CERVIX UTERI CARCINOMA

Stage IB1 (T1b1 N0 M0)

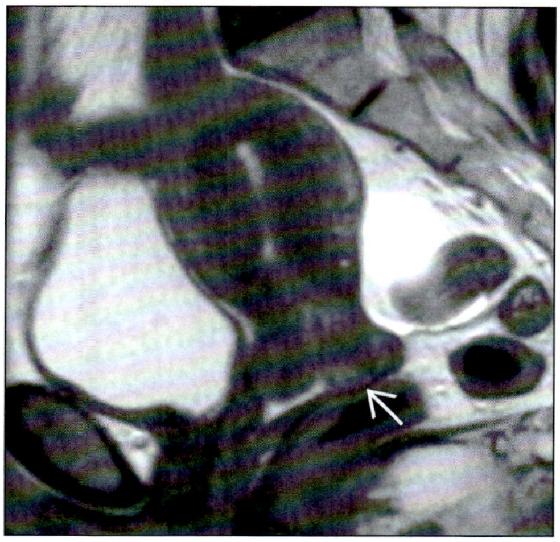

Stage IB1 (T1b1 N0 M0)

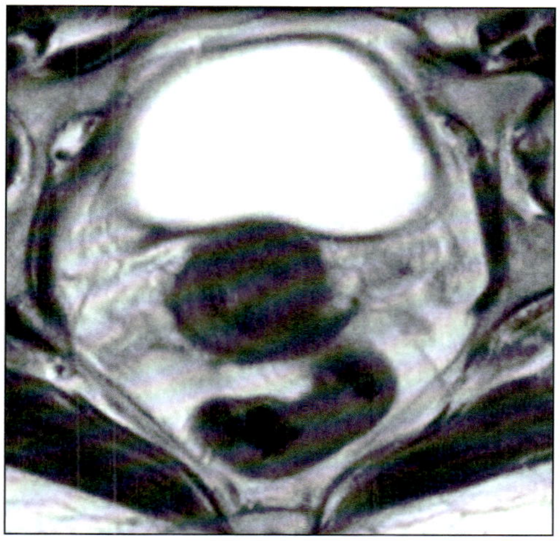

(Left) *Sagittal T2WI FSE MR shows a small hyperintense cervical mass ➡ at the expected location of the squamocolumnar junction in the ectocervix.* ***(Right)*** *Coronal oblique (short axis) T2WI FSE MR in the same patient shows the small hyperintense cervical mass.*

Stage IB1 (T1b1 N0 M0)

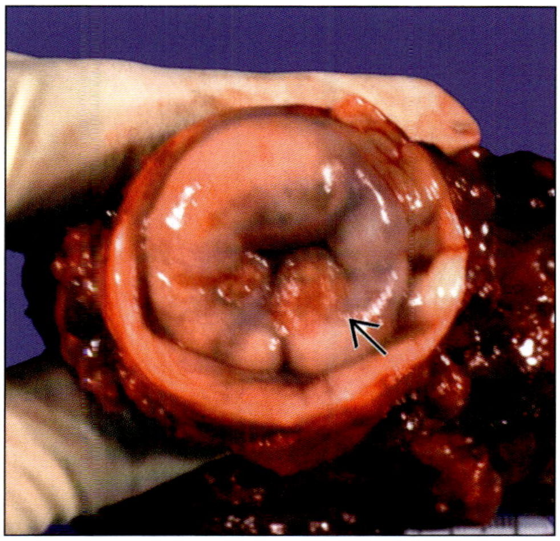

Stage IB1 (T1b1 N0 M0)

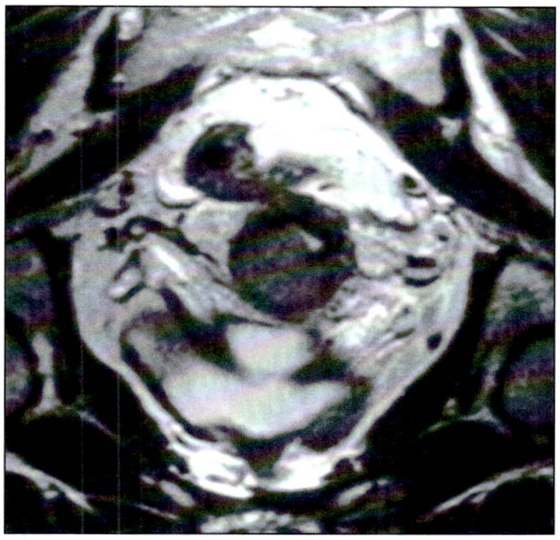

(Left) *Gross surgical specimen from the same patient shows the small exophytic mass ⇨ at the external os of the cervix arising from the expected location of the squamocolumnar junction.* ***(Right)*** *T2WI FSE MR shows a hyperintense cervical mass with preservation of a rim of normal low signal cervical stroma.*

Adenoma Malignum

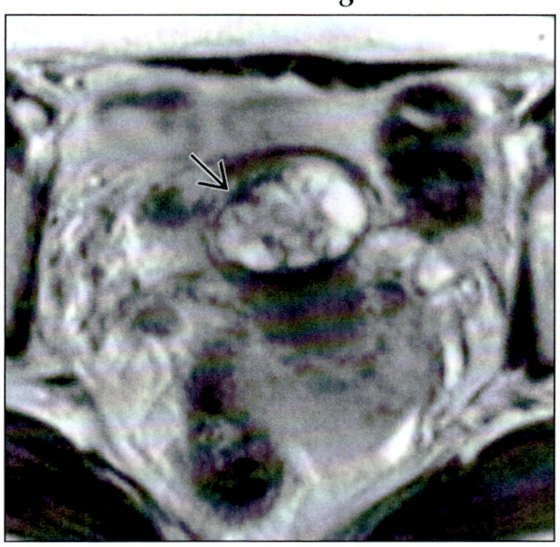

Adenoma Malignum

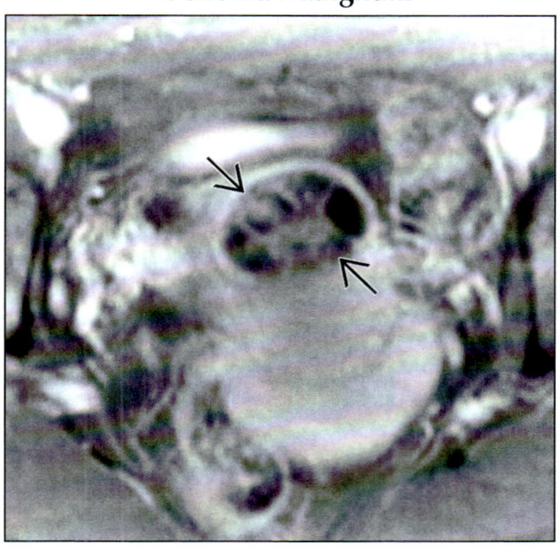

(Left) *T2WI FSE MR shows a multicystic cervical mass ⇨ penetrating deep into the cervical stroma.* ***(Right)*** *T1WI C+ FS MR in the same patient shows solid enhancing nodules ⇨ in the multicystic cervical mass.*

CERVIX UTERI CARCINOMA

Stage IB2 (T1b2 N0 M0)

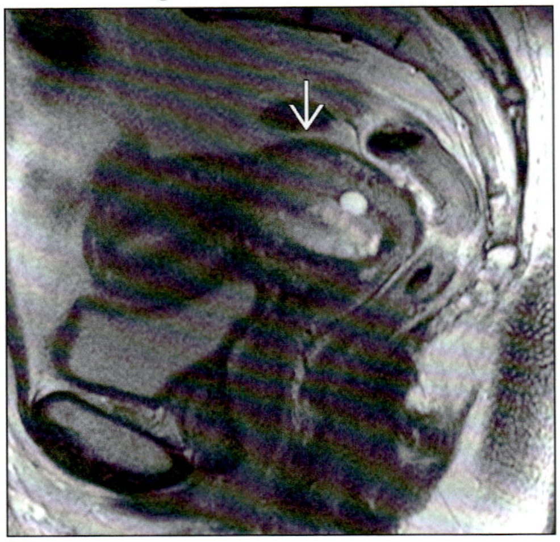

Stage IB2 (T1b2 N0 M0)

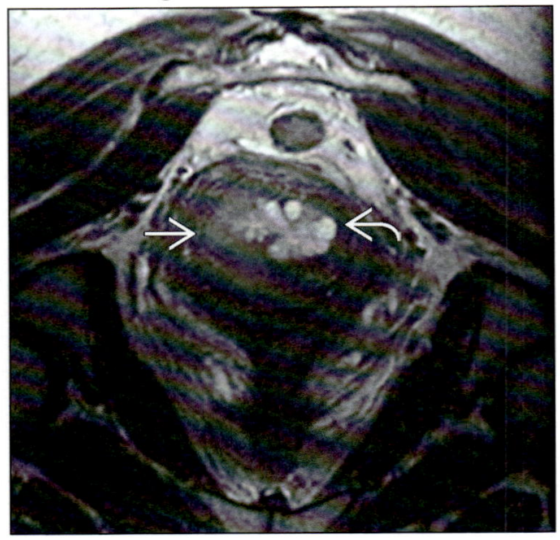

(Left) *Sagittal T2WI FSE MR shows partial thickness invasion of the posterior cervix with preservation of a rim of normal low signal stroma →.* ***(Right)*** *Coronal oblique (short axis) T2WI FSE MR in the same patient shows a hyperintense cervical mass → obliterating the normal low signal stroma. Contrast the superficial location of nabothian cysts → with the deep invasion of tumor.*

Stage IB2 (T1b2 N0 M0)

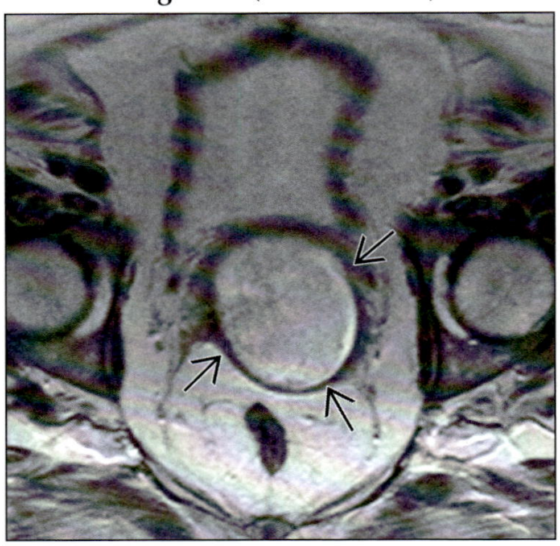

Stage IB2 (T1b2 N0 M0)

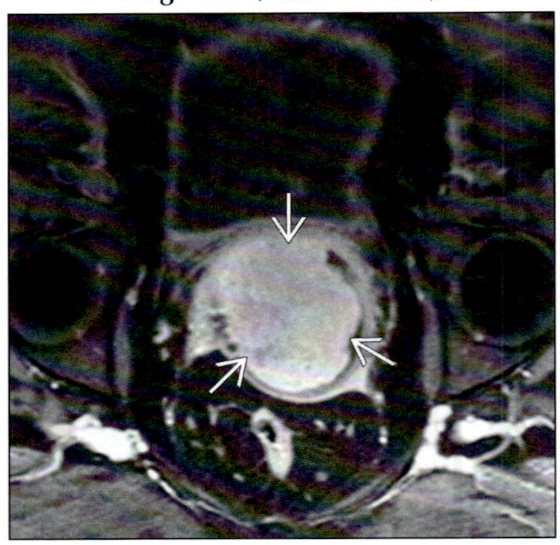

(Left) *T2WI FSE MR shows an exophytic, hyperintense cervical mass expanding the vaginal fornices →, though without disruption of the low signal vaginal wall. Despite the large size of the cervical mass, this is a stage IB tumor due to the lack of vaginal invasion.* ***(Right)*** *T1WI C+ FS MR in the same patient shows avid enhancement of the exophytic cervical mass →.*

Stage IIA1 (T2a1 N0 M0)

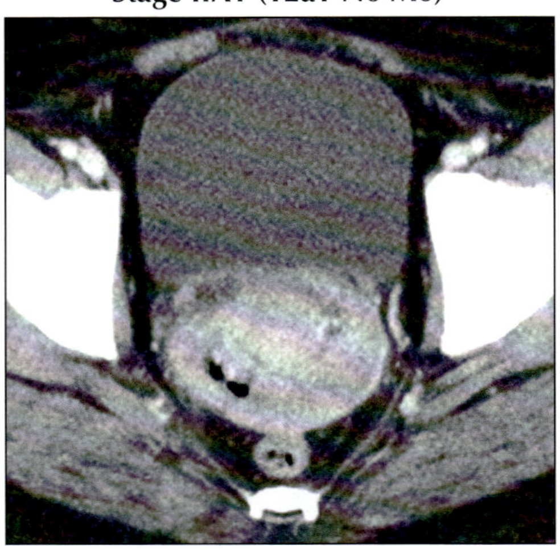

Stage IIA1 (T2a1 N0 M0)

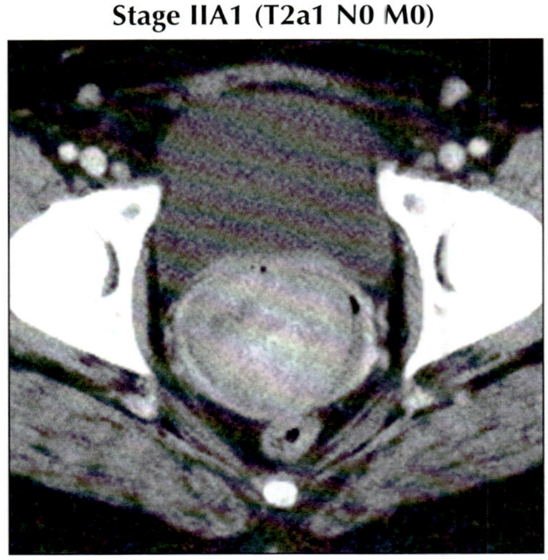

(Left) *Axial CECT shows an exophytic cervical mass invading the left and posterior vaginal wall. The parametrial fat is normal in density and symmetric, suggesting no invasion.* ***(Right)*** *Axial CECT in the same patient, slightly more caudally, shows a large exophytic cervical mass without parametrial invasion. Minimal gas and fluid surround the mass in the vaginal vault.*

Stage IIA1 (T2a1 N0 M0)

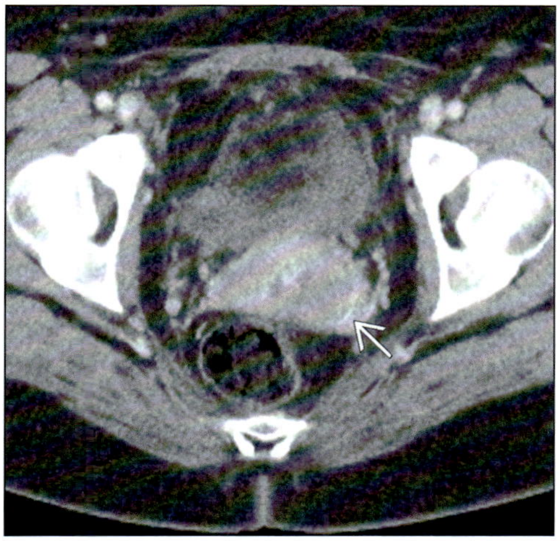

Stage IIA1 (T2a1 N0 M0)

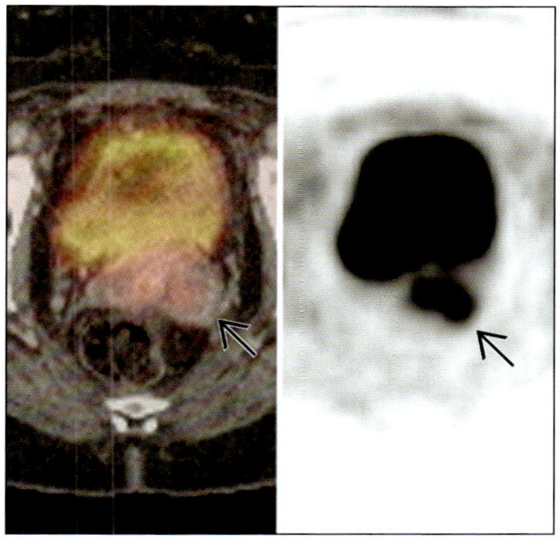

(Left) *Axial CECT shows a hypoenhancing mass ➡ in the cervix. The mass is difficult to see due to poor soft tissue contrast, typical of cervical cancer on CT.* ***(Right)*** *Axial fused PET/CT and PET in the same patient clearly demonstrate a hypermetabolic cervical mass →. No adenopathy or metastatic disease was found.*

Stage IIA1 (T2a1 N0 M0)

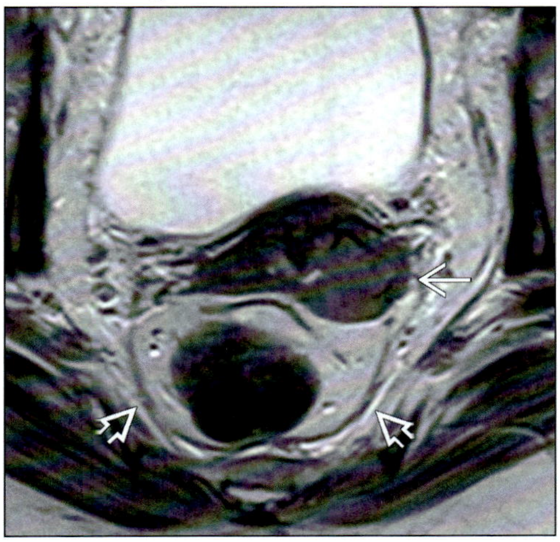

Stage IIA1 (T2a1 N0 M0)

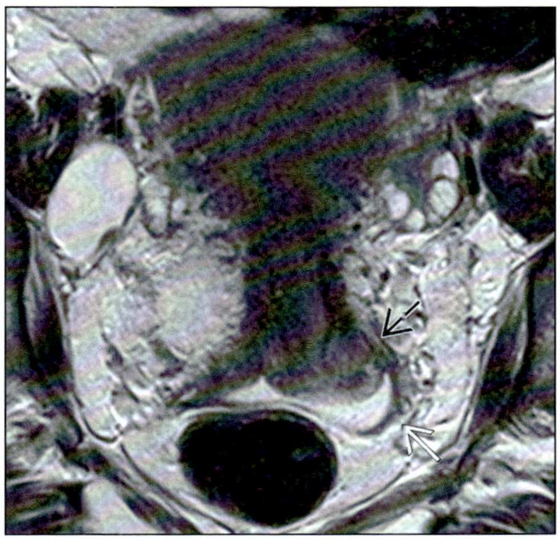

(Left) *Coronal oblique T2WI MR in the same patient shows a hyperintense, partially exophytic cervical mass ➡. Thin smooth uterosacral ligaments ➡ and normal parametrial fat indicate absence of parametrial invasion.* ***(Right)*** *Coronal oblique T2WI MR in the same patient shows a hyperintense, partially exophytic cervical mass focally invading the upper vagina →. Note preservation of the normal low signal ➡ in the remainder of the vaginal wall.*

Stage IIA1 (T2a1 N0 M0)

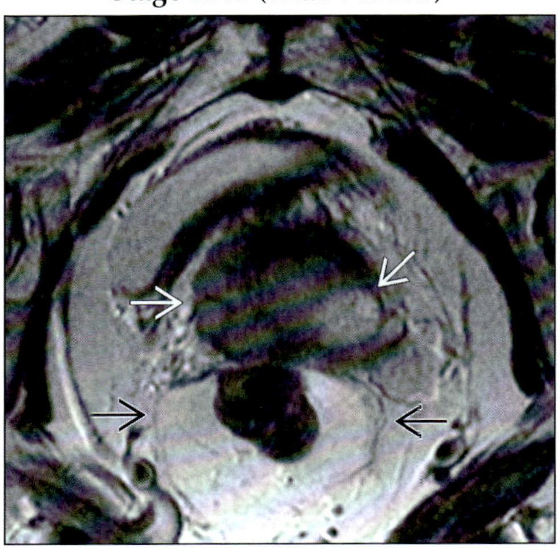

Stage IIA2 (T2a2 N0 M0)

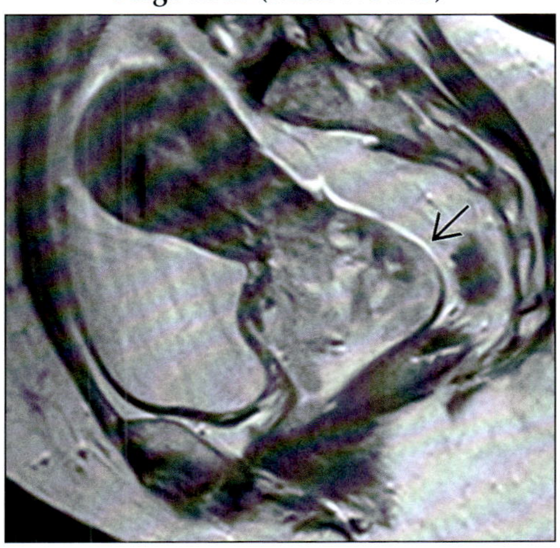

(Left) *Coronal oblique T2WI FSE MR shows a hyperintense cervical mass ➡. The parametrium-tumor interface is sharp with preservation of fat planes suggesting no invasion. Note normal thin uterosacral ligaments →.* ***(Right)*** *Sagittal T2WI FSE MR shows a large exophytic cervical mass expanding the vaginal fornices with disruption of the normal low signal vaginal wall →. The external contour of the tumor is smooth, and parametrial fat is preserved.*

CERVIX UTERI CARCINOMA

*(**Left**) Sagittal T2WI FSE MR shows a hyperintense cervical mass ➡ invading the upper anterior wall of the vagina. Note distention of the uterine cavity due to obstruction by the cervical mass. (**Right**) Gross surgical specimen from hysterectomy from the same patient shows the large exophytic cervical mass.*

Stage IIA2 (T2a2 N0 M0)

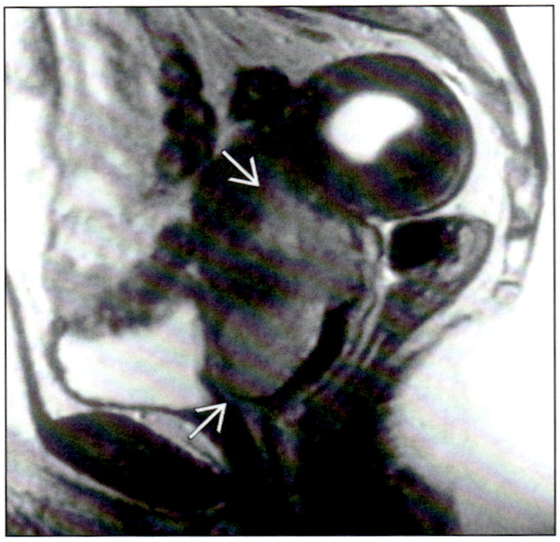

Stage IIA2 (T2a2 N0 M0)

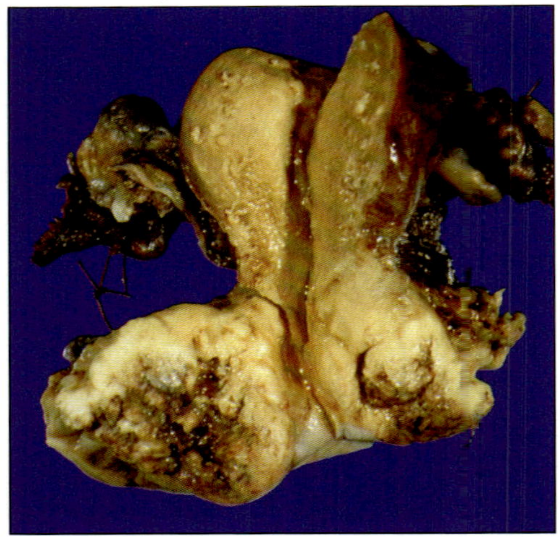

*(**Left**) Coronal oblique T2WI FSE MR shows a hyperintense mass ➡ obliterating the cervix and invading the parametrial tissues →. (**Right**) Axial CECT shows a cervical mass with full thickness cervical stromal invasion and extension into the uterus. The cervical contour is ill defined, and the paracervical fat is increased in density. These nonspecific findings can be due to parametrial inflammation or tumor invasion.*

Stage IIB (T2b N0 M0)

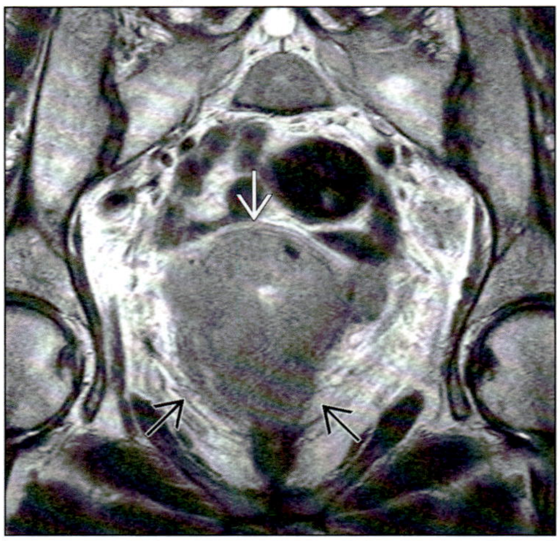

Stage IIB (T2b N0 M0)

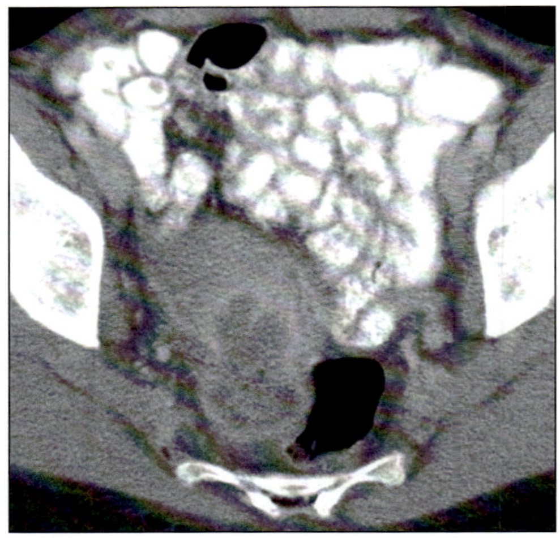

*(**Left**) Coronal oblique T2WI FSE MR (long axis) shows an exophytic cervical mass expanding the left vaginal fornix. There is full thickness invasion on the left with tumor extension into the parametrium ⇨. (**Right**) Coronal oblique T2WI FSE MR (donut view) in the same patient shows the cervical mass disrupting the normal stroma and expanding the endocervical canal. Note the contrast between the normal hypointense cervical stroma ➡ and the hyperintense mass ⇨.*

Stage IIB (T2b N0 M0)

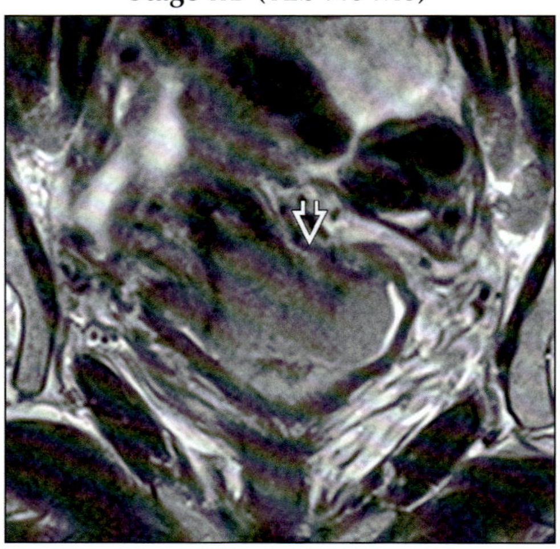

Stage IIB (T2b N0 M0)

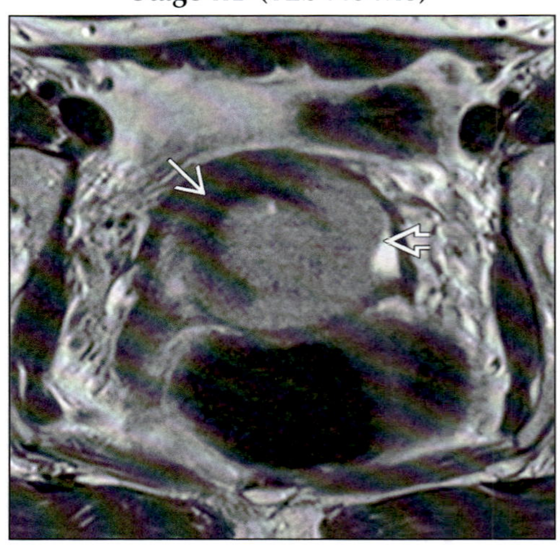

Stage IIB (T2b N0 M0)

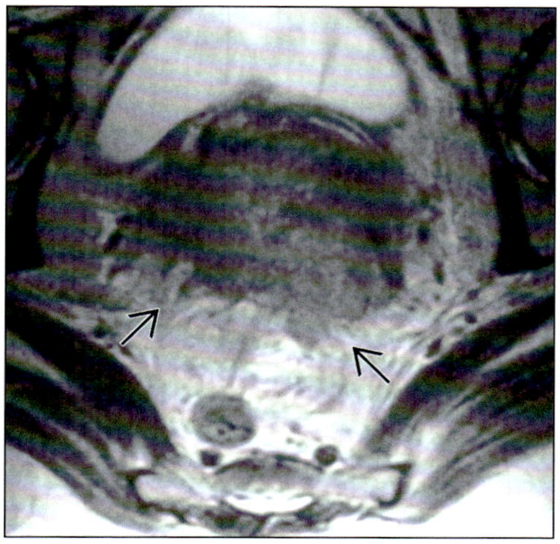

Stage IIB (T2b N0 M0)

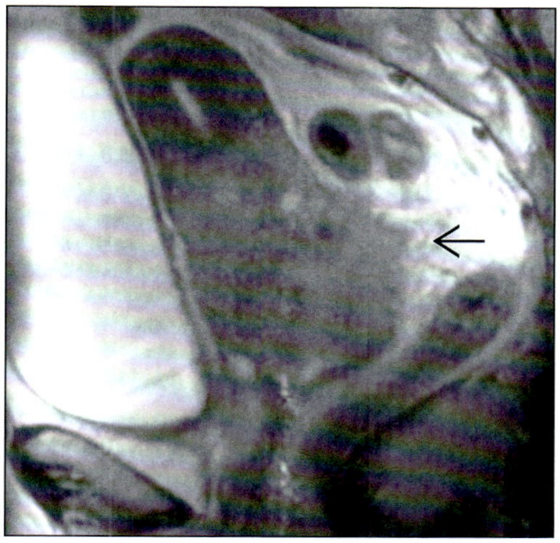

(Left) *Coronal oblique T2WI FSE MR shows full thickness invasion of the cervix by a hyperintense mass with frank tumor extension → into the parametrium bilaterally.* ***(Right)*** *Sagittal T2WI FSE MR shows a large hyperintense cervical mass that invades the parametrial fat posteriorly →, along with the lower uterine segment and upper vagina. Note preservation of an intervening fat plane between the tumor and the normal low signal urinary bladder wall and rectum.*

Stage IIIA (T3a N0 M0)

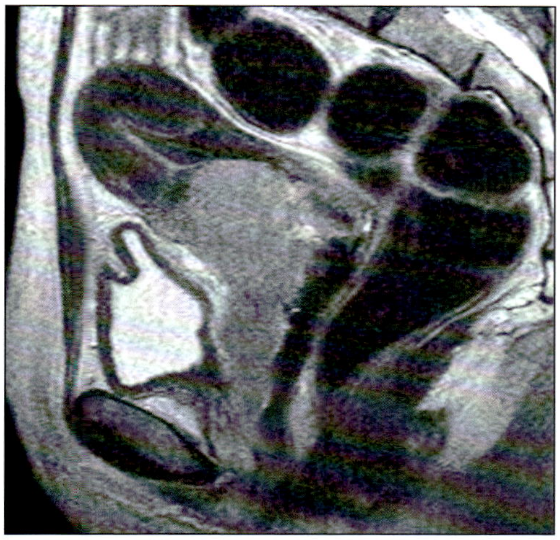

Stage IIIA (T3a N0 M0)

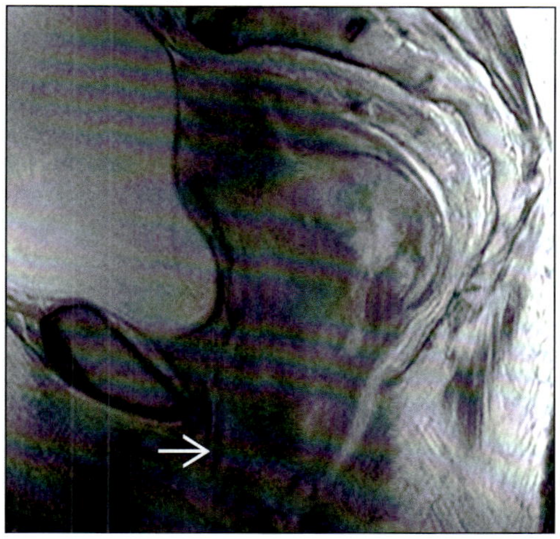

(Left) *Sagittal T2WI FSE MR shows a hyperintense cervical mass invading the anterior vaginal wall with extension to the lower 1/3 of the vagina. The low signal urinary bladder wall is intact.* ***(Right)*** *Sagittal T2WI FSE MR shows a large cervical mass expanding and invading the vagina caudally to the level of the introitus ➡.*

Stage IIIB (T1b1 N1 M0)

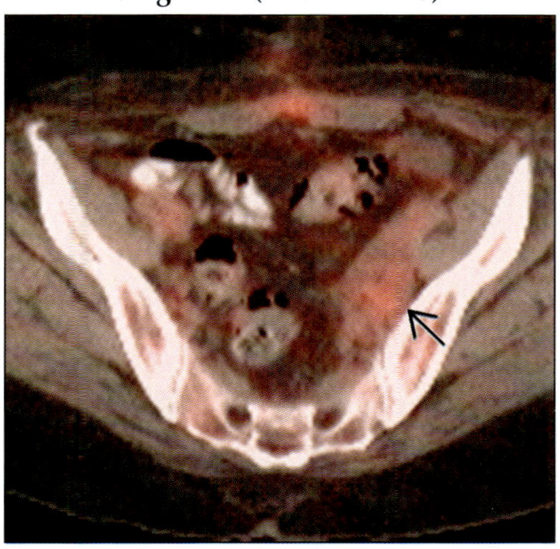

Stage IIIB (T2b N1 M0)

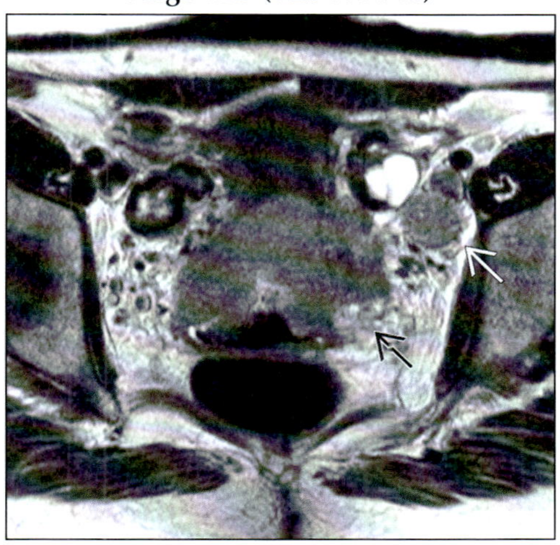

(Left) *Axial fused PET/CT in a patient with clinical stage IB disease shows enlarged left pelvic lymph nodes with increased FDG activity →. Regional lymph node metastasis upstages the patient to stage IIIB, which requires radiation and chemotherapy.* ***(Right)*** *Axial T2WI FSE MR shows enlarged spherical left external iliac lymph node ➡. Also note the T2 hyperintense cervical mass invading the vagina, lower uterine segment, and parametrial tissues →.*

CERVIX UTERI CARCINOMA

*(**Left**) Coronal CECT shows right hydronephrosis → to the level of the cervical mass →, consistent with right ureteral invasion. (**Right**) Axial CECT in the same patient shows a heterogeneous cervical mass with frank extension into the paracervical fat on the right →. There is abrupt termination of the ureteral dilation in the previous figure at this level, making this a FIGO stage IIIB tumor.*

Stage IIIB (T3b N0 M0)

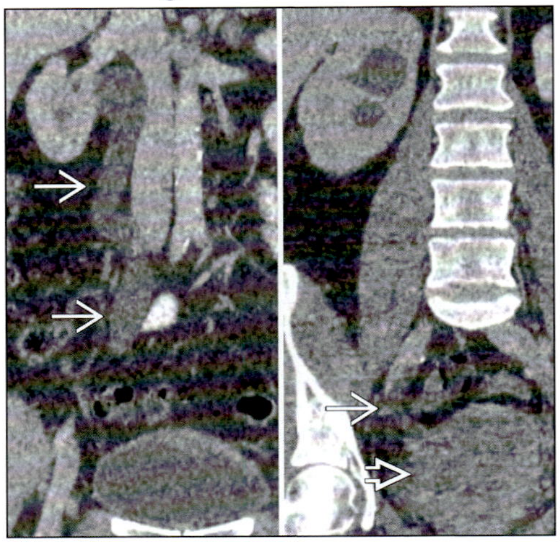

Stage IIIB (T3b N0 M0)

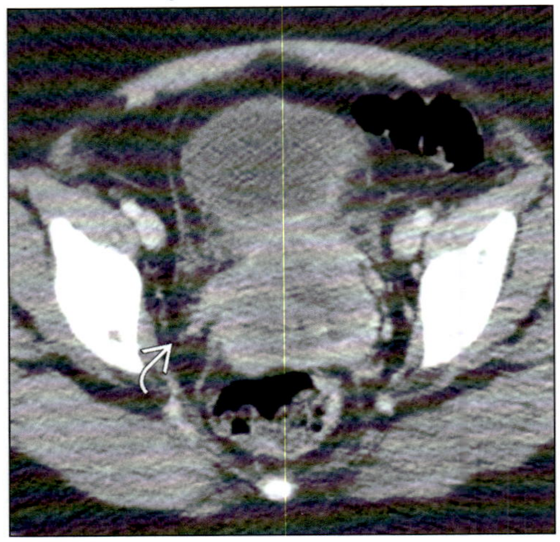

*(**Left**) Axial T2WI FSE MR in a postpartum patient shows an exophytic cervical mass extending into the vaginal vault, as well as invading the upper vagina → and the parametrial tissues on the left →. Note that the posterior vaginal wall → is intact. (**Right**) Axial T2WI FSE MR in the same patient shows left external iliac adenopathy →. Note enlarged postpartum uterus.*

Stage IIIB (T2b N1 M0)

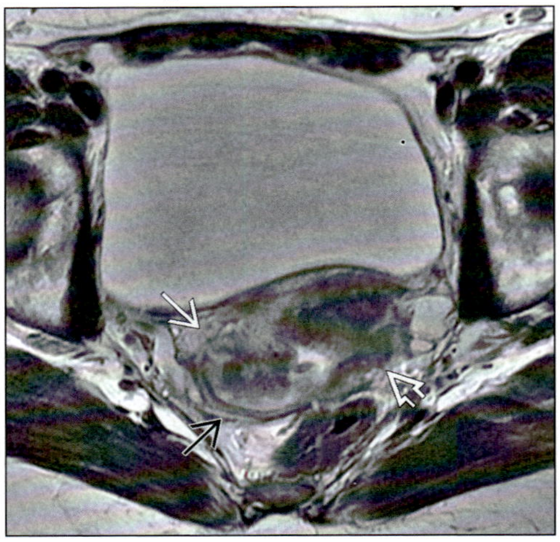

Stage IIIB (T2b N1 M0)

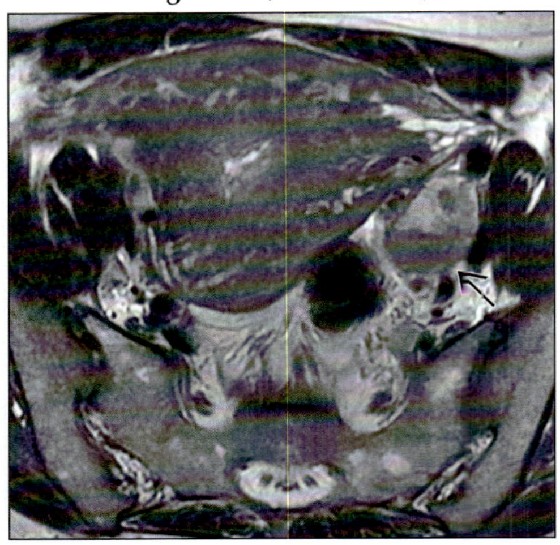

*(**Left**) Axial CECT shows a heterogeneous cervical mass → placing mass effect on the urinary bladder and rectum without definite mucosal invasion. (**Right**) Axial CECT in the same patient shows extension of the cervical mass → to encase the right external iliac artery →, consistent with pelvic sidewall invasion.*

Stage IIIB (T3b N1 M0)

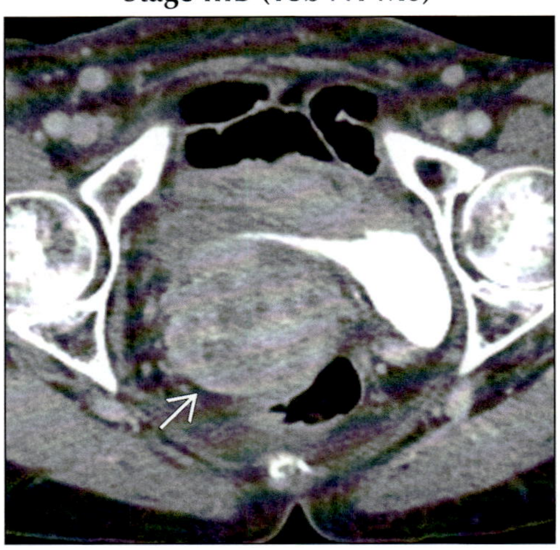

Stage IIIB (T3b N1 M0)

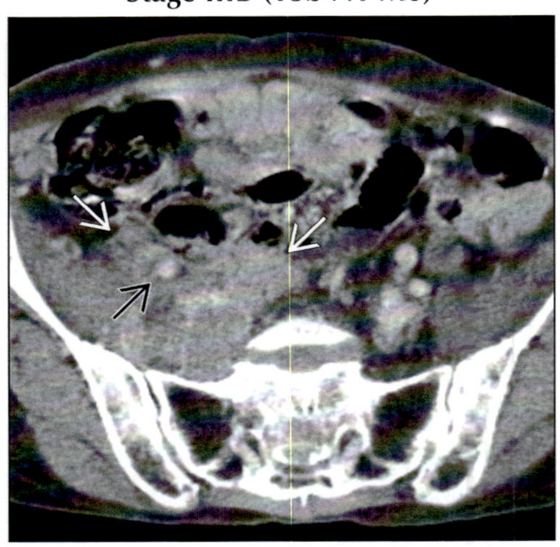

CERVIX UTERI CARCINOMA

Stage IIIB (T3b N1 M0)

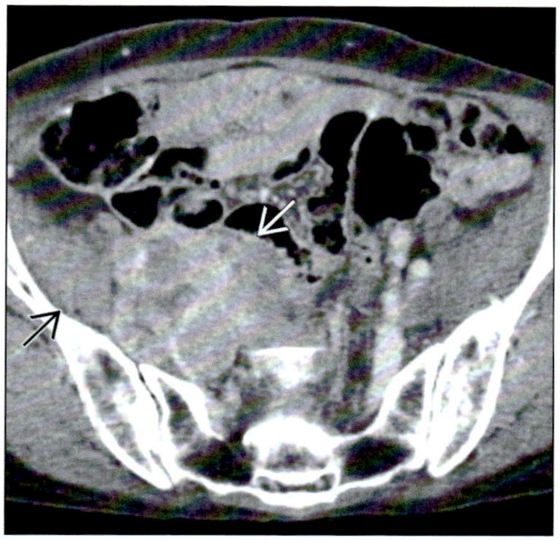

Stage IIIB (T3b N0 M0)

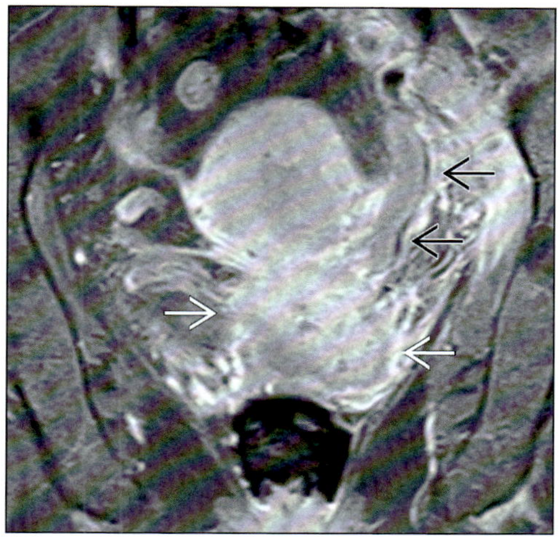

(Left) *Axial CECT in the same patient shows extension of the cervical mass → to abut the right iliacus muscle →, also indicative of pelvic sidewall invasion.* ***(Right)*** *Coronal T1WI C+ FS MR shows a cervical mass → with frank invasion into the parametrium. Dilated left ureter → descends and abruptly terminates at the level of the cervical mass, consistent with ureteral invasion and stage IIIB disease.*

Stage IIIB with Bullous Edema Sign

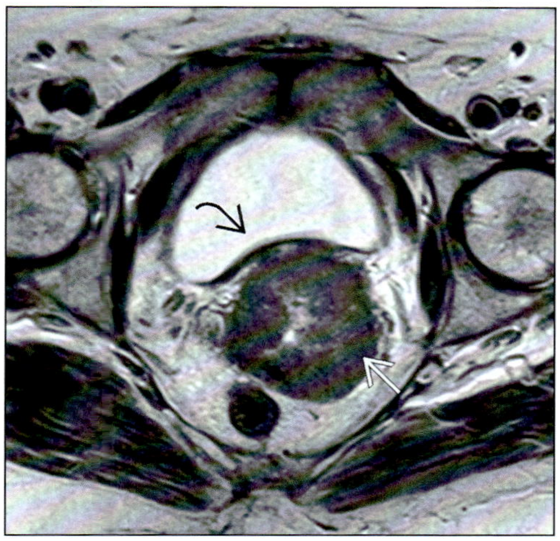

Stage IIIB with Bullous Edema Sign

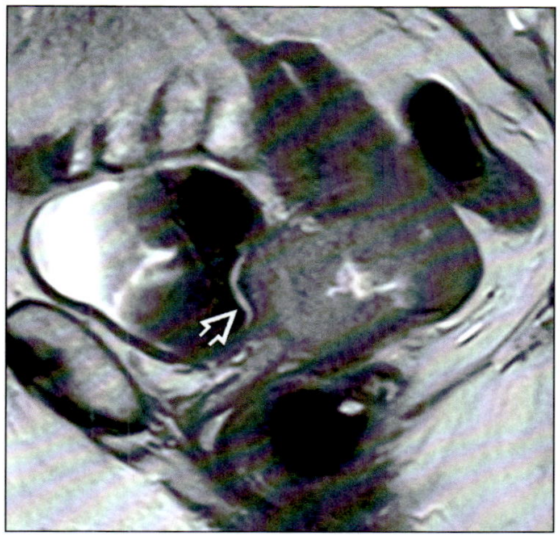

(Left) *Axial T2WI FSE MR shows hyperintense cervical mass → invading the vesicouterine ligament. There is reactive T2 hyperintense thickening of the urinary bladder mucosa →; however, no disruption of the low signal wall is present to suggest invasion. Left hydronephrosis was seen (not shown).* ***(Right)*** *Sagittal T2WI MR after intravenous contrast better demonstrates the reactive urinary bladder wall edema →, which is outlined by dense, low signal gadolinium.*

Stage IVA (T4 N0 M0)

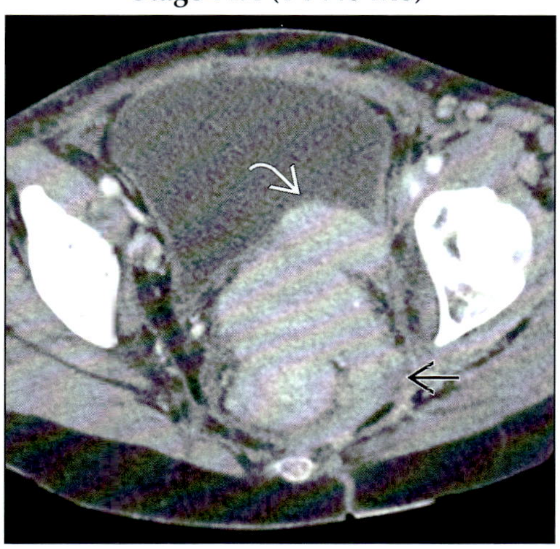

Stage IVA (T4 N0 M0)

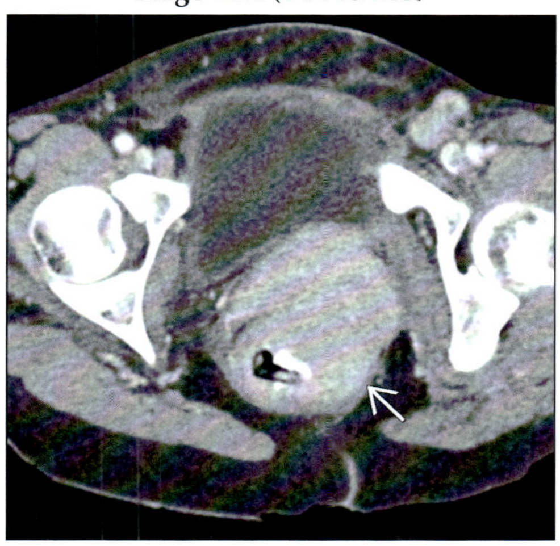

(Left) *Axial CECT shows replacement of the cervix by a mass that invades anteriorly into the urinary bladder lumen →. Note nodular thickening of the left uterosacral ligament →.* ***(Right)*** *Axial CECT in the same patient after administration of rectal contrast better shows eccentric wall thickening of the left rectum → and luminal irregularity indicative of mucosal invasion.*

CERVIX UTERI CARCINOMA

*(**Left**) Sagittal T2WI FSE MR shows a large hyperintense cervical mass extending anteriorly to invade the urinary bladder → and posteriorly to the rectal mucosa →. (**Right**) Axial CECT shows the rectum abutting the cervix with no intervening fat plane. There is a fluid- and gas-filled tract → extending from the endocervical canal to the rectum, consistent with a fistula. Note fecal material within the cervix.*

Stage IVA (T4 N0 M0)

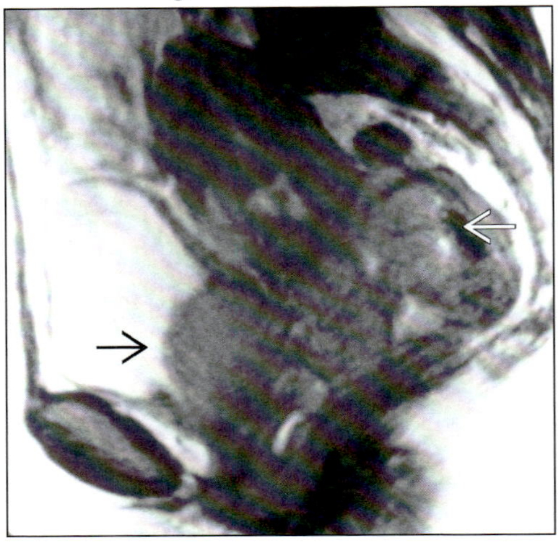

Stage IVA (T4 N0 M0)

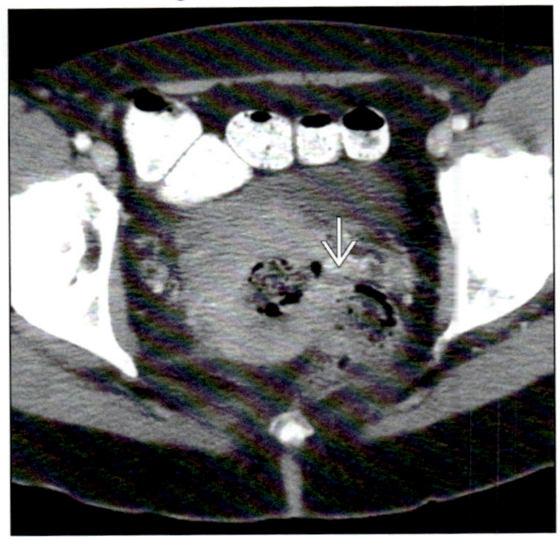

*(**Left**) Axial CECT at the level of the cervix in a patient with clinical stage IB2 disease demonstrates the limitations of CT in visualizing cervical masses. This patient had a necrotic, 5.5 cm cervical mass on physical exam. (**Right**) Axial CECT in the same patient shows fluid distension of the uterine cavity →, the only finding that suggests a cervical mass in this patient. The uterus is retroflexed.*

Stage IVB (T1b2 N1 M1)

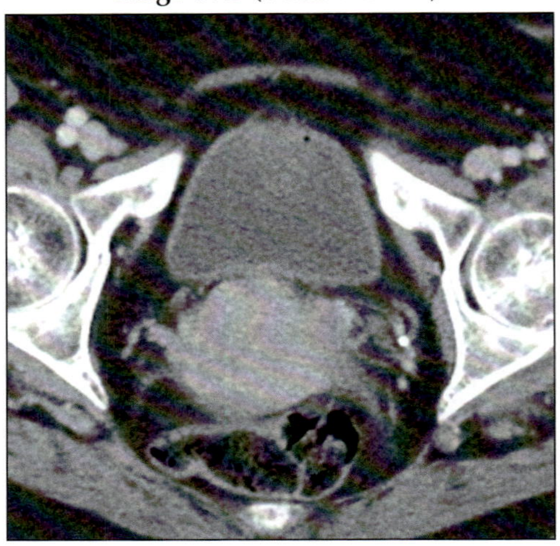

Stage IVB (T1b2 N1 M1)

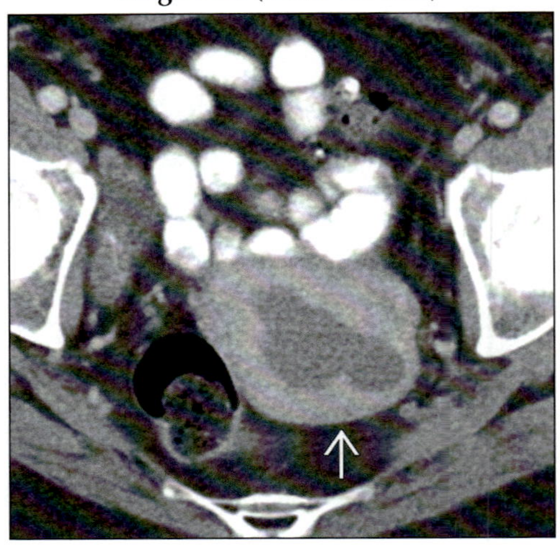

*(**Left**) Axial CECT in the same patient shows interaortocaval adenopathy →, upstaging this patient to stage IVB with metastatic disease. (**Right**) Axial CECT in the same patient shows left external iliac adenopathy → and a solid right ovarian mass →. Despite the poor performance of CT in the evaluation of the primary tumor, the examination influenced staging by revealing pelvic adenopathy and metastatic disease to the ovary and paraaortic lymph nodes.*

Stage IVB (T1b2 N1 M1)

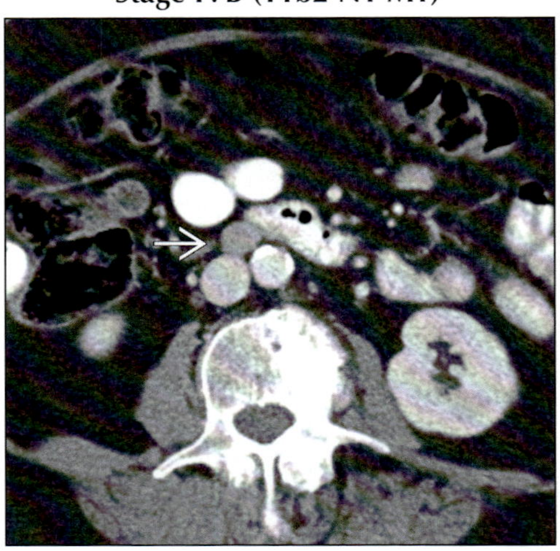

Stage IVB (T1b2 N1 M1)

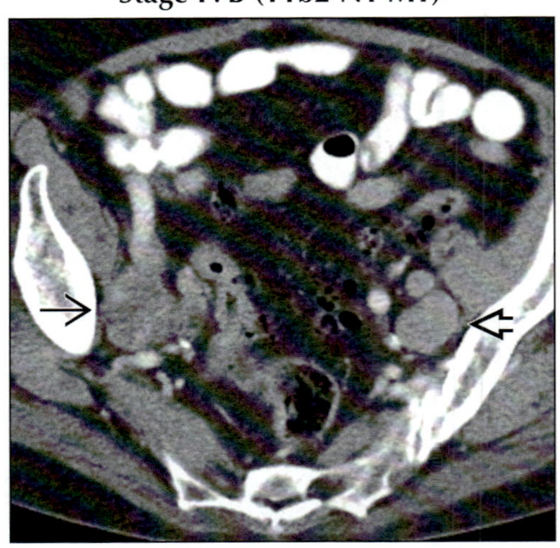

Stage IVB (T2b N1 M1)

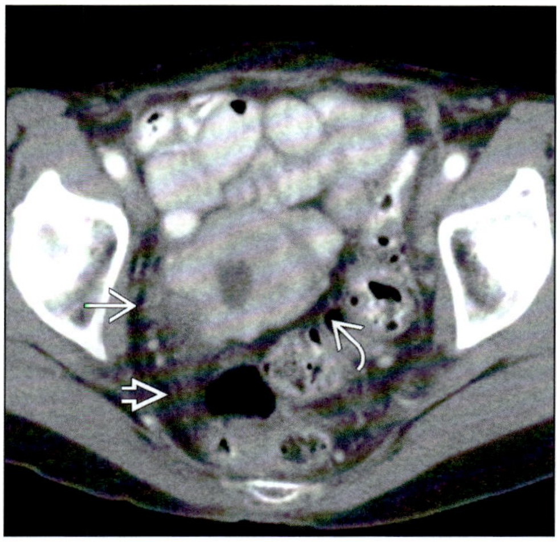

Stage IVB (T2b N1 M1)

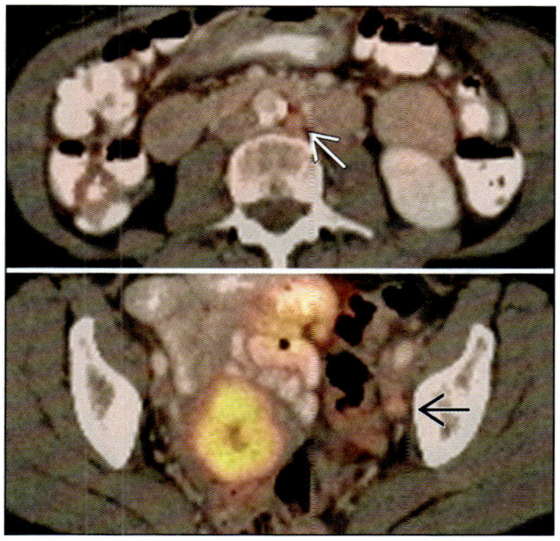

*(**Left**) Axial CECT shows a cervical mass. Irregularity of the right tumor-fat interface, increased density of the parametrial fat, and thickening of the right uterosacral ligament are consistent with parametrial invasion. The left parametrial fat is preserved. (**Right**) Axial PET/CT in the same patient shows the hypermetabolic cervical mass. Small left obturator and paraaortic nodes are not enlarged but hypermetabolic, upstaging this patient.*

Stage IVB (T2b N1 M1)

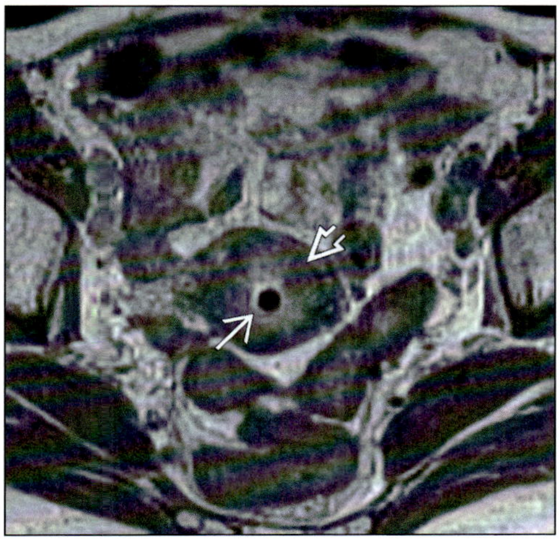

Stage IVB (T2b N1 M1)

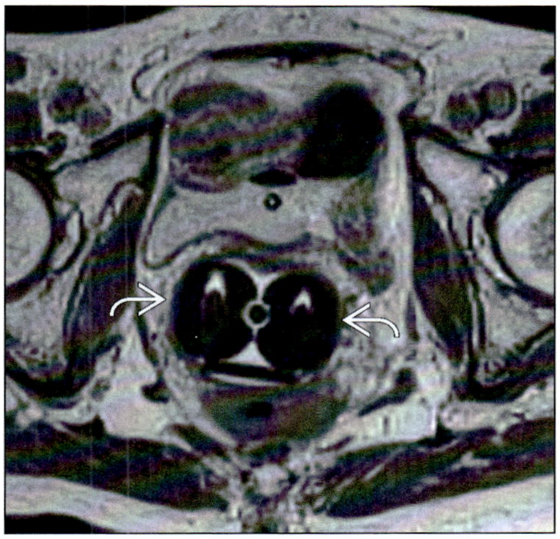

*(**Left**) MR in the same patient was performed to confirm position of tandem and ovoids and determine dose for administration of brachytherapy. Axial image shows tandem appropriately positioned in the endocervical canal and surrounded by mildly hyperintense tumor. (**Right**) Axial MR image in the same patient shows ovoids appropriately positioned in the upper vagina.*

Stage IVB (T1b2 N1 M1)

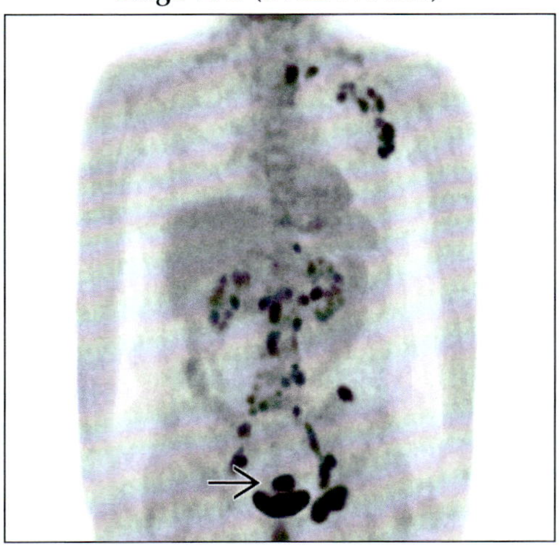

Stage IVB (T2b N0 M1)

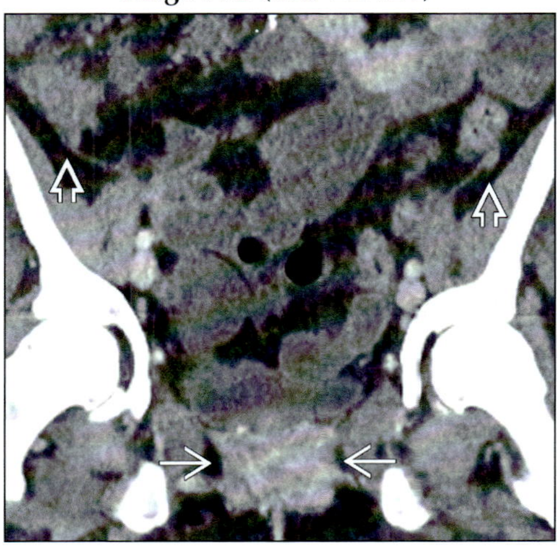

*(**Left**) Whole body PET image shows overall disease burden in a patient with metastatic cervical cancer. Note the FDG-avid primary tumor, as well as metastases in the inguinal, iliac, periaortic, supraclavicular, and axillary lymph nodes. (**Right**) Coronal CECT shows an enhancing urethral mass in a patient with metastatic cervical cancer. Also note peritoneal carcinomatosis. Numerous pulmonary nodules, although present, are not shown.*

CERVIX UTERI CARCINOMA

(Left) *Whole-body PET image shows FDG-avid, subcentimeter common iliac lymph nodes → and lung nodules ⇨. The patient was upstaged from initial clinical stage IIA to IVB, and the treatment was changed from curative to palliative.* **(Right)** *Axial fused PET/CT shows 2 focal areas of increased FDG activity in the liver ➡, compatible with hepatic metastatic disease.*

Stage IVB (T2a N1 M1)

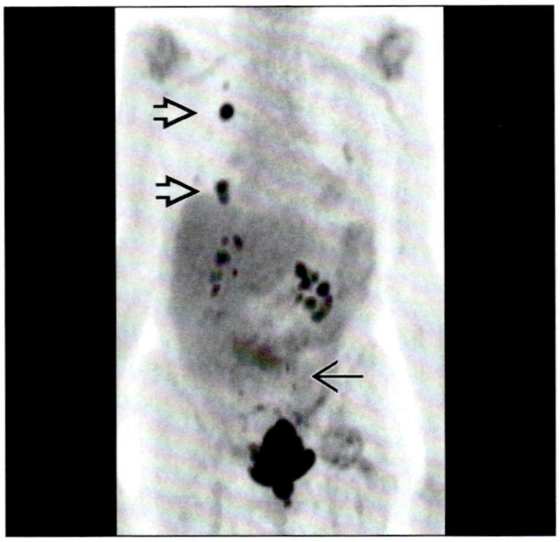

Stage IVB (T2a2 N0 M1)

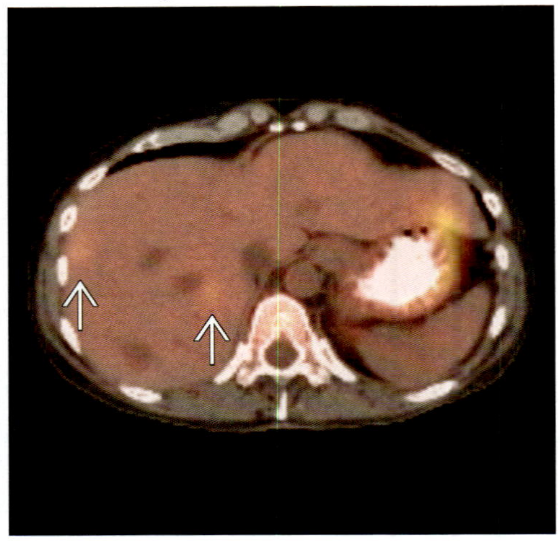

(Left) *Coronal CECT shows a mass ➡ in the right hemipelvis invading the iliacus and psoas muscles and encasing the right iliac artery. Obstruction of the ureter is not included on this image; however, hydronephrosis and a delayed right nephrogram ➡ are evident.* **(Right)** *Axial CECT in the same patient shows the uterine fundus ➡, although the cervix ➡ is absent, as is typical following radiation therapy. Right pelvic sidewall recurrence ➡ is also seen.*

Pelvic Sidewall Recurrence

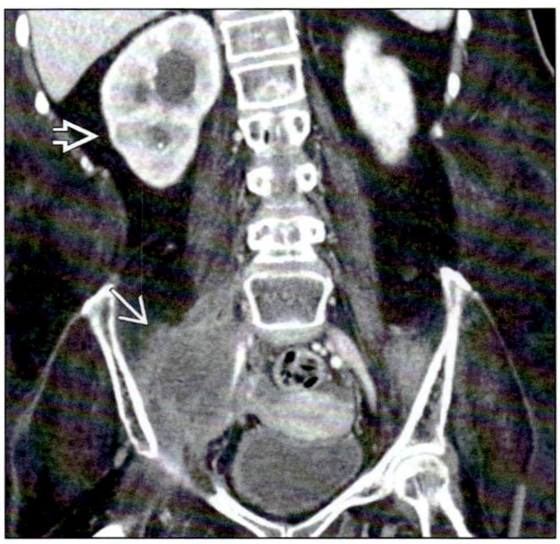

Pelvic Sidewall Recurrence

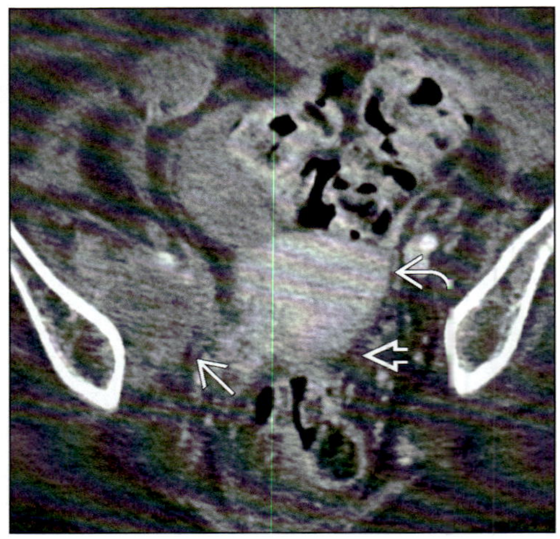

(Left) *Axial T2WI FSE MR shows 2 cystic masses ➡ at the left pelvic sidewall in this patient with cervical cancer status post remote hysterectomy.* **(Right)** *Axial CECT shows right hydronephrosis with obstruction of the ureter by an irregular enhancing mass at the right vaginal cuff. The mass ➡ extends into the parametrial tissues, up to the obturator internus muscle, to the thickened urinary bladder and rectum with loss of intervening fat planes.*

Cystic Pelvic Sidewall Recurrence

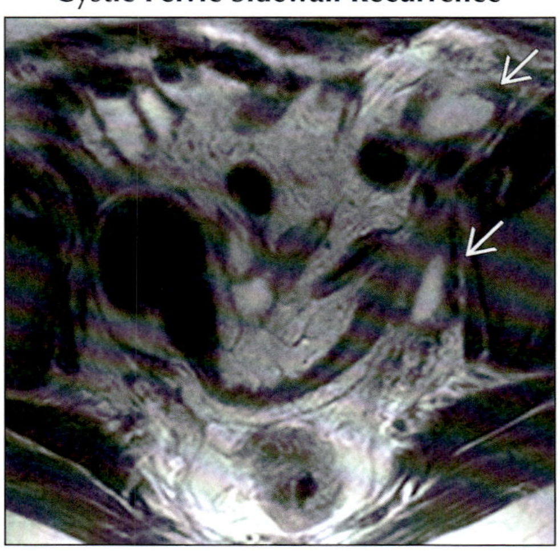

Central Recurrence

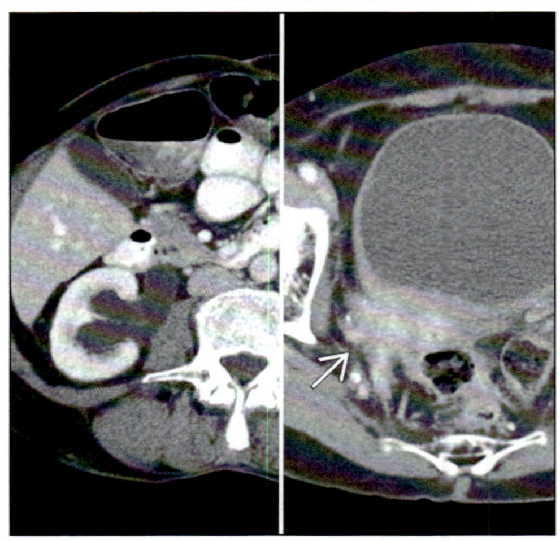

CERVIX UTERI CARCINOMA

Recurrence

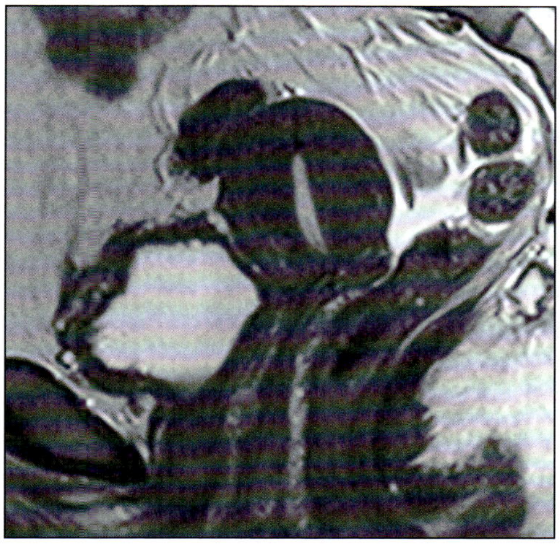

Recurrence

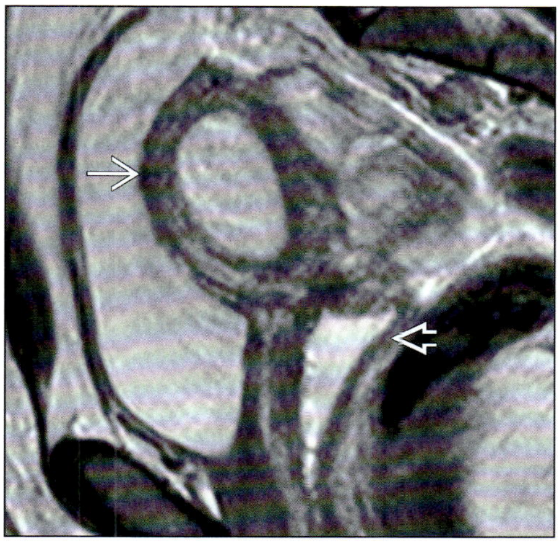

(Left) *Sagittal T2WI FSE MR in a patient with cervical cancer shows the normal post-trachelectomy appearance with absence of the cervix.* ***(Right)*** *Sagittal T2WI FSE MR in the same patient, 1 year later, demonstrates distension of the uterine cavity → with fluid, concerning for tumor recurrence and obstruction. Note distension of the vagina → with Surgilube.*

Recurrence

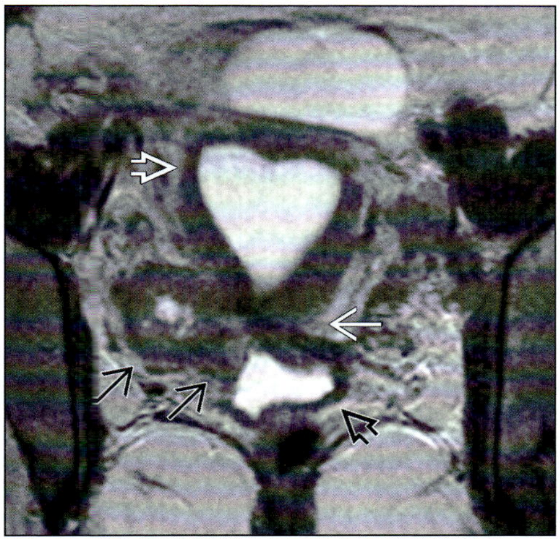

Recurrence

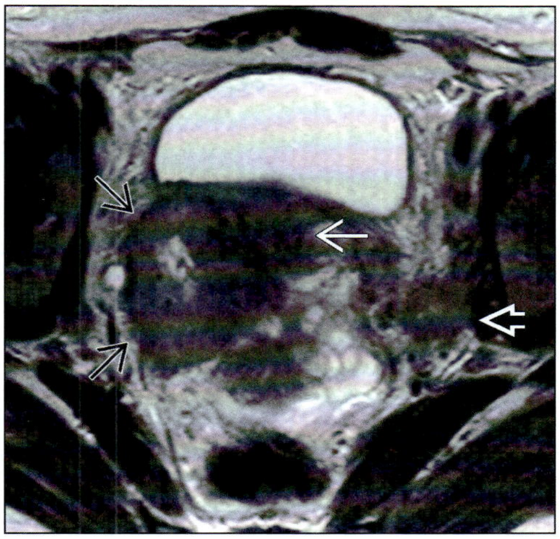

(Left) *Coronal oblique T2WI FSE MR in the same patient shows the uterine cavity distended → with fluid and stenosis → with an associated T2 hyperintense exophytic mass → at the level of the trachelectomy. Note the utility of distending the vagina → with Surgilube.* ***(Right)*** *Coronal oblique (donut) T2WI FSE MR in the same patient at the level of the stenosis → shows the exophytic recurrent tumor → and pelvic adenopathy →.*

Recurrence

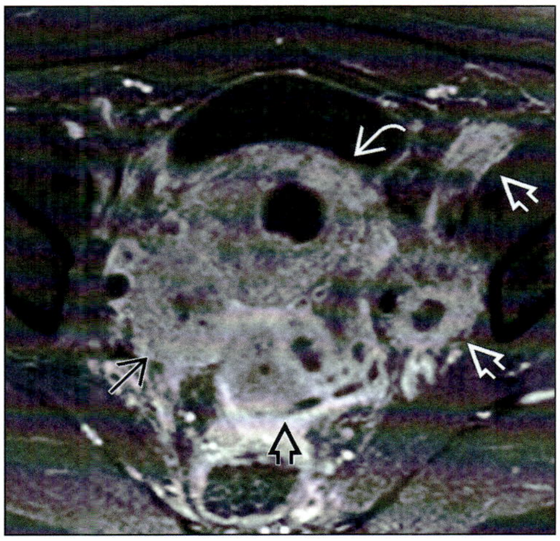

Recurrence

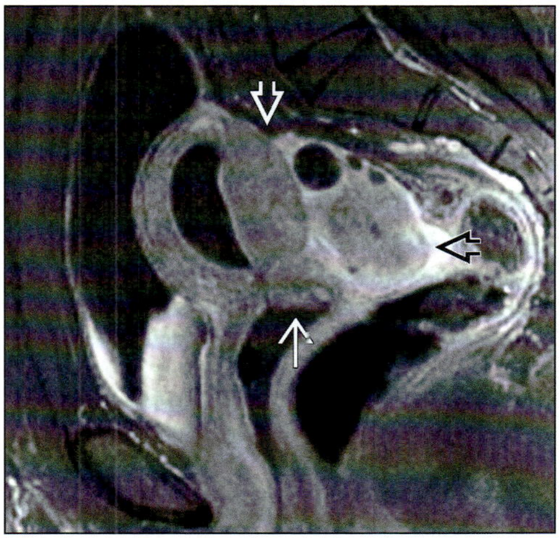

(Left) *Axial T1WI C+ FS MR shows the distended uterine cavity →, enhancing exophytic recurrent tumor →, left external iliac adenopathy →, and left ovarian metastasis →.* ***(Right)*** *Sagittal T1WI C+ FS MR shows the portion of the recurrent mass → at the trachelectomy site with invasion of the vaginal cuff and resultant stenosis. Thickening of the posterior uterine wall → is concerning for tumor infiltration. Ovarian metastasis → is again noted.*

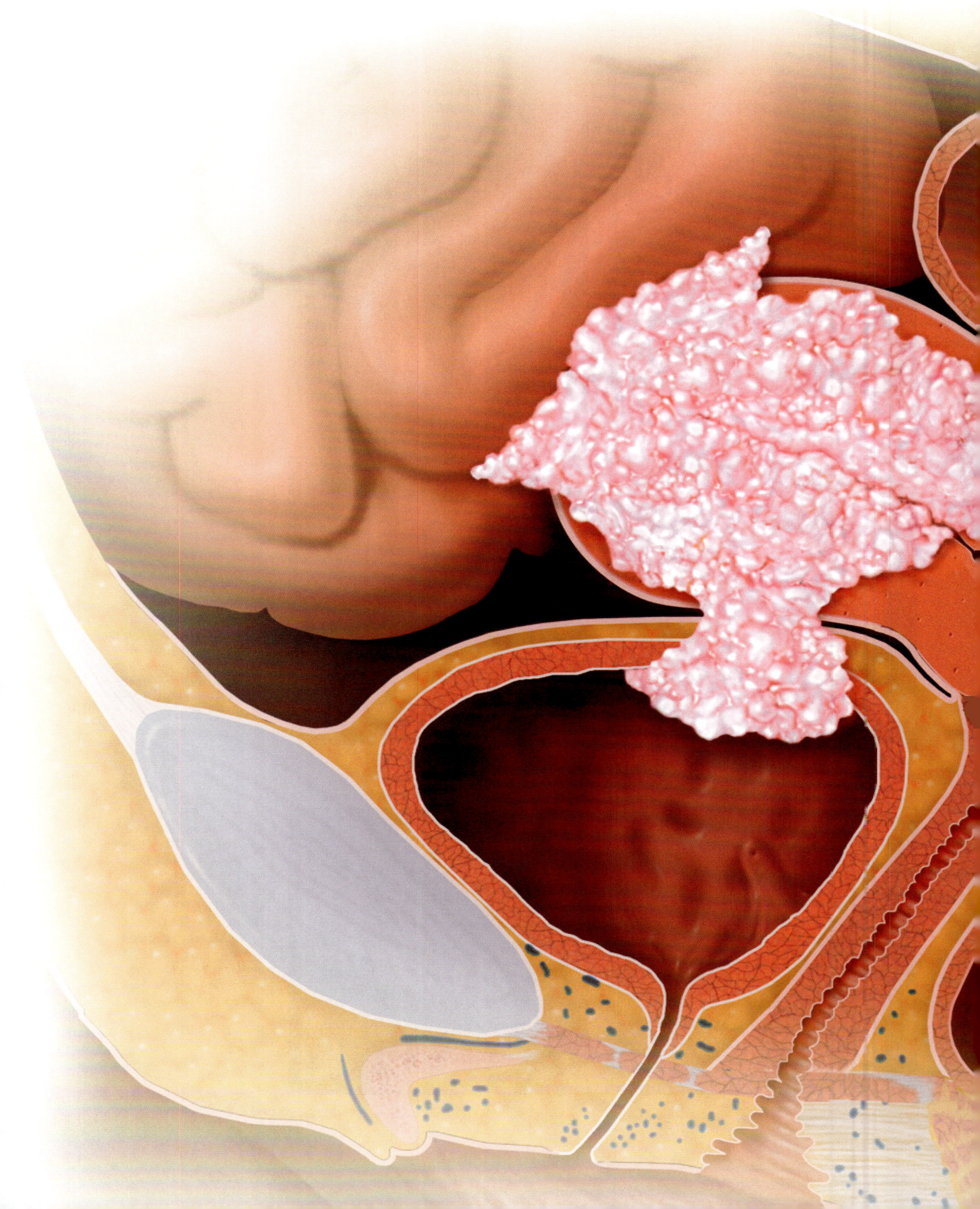

Corpus Uteri Carcinoma

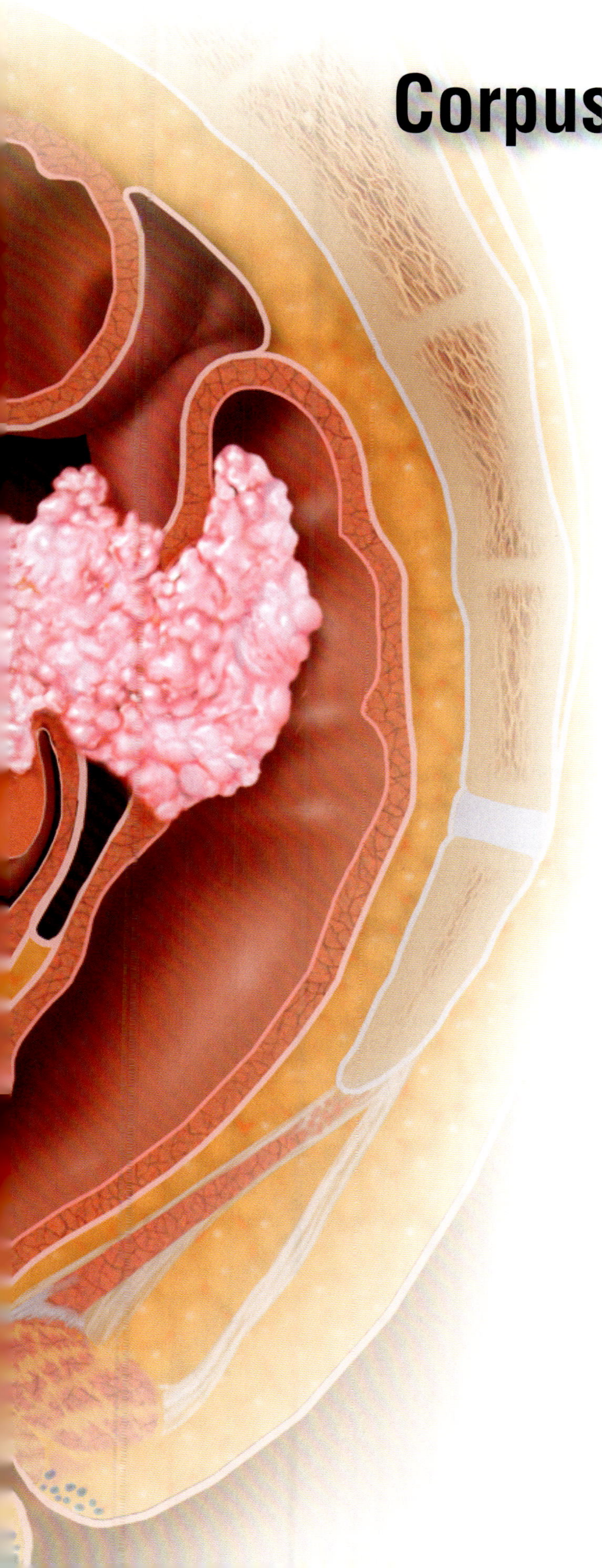

CORPUS UTERI CARCINOMA

(T) Primary Tumor for Uterine Carcinomas

Adapted from 7th edition AJCC Staging Forms.

TNM	*FIGO*	*Definitions*
TX		Primary tumor cannot be assessed
T0		No evidence of primary tumor
Tis[1]		Carcinoma in situ (preinvasive carcinoma)
T1	I	Tumor confined to corpus uteri
T1a	IA	Tumor limited to endometrium or invades < 1/2 of the myometrium
T1b	IB	Tumor invades ≥ 1/2 of the myometrium
T2	II	Tumor invades stromal connective tissue of the cervix but does not extend beyond uterus[2]
T3a	IIIA	Tumor invades serosa &/or adnexa (direct extension or metastasis)
T3b	IIIB	Vaginal involvement (direct extension or metastasis) or parametrial involvement
T4	IVA	Tumor invades bladder mucosa &/or bowel mucosa (bullous edema is not sufficient to classify a tumor as T4)

[1]*FIGO no longer includes stage 0 (Tis).* [2]*Endocervical glandular involvement only should be considered as stage I and not as stage II.*

(N) Regional Lymph Nodes for Uterine Carcinomas

Adapted from 7th edition AJCC Staging Forms.

TNM	*FIGO*	*Definitions*
NX		Regional lymph nodes cannot be assessed
N0		No regional lymph node metastasis
N1	IIIC1	Regional lymph node metastasis to pelvic lymph nodes
N2	IIIC2	Regional lymph node metastasis to paraaortic lymph nodes, with or without positive pelvic lymph nodes

(M) Distant Metastasis for Uterine Carcinomas

Adapted from 7th edition AJCC Staging Forms.

TNM	*FIGO*	*Definitions*
M0		No distant metastasis
M1	IVB	Distant metastasis (includes metastasis to inguinal lymph nodes intraperitoneal disease, or lung, liver, or bone; excludes metastasis to paraaortic lymph nodes, vagina, pelvic serosa, or adnexa)

CORPUS UTERI CARCINOMA

AJCC Stages/Prognostic Groups for Uterine Carcinomas[1]

Adapted from 7th edition AJCC Staging Forms.

Stage	*T*	*N*	*M*
0	Tis	N0	M0
I	T1	N0	M0
IA	T1a	N0	M0
IB	T1b	N0	M0
II	T2	N0	M0
III	T3	N0	M0
IIIA	T3a	N0	M0
IIIB	T3b	N0	M0
IIIC1	T1-T3	N1	M0
IIIC2	T1-T3	N2	M0
IVA	T4	Any N	M0
IVB	Any T	Any N	M1

[1]*Carcinosarcomas should be staged as carcinoma.*

(T) Primary Tumor for Leiomyosarcoma and Endometrial Stromal Sarcoma[1]

Adapted from 7th edition AJCC Staging Forms.

TNM	*FIGO*	*Definitions*
TX		Primary tumor cannot be assessed
T0		No evidence of primary tumor
T1	I	Tumor limited to the uterus
T1a	IA	Tumor ≤ 5 cm in greatest dimensions
T1b	IB	Tumor > 5 cm
T2	II	Tumor extends beyond the uterus, within the pelvis
T2a	IIA	Tumor involves adnexa
T2b	IIB	Tumor involves other pelvic tissues
T3	III[2]	Tumor infiltrates abdominal tissues
T3a	IIIA	1 site
T3b	IIB	> 1 site
T4	IVA	Tumor invades bladder or rectum

[1]*Simultaneous tumors of the uterine corpus and ovary/pelvis in association with ovarian/pelvic endometriosis should be classified as independent primary tumors.* [2]*In this stage lesions must infiltrate abdominal tissues and not just protrude into the abdominal cavity.*

(N) Regional Lymph Nodes for Leiomyosarcoma and Endometrial Stromal Sarcoma

Adapted from 7th edition AJCC Staging Forms.

TNM	*FIGO*	*Definitions*
NX		Regional lymph nodes cannot be assessed
N0		No regional lymph node metastasis
N1	IIIC	Regional lymph node metastasis

CORPUS UTERI CARCINOMA

(M) Distant Metastasis for Leiomyosarcoma and Endometrial Stromal Sarcoma

Adapted from 7th edition AJCC Staging Forms.

TNM	*FIGO*	*Definitions*
M0		No distant metastasis
M1	IVB	Distant metastasis (excluding adnexa, pelvic and abdominal tissues)

(T) Primary Tumor for Adenosarcoma[1]

Adapted from 7th edition AJCC Staging Forms.

TNM	*FIGO*	*Descriptions*
TX		Primary tumor cannot be assessed
T0		No evidence of primary tumor
T1	I	Tumor limited to the uterus
T1a	IA	Tumor limited to the endometrium/endocervix
T1b	IB	Tumor invades to < 1/2 of the myometrium
T1c	IC	Tumor invades ≥ 1/2 of the myometrium
T2	II	Tumor extends beyond the uterus, within the pelvis
T2a	IIA	Tumor involves adnexa
T2b	IIB	Tumor involves other pelvic tissues
T3	III[2]	Tumor involves abdominal tissues
T3a	IIIA	1 site
T3b	IIIB	> 1 site
T4	IVA	Tumor invades bladder or rectum

[1]*Simultaneous tumors of the uterine corpus and ovary/pelvis in association with ovarian/pelvic endometriosis should be classified as independent primary tumors.* [2]*In this stage lesions must infiltrate abdominal tissues and not just protrude into the abdominal cavity.*

(N) Regional Lymph Nodes for Adenosarcoma

Adapted from 7th edition AJCC Staging Forms.

TNM	*FIGO*	*Descriptions*
NX		Regional lymph nodes cannot be assessed
N0		No regional lymph node metastasis
N1	IIIC	Regional lymph node metastasis

(M) Distant Metastasis for Adenosarcoma

Adapted from 7th edition AJCC Staging Forms.

TNM	*FIGO*	*Definitions*
M0		No distant metastasis
M1	IVB	Distant metastasis (excluding adnexa, pelvic and abdominal tissues)

AJCC Stages/Prognostic Groups for Uterine Sarcomas

Adapted from 7th edition AJCC Staging Forms.

Stage	*T*	*N*	*M*
I	T1	N0	M0
IA[1]	T1a	N0	M0
IB[1]	T1b	N0	M0
IC[2]	T1c	N0	M0
II	T2	N0	M0
IIIA	T3a	N0	M0
IIIB	T3b	N0	M0
IIIC	T1, T2, T3	N1	M0
IVA	T4	Any N	M0
IVB	Any T	Any N	M1

[1]*Stage IA and IB differ from those applied for leiomyosarcoma and endometrial stromal sarcoma.* [2]*Stage IC does not apply for leiomyosarcoma and endometrial stromal sarcoma.*

CORPUS UTERI CARCINOMA

Stage IA-IB (T1a-T1b N0 M0)

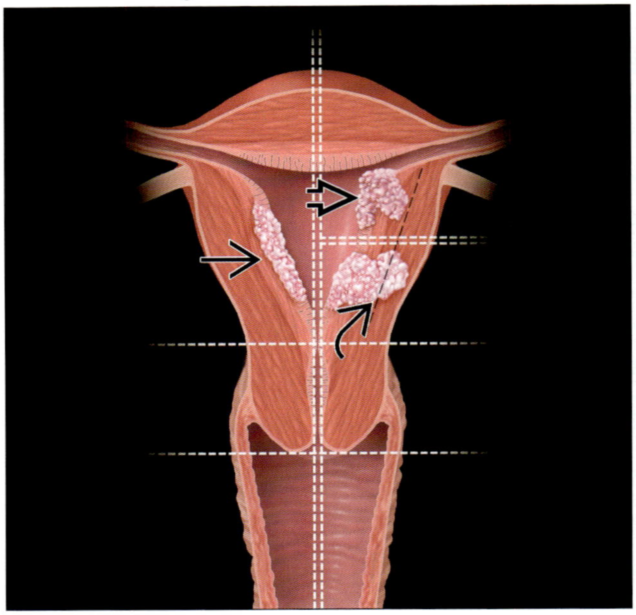

Coronal graphic shows T1 tumors, those confined to corpus uteri. T1a tumors are limited to the endometrium → or involve less than 1/2 of the myometrium →; T1b tumors invade 1/2 or more of the myometrium → indicated by the tumor traversing the dotted horizontal line, marking the halfway plane of the myometrium.

Stage II (T2 N0 M0)

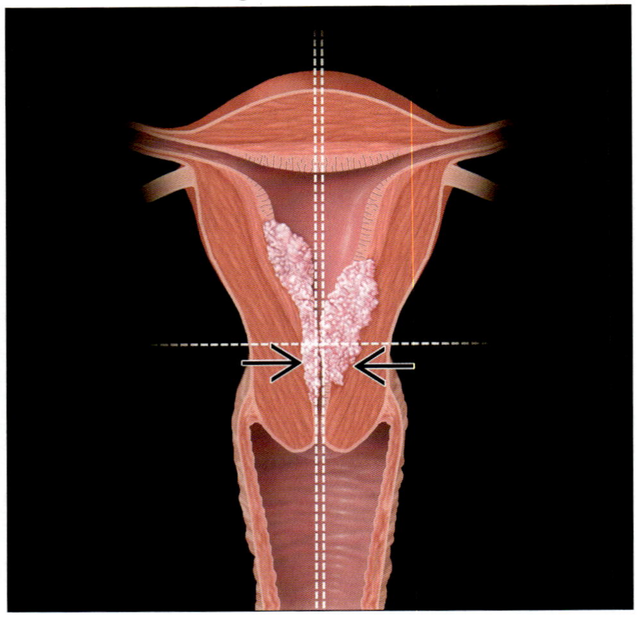

Coronal graphic shows a typical T2 tumor →, which invades the cervix but does not extend beyond the uterus. Endocervical glandular involvement only should be considered stage I and not stage II.

Stage IIIA-B (T3a-T3b N0 M0)

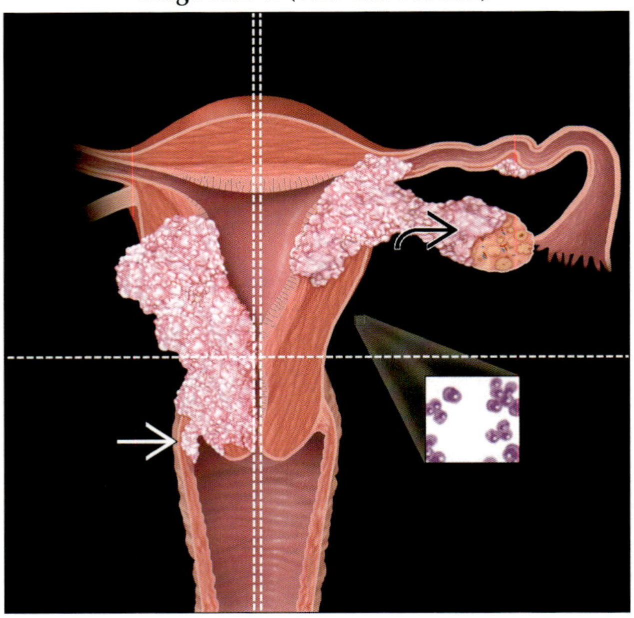

Coronal graphic shows stage III disease, both T3a, which is tumor involving the serosa &/or adnexa →, and T3b, which is tumor that involves the vagina → by direct extension or metastases or parametrial involvement.

Stage IVA (T4 N0 M0)

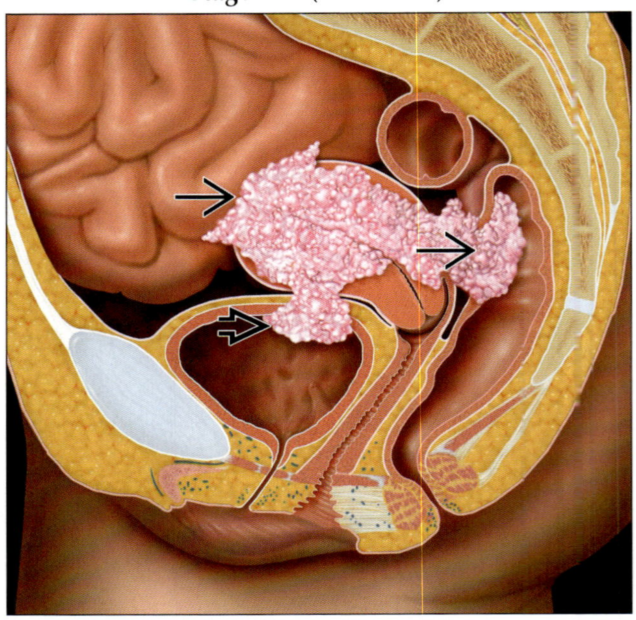

Sagittal graphic shows stage IVA disease with tumor that invades the bladder mucosa → &/or bowel mucosa →. However, bullous edema is not sufficient to classify a tumor as T4. Stage IVB is defined as distant metastasis, including metastasis to inguinal lymph nodes, peritoneum, lung, liver, or bone.

N1

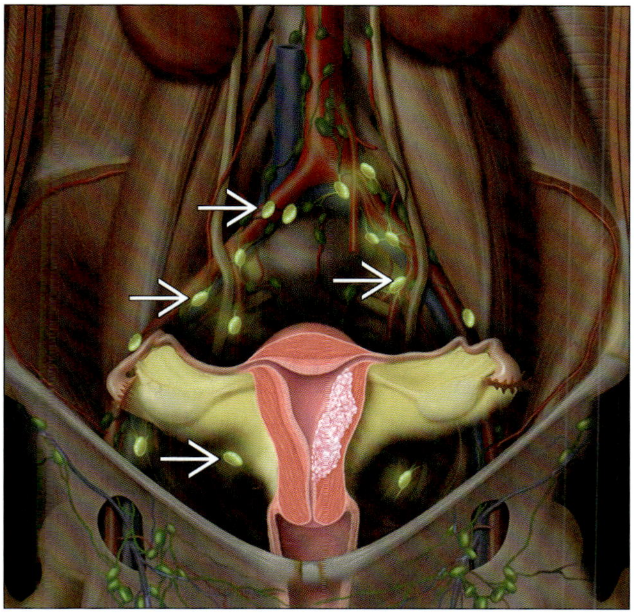

Coronal graphic shows an example of N1 disease, defined as regional lymph node metastasis to pelvic lymph nodes ➔.

N2

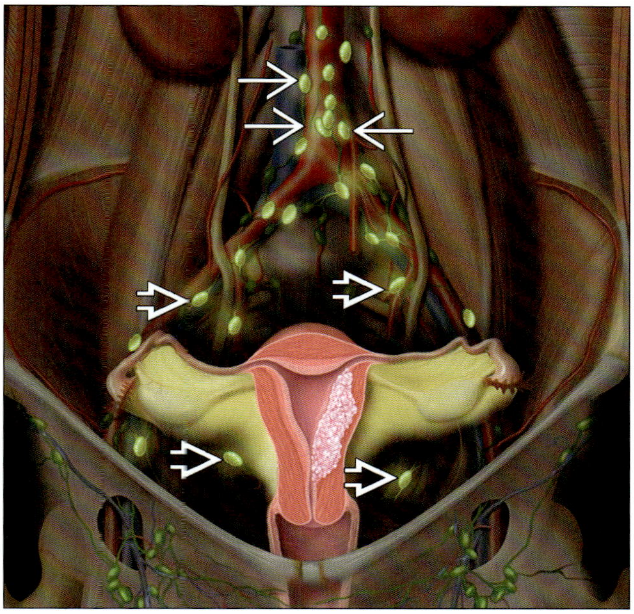

Coronal graphic shows an example of N2 disease, defined as regional lymph node metastasis to paraaortic lymph nodes ➔ with or without positive pelvic lymph nodes ➯.

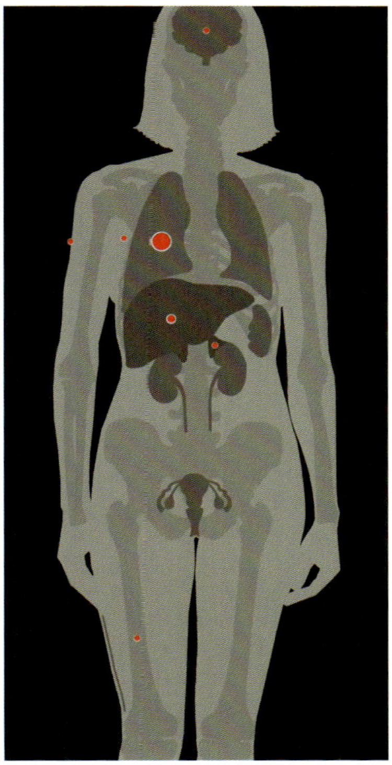

METASTASES, ORGAN FREQUENCY

Lung	32%
Liver	7%
Other sites (adrenals, breast, brain, bone, skin)	4%

CORPUS UTERI CARCINOMA

OVERVIEW

General Comments

- Corpus uteri carcinoma is the most common gynecologic cancer in USA
  - Also most common gynecologic cancer in many other developed countries
- 95% of uterine malignancies are endometrial carcinomas
- Malignancies of uterine corpus
  - Cancers above level of the cervical os involving upper 2/3 of uterus
- Endometrial cancer can be divided into 2 types
  - **Type I**
    - Endometrioid histology
    - Includes the very common endometrioid adenocarcinoma
    - Makes up to 70-80% of new diagnoses in USA
    - Association with chronic estrogen exposure
    - Premalignant disease, such as endometrial hyperplasia, often precedes cancer
  - **Type II**
    - Nonendometrioid histology
    - Includes papillary serous and clear cell carcinomas
    - Aggressive clinical course
    - No association with estrogen exposure has been identified
    - Not associated with readily observable premalignant disease

Classification

- **Primary malignant tumors (WHO classification)**
  - **Endometrial carcinoma**
    - Endometrioid adenocarcinoma
      - Several forms
    - Mucinous adenocarcinoma
    - Serous adenocarcinoma
    - Clear cell adenocarcinoma
    - Mixed cell adenocarcinoma
    - Squamous cell carcinoma
    - Transitional cell carcinoma
    - Small cell carcinoma
    - Others
  - **Mesenchymal tumors**
    - Endometrial stromal and related tumors
      - Endometrial stromal sarcoma, low grade
      - Endometrial stromal nodule
      - Undifferentiated endometrial sarcoma
    - Smooth muscle tumors
      - Leiomyosarcoma (epithelioid and myxoid variants)
      - Smooth muscle tumor of uncertain malignant potential
      - Leiomyoma, not otherwise specified
    - Miscellaneous mesenchymal tumors
  - **Mixed epithelial and mesenchymal tumors**
    - Carcinosarcoma
    - Adenosarcoma
    - Carcinofibroma
    - Adenofibroma
    - Adenomyoma
  - **Gestational trophoblastic disease**
    - Trophoblastic neoplasms
      - Choriocarcinoma
      - Placental site trophoblastic tumor
      - Epithelioid trophoblastic tumor
    - Molar pregnancies
      - Hydatiform mole
    - Nonneoplastic
      - Nonmolar trophoblastic lesions
  - **Miscellaneous tumors**
    - Sex cord-like tumors
    - Neuroectodermal tumors
    - Melanotic paraganglioma
    - Tumors of germ cell type
    - Others
  - **Lymphoid and hematopoietic tumors**
    - Malignant lymphoma
    - Leukemia

PATHOLOGY

Routes of Spread

- **Direct extension**
  - Most common
- **Lymphatic spread**
  - Common nodes include
    - Pelvic (N1)
    - Paraaortic (N2)
    - Inguinal nodes (less common)
- **Hematogenous spread**
  - Lungs
  - Liver
  - Bone
  - Skin
  - Brain (uncommon)
- **Peritoneal spread**
  - Intraperitoneal implants
  - Common in papillary serous carcinoma

General Features

- Comments
  - Endometrioid adenocarcinoma
    - Represents 75-80% of endometrial cancers
- Genetics
  - Rare hereditary form
    - Lynch II family cancer syndrome
      - Nonpolyposis colorectal cancer
      - Ovarian cancer
      - Endometrial cancer
  - **Type I endometrial cancers**
    - Microsatellite instability
    - *KRAS* mutations
    - *PTEN* mutations
    - DNA mismatch repair defects
    - Mutations in *p53*
      - Less frequent
      - Late occurrence in development (differing from type II cancers)
  - **Type II endometrial cancers**
    - Mutations in *p53*
      - Common mutation
    - Nondiploid karyotype
    - Her-2/neu (c-erB-2) overexpression
- Etiology
  - Carcinoma that spontaneously arises from endometrium that is atrophic or inert
- Epidemiology & cancer incidence

CORPUS UTERI CARCINOMA

- Estimated 2009 statistics in USA for endometrial cancer overall
  - 42,160 new cases
  - 7,780 deaths
- Represents 6% of all cancers in women
- **Risk factors**
  - Estrogen hormone replacement therapy
    - Increases risk 2-10x
  - Obesity
    - Increases risk 2-20x
  - Polycystic ovarian syndrome (PCOS)
    - Increases risk 3x
  - Chronic anovulation
    - Increases risk 3x
  - Tamoxifen
    - Increases risk 2-3x
  - Nulliparity
    - Increases risk 2-3x
  - Early menarche
    - Increases risk 2-3x
  - Late menopause
    - Increases risk 2-3x
  - Hypertension
    - Increases risk 2-3x
  - Diabetes
    - Increases risk 2-3x
- Demographics
  - **Age**
    - Most common in 6th and 7th decades of life
  - **Ethnicity**
    - Common in Eastern Europe and USA
    - Uncommon in Asia
- Associated diseases, abnormalities
  - Endometrial hyperplasia
    - Associated with 20-40%

Microscopic Pathology

- H&E
  - Histological patterns can be broadly divided into type I and type II endometrial cancers
    - Endometrioid histology
    - Nonendometrioid histology
  - Histopathologic types
    - Endometrioid carcinomas
      - Most common endometrial cancer (75-80% of cases)
      - Most are well differentiated
      - Back-to-back glandular proliferation of endometrium lacking intervening stroma
    - Villoglandular adenocarcinoma
      - Many villous fronds
      - Delicate central fibrovascular cores of villi and simpler branching pattern differentiates it from papillary serous carcinoma
    - Adenocarcinoma with benign squamous elements, squamous metaplasia, or squamous differentiation (adenoacanthoma)
    - Adenosquamous carcinoma (mixed adenocarcinoma and squamous cell carcinoma)
    - Mucinous adenocarcinoma
    - Serous adenocarcinoma (papillary serous)
      - Bizarre nuclei
      - Scant cytoplasm
      - Nuclear stratification
      - Marked nuclear atypia
      - Complex papillary architecture
      - Psammoma bodies (seen in 30% of cases)
      - Aggressive nature
      - Often presents late
    - Clear cell carcinoma
      - Possible patterns include tubulocystic, papillary, or solid
      - Psammoma bodies may be present but not as commonly as in papillary serous tumors
      - Clear cell appearance due to glycogen
      - Myometrial invasion is common (80% of carcinomas)
      - Aggressive nature
      - Often presents late
    - Squamous cell carcinoma
    - Undifferentiated carcinoma
    - Malignant mixed mesodermal tumors

IMAGING FINDINGS

Detection

- **Key diagnostic clues**
  - Endometrial mass resulting in uterine cavity expansion
  - Localized tumors
    - Polypoid masses superficially attached to the endometrium
  - Diffuse tumors
    - Extensive endometrial invasion
- **Location**
  - Uterine cavity
  - Invasion into myometrium, cervix, or adjacent structures may be seen in some patients
- **Size**
  - Varies from small to large tumors
- **Morphology**
  - Polypoid masses or diffuse thickening of endometrium
- **General T staging imaging characteristics**
  - **Ultrasound**
    - Variable appearance
      - Typically nonspecific
    - Thickened endometrial complex
      - Hyperechoic with well-defined borders
    - Areas of decreased echogenicity can be seen within thickened endometrial complex
    - Mass-like lesion may be heterogeneous or homogeneous
    - Subendometrial halo intact
    - Margins irregular or ill defined
    - Extension of normal echogenicity into inner myometrium
    - Disruption of subendometrial halo may be focal or diffuse
    - 3D ultrasound
      - May offer superior endometrial cancer volume measurement as compared to thickness measurement in detecting endometrial cancer
    - Transvaginal ultrasound (TVS) findings
      - Subendometrial halo disruption is suggestive of myometrial invasion
      - Uterine cancer appears as a polypoid mass or diffuse thickening in endometrial cavity

CORPUS UTERI CARCINOMA

- Evaluation of cervix, parametrium, and lymph nodes is limited in TVS

- CT
  - NECT
    - Difficult to differentiate between cancer and normal uterine tissue
  - CECT
    - Diffuse thickening or a discrete mass may be visualized in uterine cavity
    - Compared to myometrium, uterine carcinoma is relatively low attenuation
    - Myometrial invasion is indicated by irregular tumor-myometrial border
    - Local staging limited due to lack of accurate demonstration of deep myometrial invasion and cervical involvement
- MR
  - Frequently used modality in assessing lymphadenopathy and distant metastases
  - T2WI
    - Heterogeneous intermediate signal intensity compared to normal endometrium
      - Deep myometrial invasion can be excluded if junctional zone is intact
      - If junctional zone not well seen, as in postmenopausal women, then irregular endometrium/myometrium border is suggestive of myometrial invasion
  - T1WI C+
    - Endometrial cancer less avidly enhancing relative to myometrium and cervix
    - Dynamic post-contrast images
      - Highly valuable in visualizing myometrial and cervical invasion
    - Noncontrast images
      - Valuable in differentiating endometrial cancer from fluid or blood in uterine cavity
  - DWI
    - Increased water restriction in malignancies relative to myometrium due to greater cellularity of tumors
    - Decreased apparent diffusion coefficient values
      - Corresponds to high signal intensity on DWI images
- PET
  - F18 FDG PET valuable in detection of metastases and surveillance for recurrences
  - Not helpful for evaluating primary tumor or for assessing myometrial or cervical involvement
- **Recommendations**
  - Best imaging tool
    - TVS can be used in initial evaluation, particularly in cases of abnormal bleeding
      - Most common modality for detection
      - Endometrial sampling should be performed in presentation of postmenopausal bleeding with an endometrial complex > 5 mm in size
    - CT and MR determine cancer stage for treatment planning after diagnosis has been made
  - Protocol advice
    - MR imaging protocol should include
      - T1WI: Axial, large field of view, including entire pelvis
      - T2WI: Axial, sagittal, and coronal small field of view
      - T1WI C+: Dynamic and sagittal

Staging

- **Primary**
  - **Ultrasound**
    - Greatest accuracy in early stage disease with small tumors
    - Overstaging can be seen in large, polypoid lesions
    - Early stages
      - Pulsed Doppler: Benign and malignant thickening of endometrium show significant overlap in resistive index and pulsatility
      - Color Doppler: Mild to moderate vascularity with multiple feeding vessels
  - CECT
    - Early stages
      - Focal/diffuse thickening of the endometrium
      - Tumor mass hypodense to myometrium
      - Mass located centrally
      - Lack of zonal anatomy results in decreased accuracy (65-75%)
  - MR
    - Most accurate imaging modality in local staging
    - Zonal anatomy loss in postmenopausal women: Potential problem in staging and decreases MR accuracy
    - Early stages
      - T1WI: Hypointense to isointense relative to endometrium or myometrium and detects hematometra
      - T2WI: Hypointense or isointense relative to endometrium (100%) and isointense or hyperintense relative to outer myometrium (70%)
- **Nodal**
  - Criteria in defining lymph nodes as pathologic
    - Oval nodes ≥ 1 cm in short axis
    - Round nodes ≥ 0.8 cm in diameter
  - Enhancement of nodes or node signal is not predictive of metastatic lymphadenopathy
  - CT and MR show equal accuracy in assessing involvement of pelvic and paraaortic lymph nodes
  - Nodal metastases may skip
    - Metastasizes to paraaortic lymph nodes through the ovarian lymphatics without pelvic lymphadenopathy
  - CT
    - CECT detects adenopathy
    - CT and MR are chosen modalities in detecting adenopathy
      - 60-90% accuracy
  - MR
    - **T1WI**
      - Detects adenopathy
    - **T2WI**
      - Detects pelvic &/or paraaortic adenopathy
    - Increased sensitivity for nodal metastases with MR enhanced by ultrasmall superparamagnetic iron oxide (USPIO)
    - CT and MR are chosen modalities in detecting adenopathy
      - 60-90% accuracy
  - PET

- Increased sensitivity for nodal metastases with F18 FDG PET
- Insensitive for small nodal metastases < 6-7 mm
  - Below resolution of most PET cameras
- High positive predictive value when nodes 7-15 mm demonstrate increased activity

- **Metastatic disease**
  - CT
    - Most common modality for serial evaluation of patients with uterine malignancies
    - **CECT**
      - Frequently used modality in assessing distant metastases
  - **MR**
    - More often used as problem-solving tool for indeterminate lesions seen on US or CT
  - **PET/CT**
    - PET/CT valuable in detecting lesions in organs as well as nodes
    - Some uterine malignancies are not FDG avid or less FDG avid (leiomyosarcoma)
    - Metastatic lesions may also have variable FDG activity compared to FDG activity of primary tumor

Restaging

- **CT**
  - Most frequently used modality for restaging patients
  - Helpful for differentiating scar vs. residual/recurrent tumor
  - More sensitive than PET for detecting early carcinomatosis or peritoneal spread
- **MR**
  - Used for problem solving or indeterminate lesions on other modalities
- **PET/CT**
  - Can be helpful for detecting occult disease
  - Pitfalls
    - Inability to detect early carcinomatosis and occasionally non-FDG-avid lesions on PET
    - Need to look at CT images even if performed at low dose to look for peritoneal involvement

CLINICAL ISSUES

Presentation

- Abnormal vaginal bleeding
  - 75-90% of patients present with postmenopausal bleeding
  - May also present with leukorrhea
- Other signs and symptoms resulting from metastatic disease in more advanced cancers may occur
  - Dysuria
  - Constipation
  - Pain
- Clinical profile
  - Abnormal vaginal bleeding in postmenopausal woman
- Dilatation and curettage used clinically to make diagnosis

Cancer Natural History & Prognosis

- Typically diagnosed earlier as majority of women seek evaluation following vaginal bleeding, which is seen in most cases
- Majority of patients diagnosed with surgical stage I disease (70-75% of cases)
- **Prognostic factors**
  - Histologic grade of tumor
  - Depth of myometrial invasion
  - Stage of disease
  - Lymph node involvement
- **5-year survival rates**
  - Stage I (90%)
  - Stage II (80%)
  - Stages III and IV (15-20%)
- **5-year survival rates specific to endometrial adenocarcinoma**
  - Stage IA (99%)
  - Stage IB (99%)
  - Stage IC (92%)
  - Stage II (80%)
  - Stage III (60%)
  - Stage IV (30%)

Treatment Options

- Major treatment alternatives
  - Multimodality treatment plan based on disease stage
    - Surgery
      - Total abdominal hysterectomy (TAH) and bilateral salpingo-oophorectomy (BSO)
    - Radiation treatment given preoperatively or postoperatively
    - Chemotherapy
    - Hormonal treatments
      - Commonly include progestational agents
- Major treatment roadblocks
  - Recurrence
    - Up to 23% at mean follow-up of 70+ months
- Treatment options by stage
  - **Stage I**
    - Total abdominal hysterectomy and bilateral salpingo-oophorectomy
    - Possible removal of certain pelvic lymph nodes can be performed in cases that meet the following criteria
      - Well or moderately differentiated
      - Upper 2/3 of corpus is involved
      - Peritoneal cytology is negative
      - Vascular space invasion not present
      - < 50% myometrial invasion
    - In all other cases, total abdominal hysterectomy and bilateral salpingo-oophorectomy
    - Combined with sampling of periaortic and selected pelvic lymph nodes
      - If nodes are positive for disease, further treatment should be given, typically involving radiation therapy and possibly chemotherapy and surgery as well
  - **Stage II**
    - Standard surgical approach of hysterectomy and bilateral salpingo-oophorectomy

- May be combined with intracavity and external-beam radiation therapy given preoperatively, with paraaortic nodes biopsied during surgery
- Radiation therapy should be given postoperatively if microscopic cervical involvement is found

- **Stage III**
  - Generally treated with surgery and radiation therapy
    - Typical radiation therapy treatment plan consists of combination of intracavitary and external-beam radiation therapy
  - Progestational agents may also be considered in patients who are not candidates for surgery or radiation therapy
- **Stage IV**
  - Treatment plan guided by sites of metastatic lesions and resulting symptoms
  - Bulky pelvic lesions are treated with radiation therapy consisting of intracavity and external-beam radiation therapy combined
  - Hormonal therapy is indicated in distant metastatic disease, particularly in pulmonary metastases

REPORTING CHECKLIST

T Staging

- Report involvement or noninvolvement of endocervical mucosa &/or stroma of endocervix
- Report depth of myometrium involvement and if there is extension through myometrial wall into parametrium
- Report any potential involvement of ovaries or extension into vagina

N Staging

- Enlarged nodes should be reported, particularly paraaortic and obturator nodes, as they will likely be targeted for sampling
  - Also note whether or not likely accessible to percutaneous biopsy
- Inguinal nodes common and often nonspecific, but enlarged pelvic nodes should be reported as suspicious
- Look for and comment on usual abnormal characteristics that would make a node more suspicious
  - Enhancement
  - Enlargement
  - Necrosis

M Staging

- Report involvement of
  - Vagina
  - Lungs
  - Intraabdominal organs &/or peritoneal areas

SELECTED REFERENCES

1. American Joint Committee on Cancer: AJCC Cancer Staging Manual. 7th ed. New York: Springer, 2010
2. Basu S et al: PET and PET-CT imaging of gynecological malignancies: present role and future promise. Expert Rev Anticancer Ther. 9(1):75-96, 2009
3. Bernardini MQ et al: Issues surrounding lymphadenectomy in the management of endometrial cancer. J Surg Oncol. 99(4):232-41, 2009
4. De Gaetano AM et al: Imaging of gynecologic malignancies with FDG PET-CT: case examples, physiologic activity, and pitfalls. Abdom Imaging. 34(6):696-711, 2009
5. Grigsby PW: Role of PET in gynecologic malignancy. Curr Opin Oncol. 21(5):420-4, 2009
6. Holalkere NS et al: Issues in imaging malignant neoplasms of the female reproductive system. Curr Probl Diagn Radiol. 38(1):1-16, 2009
7. Hunn J et al: Endometrial cancer--current state of the art therapies and unmet clinical needs: the role of surgery and preoperative radiographic assessment. Adv Drug Deliv Rev. 61(10):890-5, 2009
8. Maffione AM et al: Positron-emission tomography in gynaecologic malignancies. Arch Gynecol Obstet. 280(4):521-8, 2009
9. Peungjesada S et al: Magnetic resonance imaging of endometrial carcinoma. J Comput Assist Tomogr. 33(4):601-8, 2009
10. Whittaker CS et al: Diffusion-weighted MR imaging of female pelvic tumors: a pictorial review. Radiographics. 29(3):759-74; discussion 774-8, 2009
11. Bakkum-Gamez JN et al: Current issues in the management of endometrial cancer. Mayo Clin Proc. 83(1):97-112, 2008
12. Selman TJ et al: A systematic review of tests for lymph node status in primary endometrial cancer. BMC Womens Health. 8:8, 2008
13. Sorosky JI: Endometrial cancer. Obstet Gynecol. 111(2 Pt 1):436-47, 2008
14. Whitcomb BP: Gynecologic malignancies. Surg Clin North Am. 88(2):301-17, vi, 2008
15. Akin O et al: Imaging of uterine cancer. Radiol Clin North Am. 45(1):167-82, 2007
16. Iyer RB et al: PET/CT and cross sectional imaging of gynecologic malignancy. Cancer Imaging. 7 Spec No A:S130-8, 2007
17. Koyama T et al: Staging of carcinoma of the uterine cervix and endometrium. Eur Radiol. 17(8):2009-19, 2007
18. Lai CH et al: Positron emission tomography imaging for gynecologic malignancy. Curr Opin Obstet Gynecol. 19(1):37-41, 2007
19. Sala E et al: MRI of malignant neoplasms of the uterine corpus and cervix. AJR Am J Roentgenol. 188(6):1577-87, 2007
20. Barwick TD et al: Imaging of endometrial adenocarcinoma. Clin Radiol. 61(7):545-55, 2006
21. Brown MA et al: MR imaging of malignant uterine disease. Magn Reson Imaging Clin N Am. 14(4):455-69, v-vi, 2006
22. Kumar R et al: Positron emission tomography in gynecological malignancies. Expert Rev Anticancer Ther. 6(7):1033-44, 2006
23. Messiou C et al: MR staging of endometrial carcinoma. Clin Radiol. 61(10):822-32, 2006
24. Whitten CR et al: Magnetic resonance imaging of uterine malignancies. Top Magn Reson Imaging. 17(6):365-77, 2006
25. Amant F et al: Endometrial cancer. Lancet. 366(9484):491-505, 2005
26. Ascher SM et al: Imaging of cancer of the endometrium. Radiol Clin North Am. 40(3):563-76, 2002
27. Kinkel K et al: Radiologic staging in patients with endometrial cancer: a meta-analysis. Radiology. 212(3):711-8, 1999

Stage IA (T1a N0 M0), Endometrial

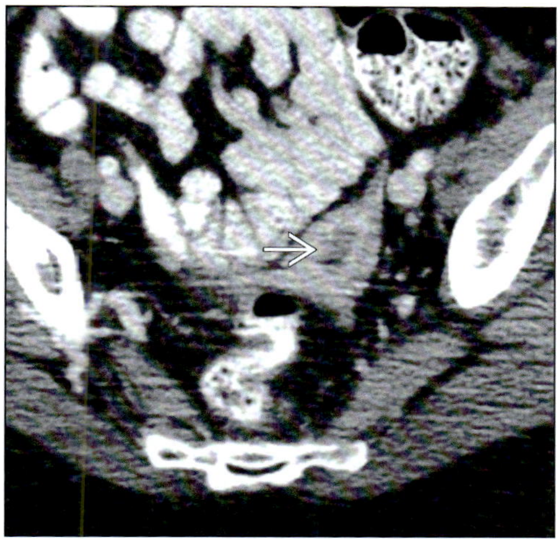

Stage IA (T1a N0 M0), Endometrial

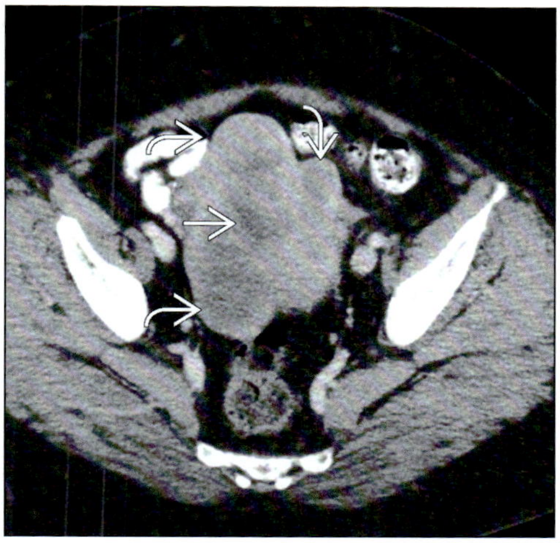

(Left) *Axial CECT shows nonspecific mild thickening of the endometrium* ⇒ *in this patient with recently diagnosed stage IA endometrial carcinoma.* ***(Right)*** *Axial CECT shows an enlarged uterus with multiple leiomyomas* ⇒ *and a slightly prominent endometrium* ⇒ *in this patient with recently diagnosed endometrial carcinoma. Pathology revealed a 2 cm mass that did not involve the myometrium, compatible with stage IA.*

Stage IA (T1a N0 M0), Endometrial

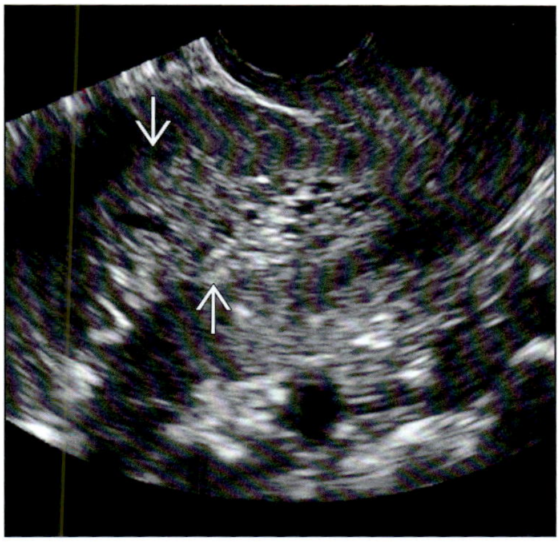

Stage IA (T1a N0 M0), Endometrial

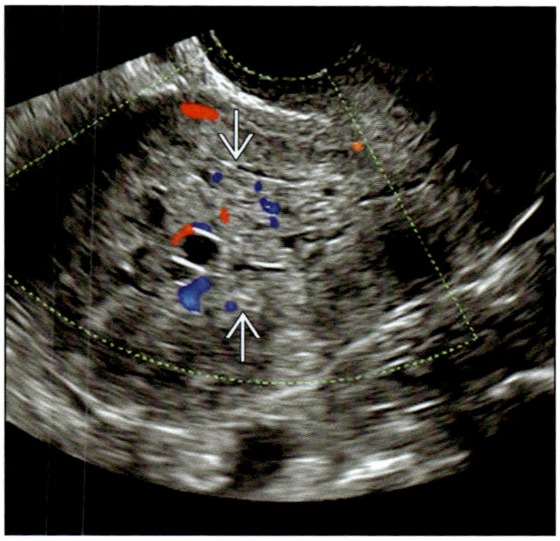

(Left) *Longitudinal transvaginal grayscale ultrasound shows a thickened heterogeneous endometrium* ⇒ *with multiple cysts.* ***(Right)*** *Color Doppler ultrasound shows areas of increased color (blood flow) to the thickened endometrium* ⇒*. Pathology revealed endometrial carcinoma that had developed within a polyp in this patient that had been on tamoxifen. Disease limited to the endometrium would be stage IA.*

Stage IA (T1a N0 M0), Endometrial

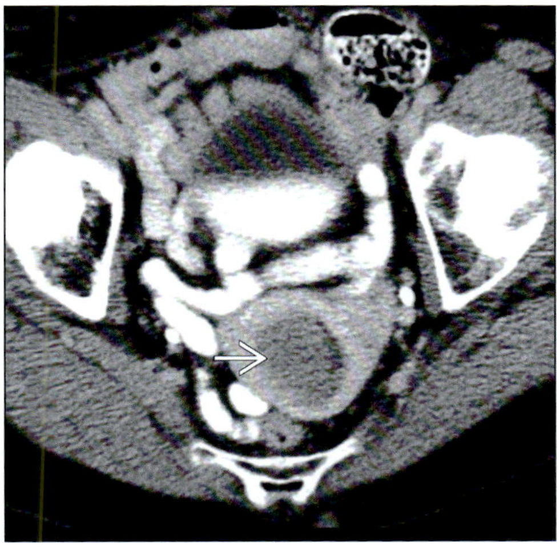

Stage IA (T1a N0 M0), Endometrial

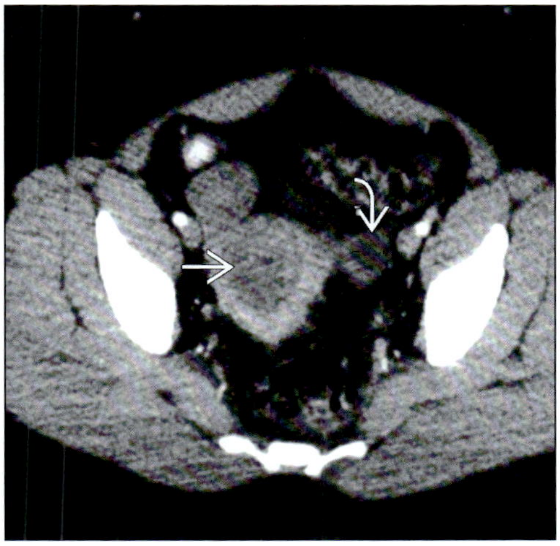

(Left) *Axial CECT shows an enlarged endometrium* ⇒ *in a patient with recently diagnosed endometrial carcinoma. Pathology showed less than 50% myometrial involvement, making this a T1a lesion and overall stage IA.* ***(Right)*** *Axial CECT shows nonspecific endometrial enlargement* ⇒ *and a left ovarian cyst* ⇒ *in this patient with recently diagnosed stage IA endometrial carcinoma.*

CORPUS UTERI CARCINOMA

*(**Left**) Axial CECT shows enlargement and abnormal enhancement of the endometrium. Outside MR showed more than 1/2 thickness involvement of the myometrium or a T1b lesion. (**Right**) Axial CECT in the same patient shows prominence/irregularity of the endometrial cavity shown by the low-attenuation center with heterogeneous enhancement of the thickened endometrium/ myometrium. This patient was diagnosed with endometrial carcinoma.*

Stage IB (T1b N0 M0), Endometrial

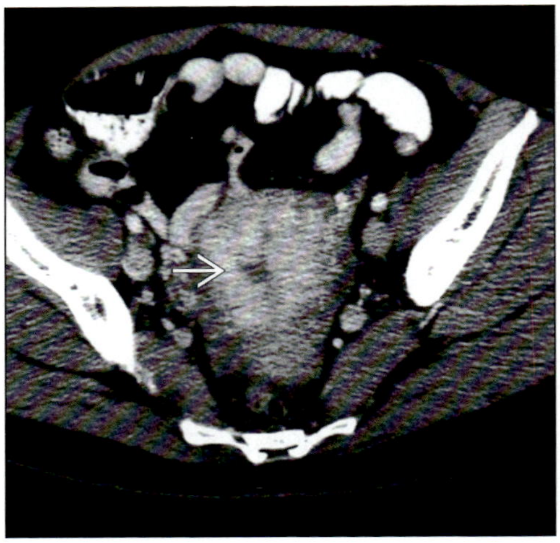

Stage IB (T1b N0 M0), Endometrial

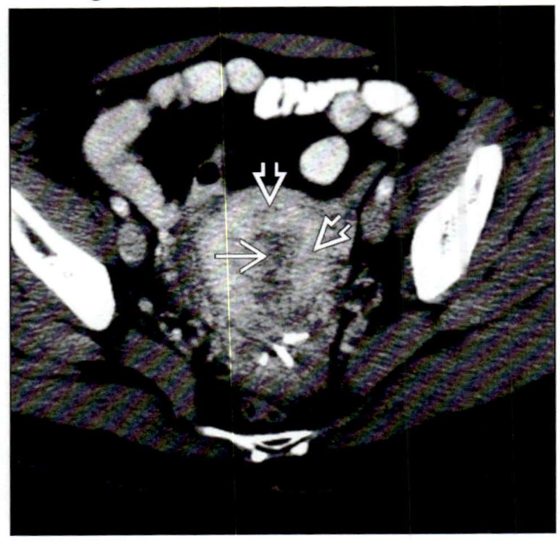

*(**Left**) Axial CECT shows an expanded fluid- and debris-filled endometrial cavity in this patient with newly diagnosed endometrial carcinoma. (**Right**) Axial CECT in the same patient shows an enhancing mass along the right lateral border of the endometrium and fluid-filled endometrial cavity. Pathology showed the lesion involving almost the full thickness of the myometrium, making this a T1b lesion and overall stage IB.*

Stage IB (T1b N0 M0), Endometrial

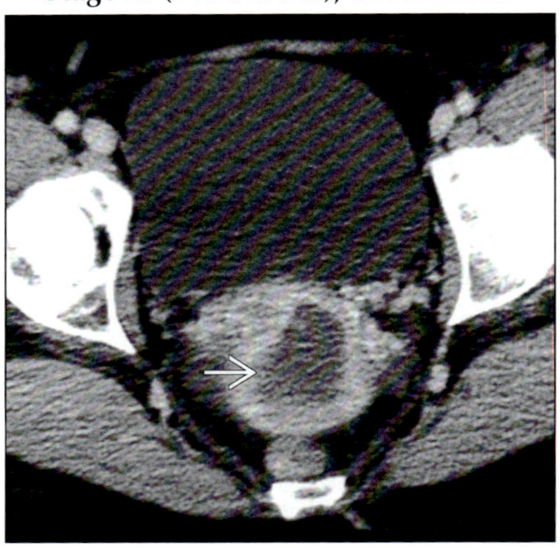

Stage IB (T1b N0 M0), Endometrial

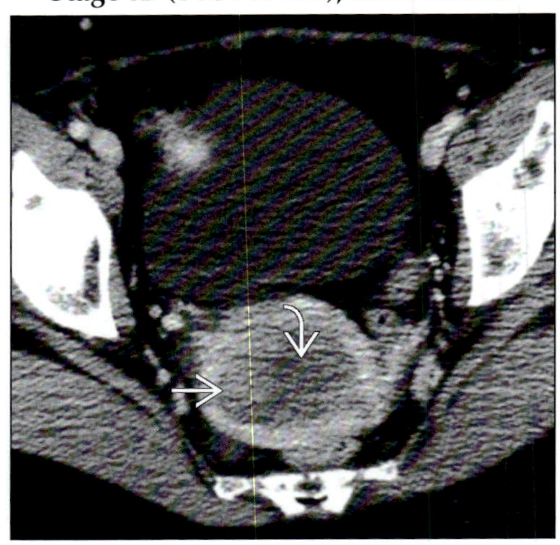

*(**Left**) Axial CECT shows irregularly thickened endometrium with some fluid/debris in the endometrial canal in this patient with postmenopausal bleeding. (**Right**) Axial PET/ CT in the same patient shows intense FDG activity in the thickened endometrium compatible with recently diagnosed endometrial carcinoma. FDG activity in the endometrium in a postmenopausal woman should be further evaluated to exclude carcinoma.*

Stage IB (T1b N0 M0), Endometrial

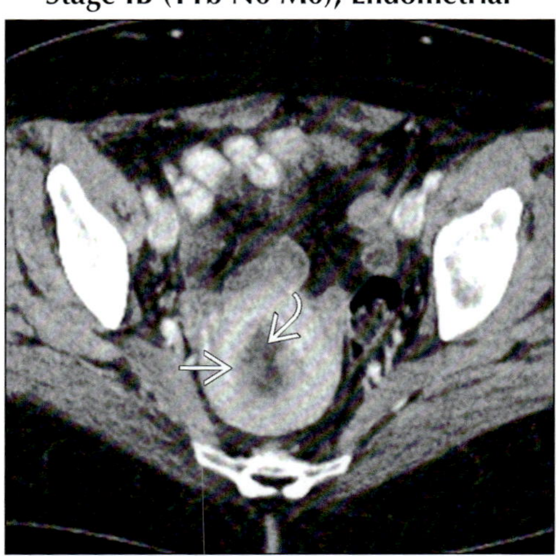

Stage IB (T1b N0 M0), Endometrial

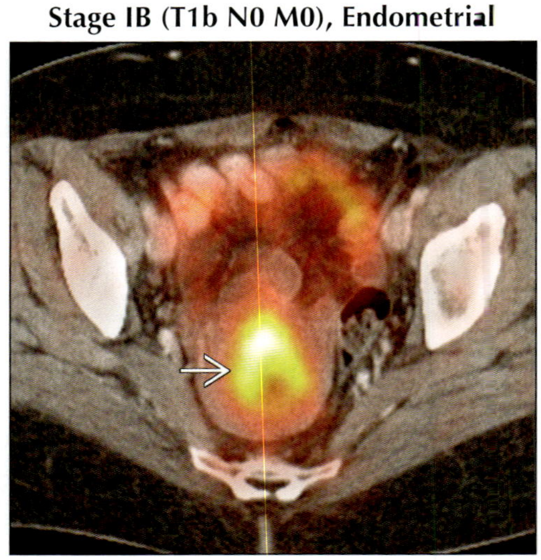

CORPUS UTERI CARCINOMA

Stage IB (T1b N0 M0), Endometrial

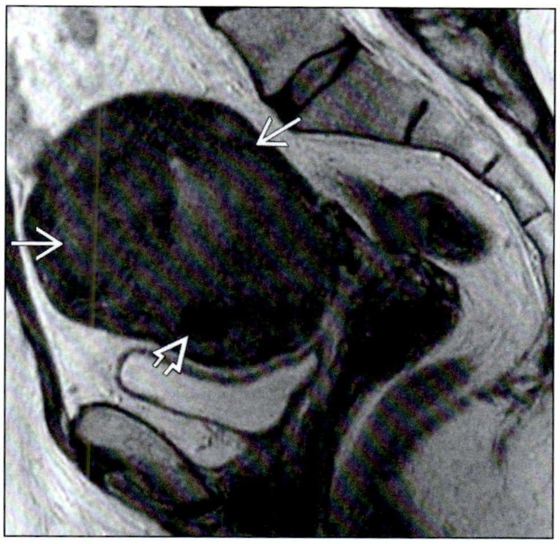

Stage IB (T1b N0 M0), Endometrial

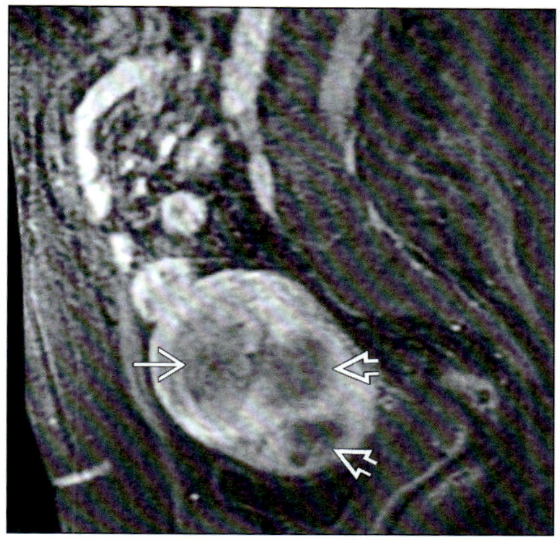

(Left) *Sagittal T1WI C+ MR shows a tumor ➡ in a bulky uterus with multiple leiomyomas ⇨ with an indistinct junctional zone, raising the suspicion of myometrial invasion.* ***(Right)*** *Sagittal T2WI FS MR in the same patient shows the higher signal mass ➡ in a bulky uterus with a better view of the multiple low signal intensity leiomyomas ⇨.*

Stage IB (T1b N0 M0), Endometrial

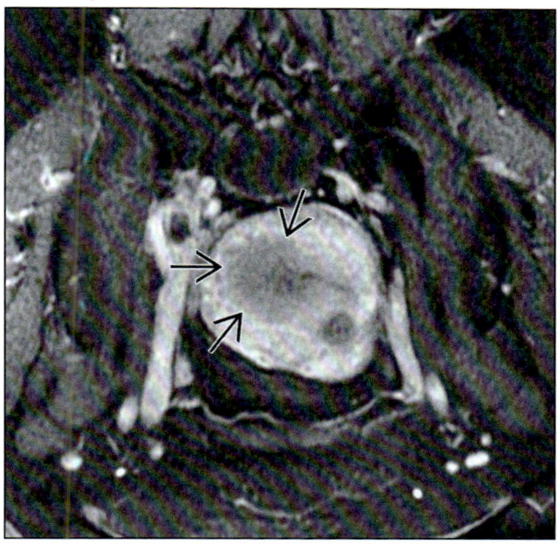

Stage IB (T1b N0 M0), Endometrial

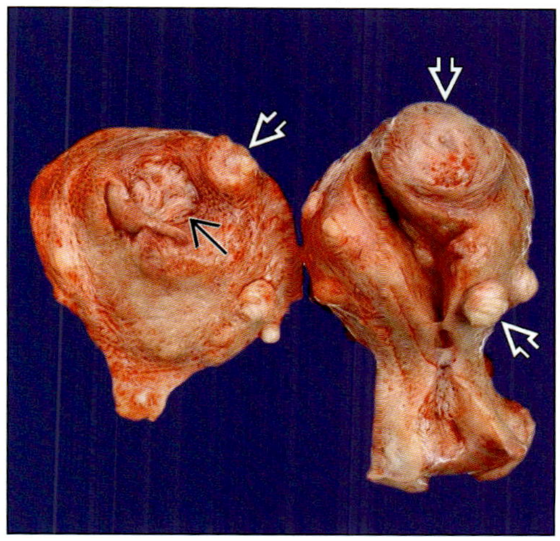

(Left) *Axial T1WI C+ FS MR post gadolinium administration in the same patient shows that the tumor → involves more than 50% of the myometrium, making this a T1b lesion or stage IB.* ***(Right)*** *Cut gross hysterectomy specimen from the same patient shows the presence of stage IB endometrial cancer →. Also note multiple leiomyomata ⇨.*

Stage II (T2 N0 M0), Endometrial

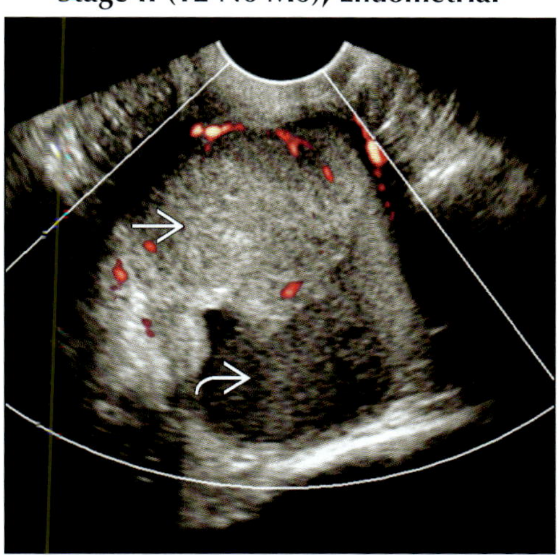

Stage II (T2 N0 M0), Endometrial

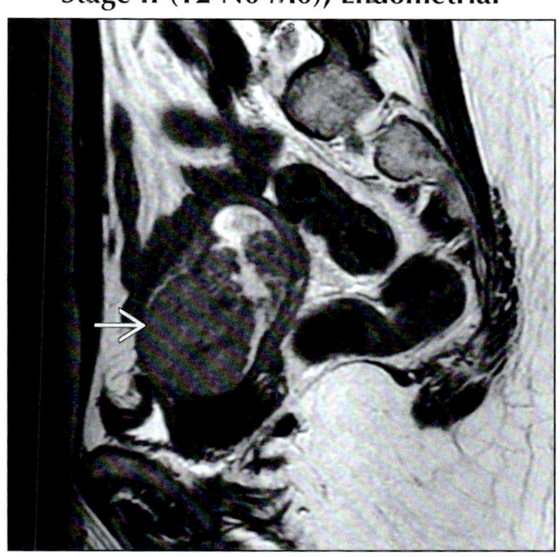

(Left) *Transverse color Doppler transvaginal ultrasound shows a large irregular mass ➡ along the endometrium with blood/ debris ↪ in the endometrial canal.* ***(Right)*** *Sagittal T1WI MR in the same patient shows an endometrial mass ➡ with extension into the endocervical canal. The low signal intensity junctional zone is disrupted anteriorly, compatible with more than 50% myometrial extension. Pathology showed invasion of cervical stromal tissue.*

CORPUS UTERI CARCINOMA

(Left) *Axial CECT shows marked expansion of the endometrial cavity with an enhancing mass* ➔ *compared to normal uterus* ⮫ *in this patient with recently diagnosed endometrial carcinoma.* ***(Right)*** *Axial PET/CT in the same patient shows intense FDG activity* ➔ *correlating with the bulky endometrial mass. Although not routinely used to evaluate the primary mass, PET/CT can be used for initial treatment decision making.*

Stage II (T2 N0 M0), Endometrial

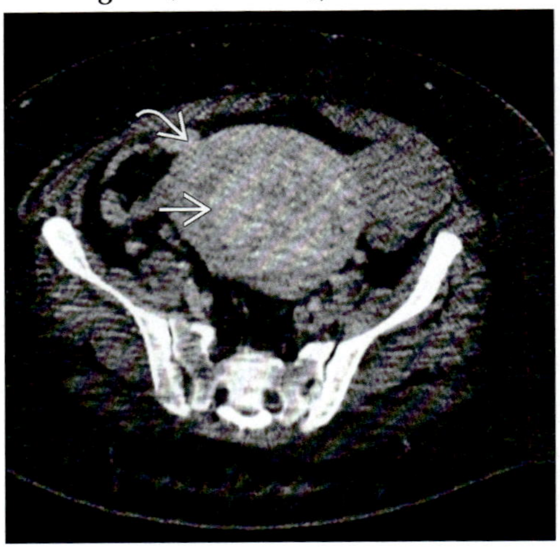

Stage II (T2 N0 M0), Endometrial

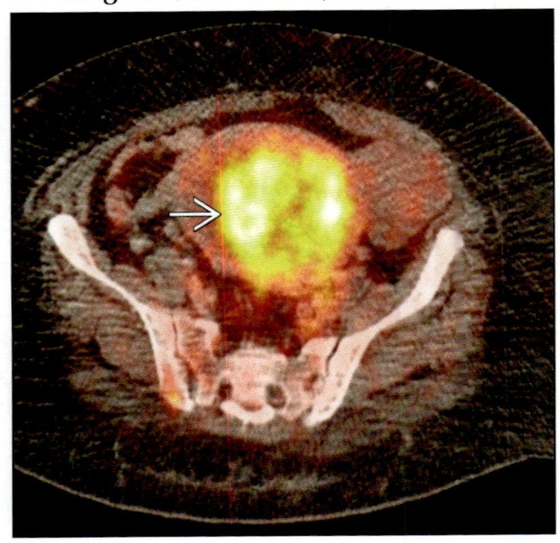

(Left) *Axial CECT shows a large heterogeneously enhancing mass* ➔ *with an enlarged uterus in this patient with recently diagnosed endometrial carcinoma.* ***(Right)*** *Axial PET/CT in the same patient shows diffuse intense FDG activity in the large endometrial mass* ➔ *occupying the whole uterus. Involvement of the vagina makes this a T3b lesion. FDG activity anteriorly* ⮫ *is normal excretory FDG in the bladder.*

Stage IIIB (T3b N0 M0), Endometrial

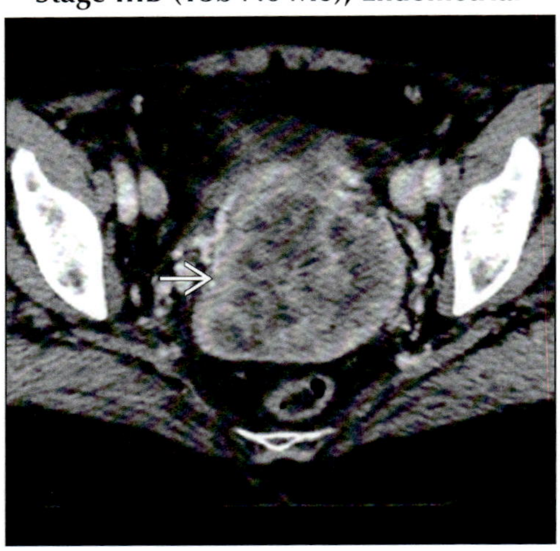

Stage IIIB (T3b N0 M0), Endometrial

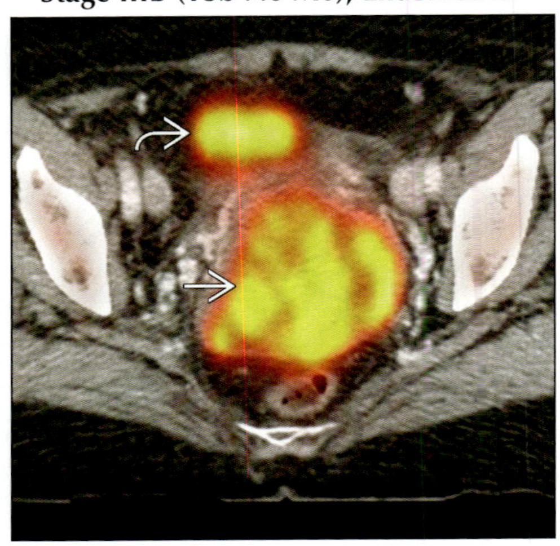

(Left) *Sagittal T1WI C+ FS MR shows a large mass* ➔ *involving the majority of the endometrium and appearing to extend into the endocervix* ⮫ *and involve more than 50% of the myometrium.* ***(Right)*** *Sagittal T1WI C+ FS MR smaller field of view image in the same patient shows the primary mass* ➔ *with obvious abnormal enhancement of the posterior wall of the bladder* ⮫*, compatible with a T4 lesion or stage IVA.*

Stage IVA (T4 N0 M0), Endometrial

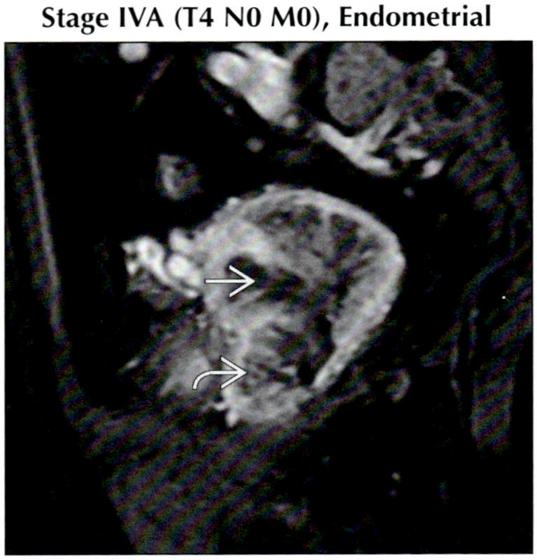

Stage IVA (T4 N0 M0), Endometrial

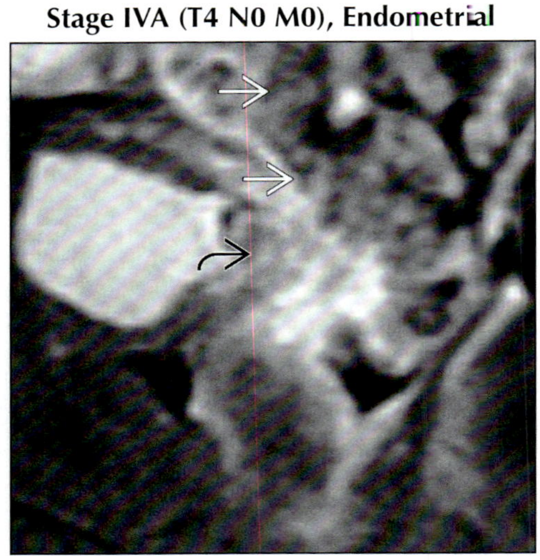

CORPUS UTERI CARCINOMA

Stage IVA (T4 N0 M0), Endometrial

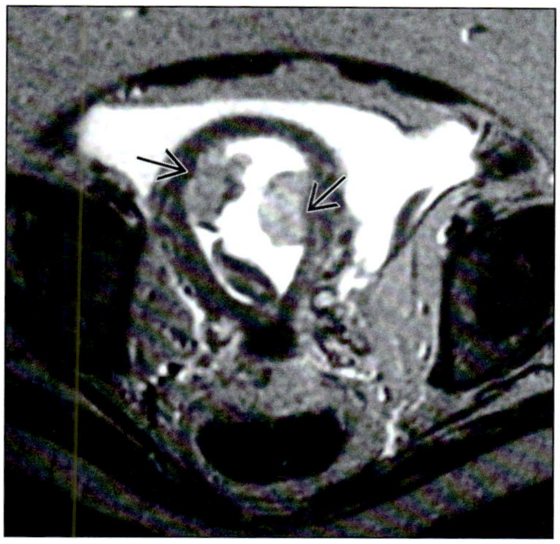

Stage IVA (T4 N0 M0), Endometrial

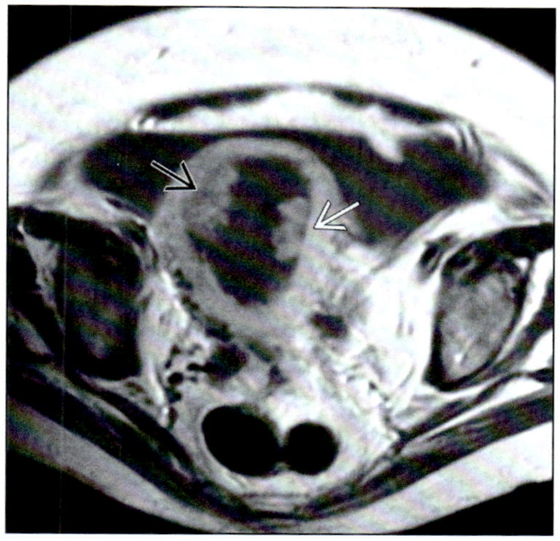

(Left) *Axial T2WI MR shows the uterus markedly distended with fluid and enhancing polypoid tumor masses* ⇨*. No deep invasion of the myometrium is evident.* ***(Right)*** *Axial T1WI C+ MR in the same patient shows the polypoid masses* ⇨ *and irregular enhancing outer uterine wall* ➡ *indicating serosal extension.*

Stage IVA (T4 N1 M0), Endometrial

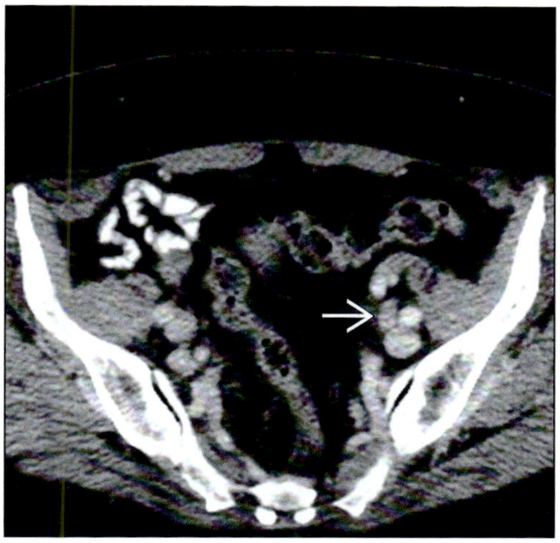

Stage IVA (T4 N1 M0), Endometrial

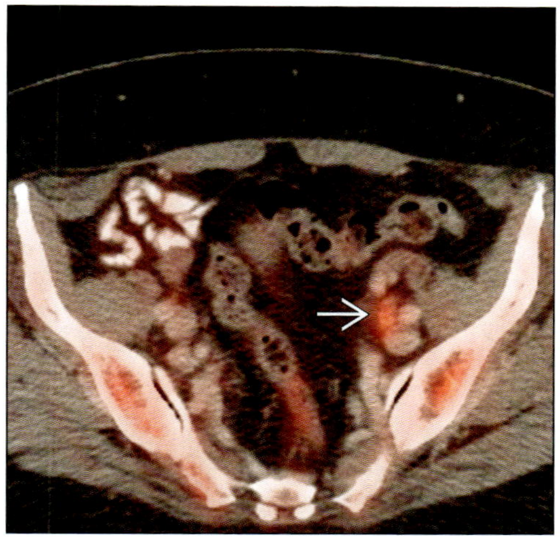

(Left) *Axial CECT shows a subtle borderline enlarged but nonspecific left external iliac node* ➡ *without any additional specific features to suggest malignancy in this patient with a newly diagnosed endometrial carcinoma (T4 lesion).* ***(Right)*** *Axial PET/CT in the same patient shows mild FDG activity within the lymph node* ➡*. Subsequent follow-up scan showed interval enlargement of the node, compatible with a malignant node.*

Stage IVA (T4 N1 M0), Endometrial

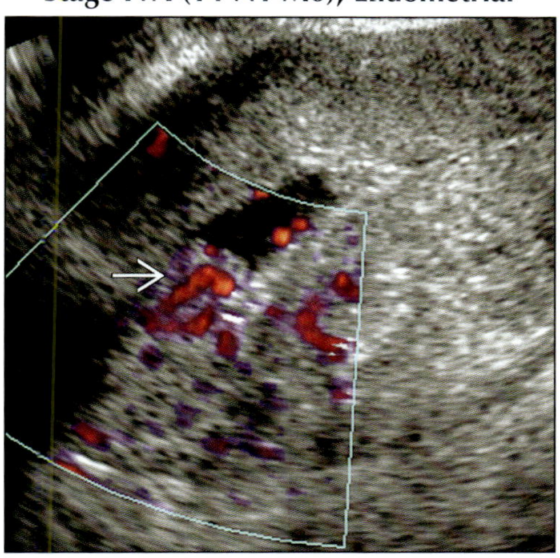

Stage IVA (T4 N1 M0), Endometrial

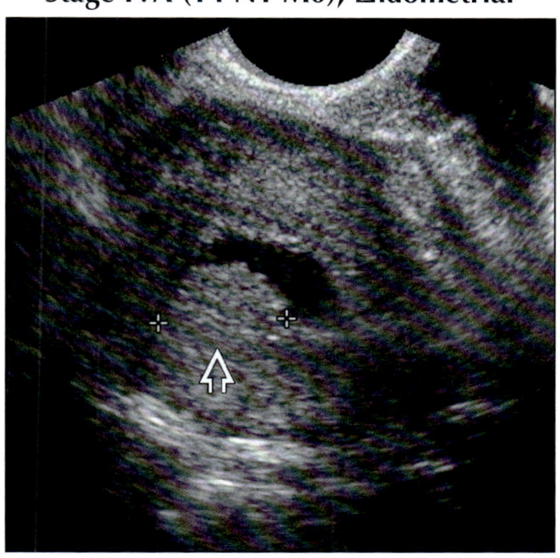

(Left) *Longitudinal power Doppler ultrasound again shows the polypoid endometrial mass* ➡ *with increased blood flow worrisome for endometrial carcinoma.* ***(Right)*** *Transverse transvaginal ultrasound in the same patient shows a focal broad-based mass* ➡ *in the fundal-posterior region of the endometrium.*

CORPUS UTERI CARCINOMA

*(**Left**) Axial T1WI C+ FS MR shows a cystic mass → surrounding the proximal common iliac vessels. The mass shows abnormally enhancing wall with central necrosis, compatible with metastatic disease. (**Right**) FDG PET scan in the same patient shows abnormal rim-like intense FDG activity → correlating with the mass surrounding the proximal common iliac vessels, compatible with metastatic disease.*

Stage IVA (T4 N1 M0), Endometrial

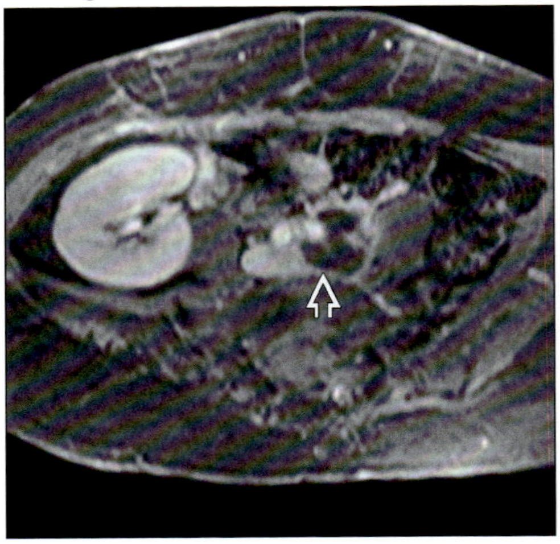

Stage IVA (T4 N1 M0), Endometrial

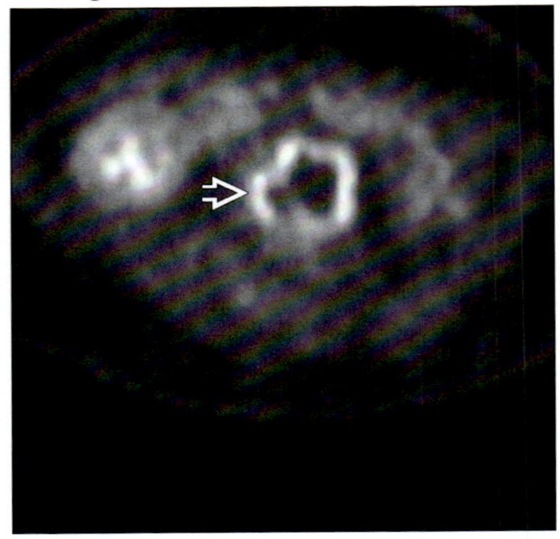

*(**Left**) Axial CECT shows an enlarged uterus with a mass → that has central low attenuation and mild enhancement peripherally in this patient with recently diagnosed endometrial carcinoma. (**Right**) Axial CECT shows a mass → with rim enhancement and central low attenuation (necrosis) centered along the greater omentum and invading the anterior abdominal wall musculature, compatible with metastatic disease.*

Stage IVA (T4 N1 M0), Endometrial

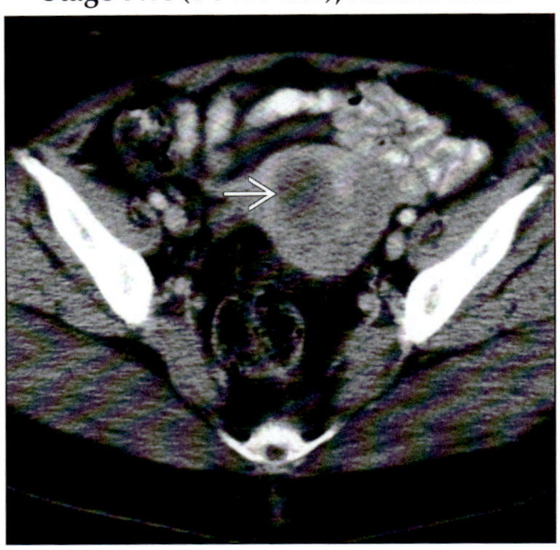

Stage IVB (T4 N1 M1), Endometrial

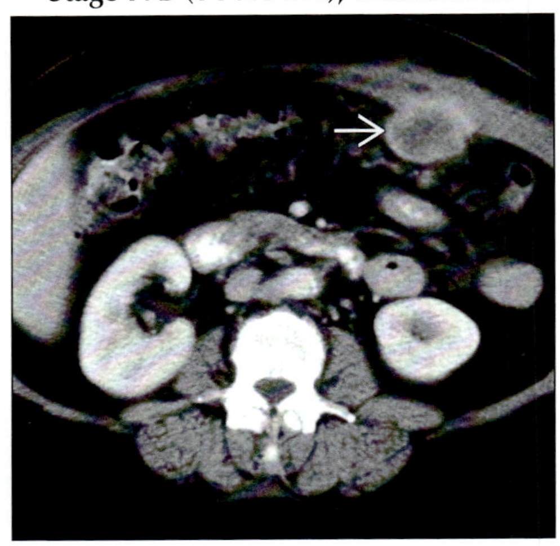

*(**Left**) Axial CECT shows a uterine mass more than 5 cm with thickened enhancing walls → and extensive central necrosis ↗ in this patient with newly diagnosed uterine leiomyosarcoma. (**Right**) Axial CECT in the same patient shows more irregularity and thickening to the uterine wall → with extensive necrosis ↗, a characteristic finding of sarcomas.*

Stage IB (T1b N0 M0), Leiomyosarcoma

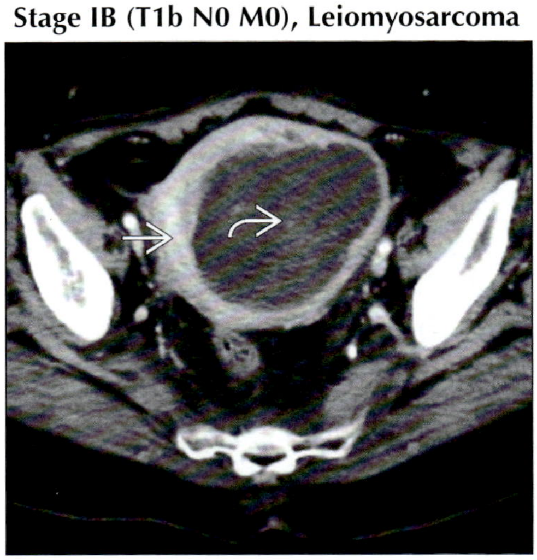

Stage IB (T1b N0 M0), Leiomyosarcoma

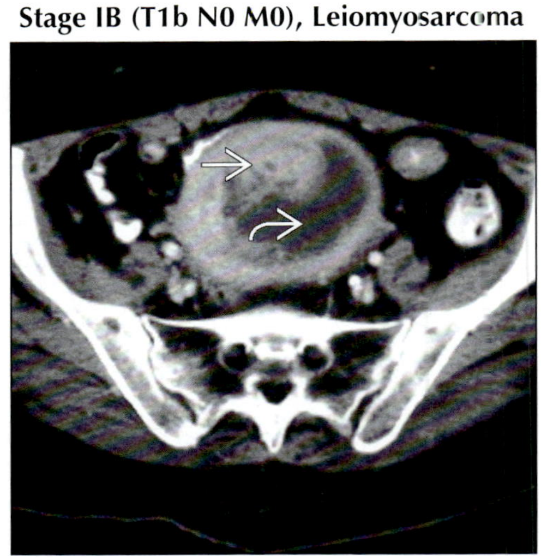

CORPUS UTERI CARCINOMA

Stage IB (T1b N0 M0), Leiomyosarcoma

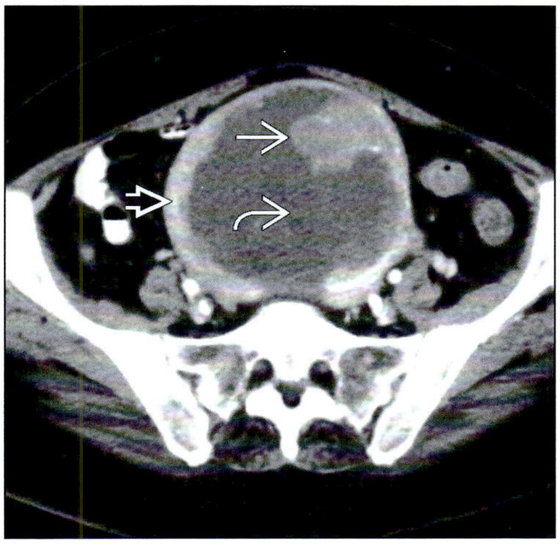

Stage IB (T1b N0 M0), Leiomyosarcoma

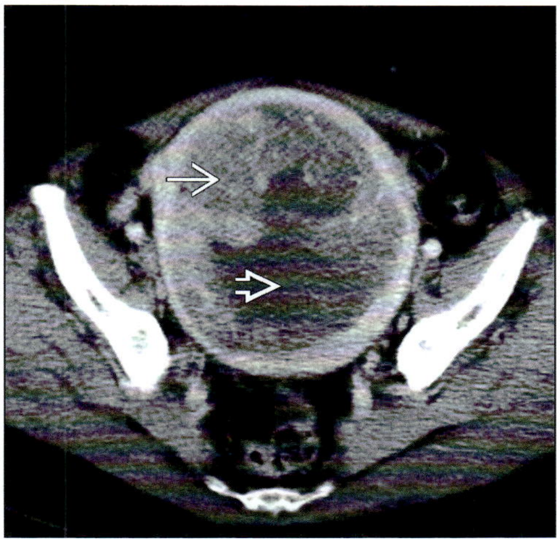

(Left) *Axial CECT in a patient with newly diagnosed uterine leiomyosarcoma measuring more than 5 cm shows uterine wall thickening, areas of polypoid abnormal enhancing soft tissue, and extensive central necrosis.* ***(Right)*** *Axial CECT in another patient with newly diagnosed uterine leiomyosarcoma measuring more than 5 cm also shows irregular enhancing uterine wall thickening and extensive central necrosis.*

Stage IB (T1b N0 M0), Leiomyosarcoma

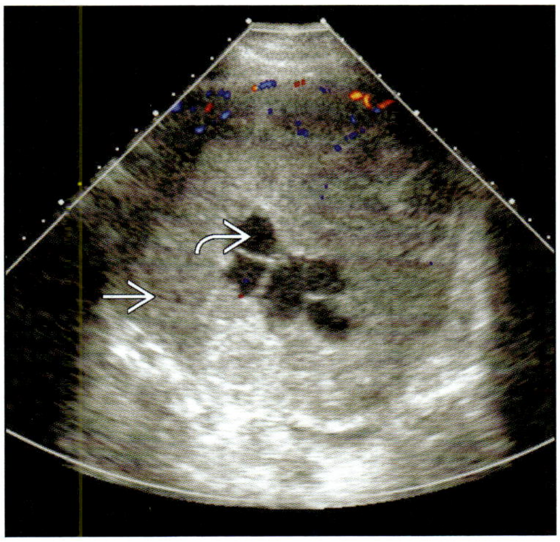

Stage IB (T1b N0 M0), Leiomyosarcoma

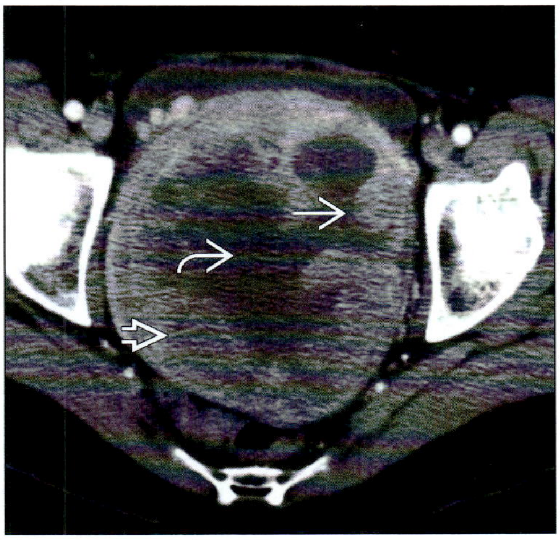

(Left) *Transverse color Doppler ultrasound shows a heterogeneous mass with central hypoechogenic areas of necrosis in a patient with abdominopelvic pain.* ***(Right)*** *Axial CECT in the same patient shows irregular uterine wall thickening, areas of polypoid abnormal enhancing soft tissue, and extensive central necrosis, all findings frequently seen with sarcomas. Surgery revealed uterine leiomyosarcoma.*

Stage IB (T1b N0 M0), Leiomyosarcoma

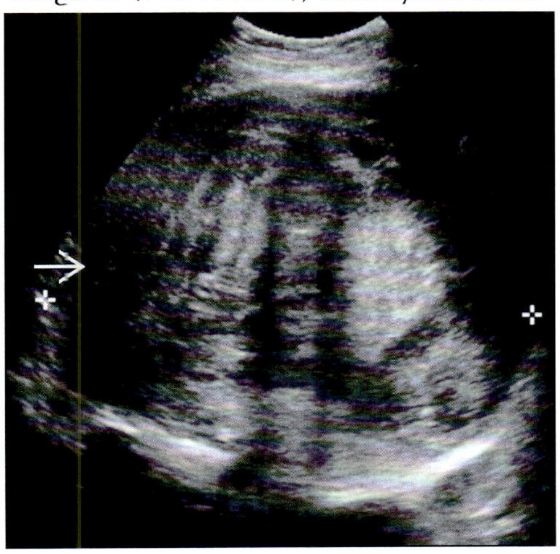

Stage IB (T1b N0 M0), Leiomyosarcoma

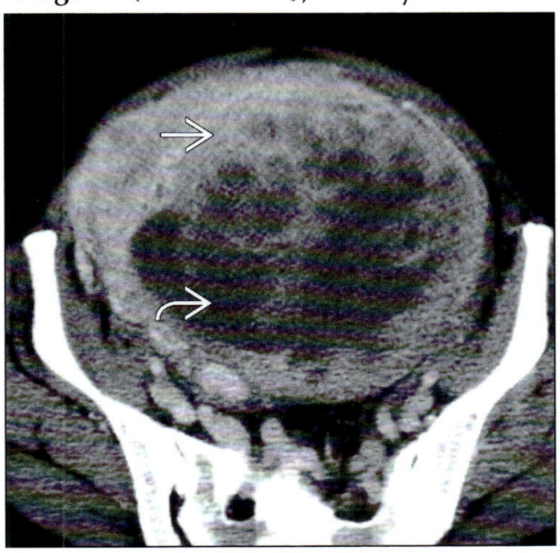

(Left) *Transverse transabdominal ultrasound shows an extremely large, heterogeneously echogenic mass filling most of the abdominopelvic cavity in this patient complaining of abdominal bloating/weight gain.* ***(Right)*** *Axial CECT in the same patient shows marked irregular uterine wall thickening and heterogeneous enhancement with extensive central necrosis, compatible with recently diagnosed uterine leiomyosarcoma.*

CORPUS UTERI CARCINOMA

Stage IB (T1b N0 M0), Leiomyosarcoma

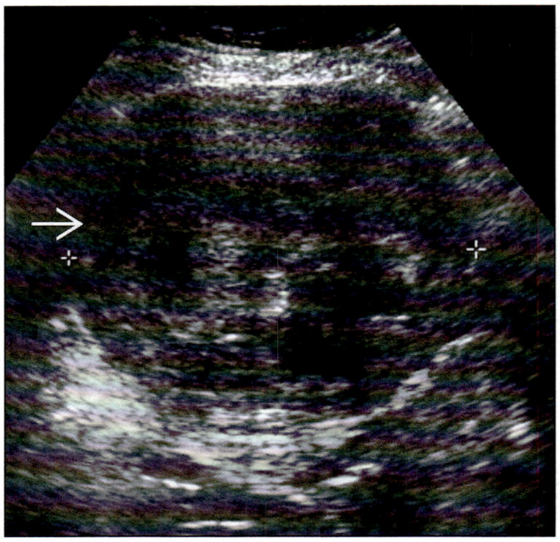

Stage IB (T1b N0 M0), Leiomyosarcoma

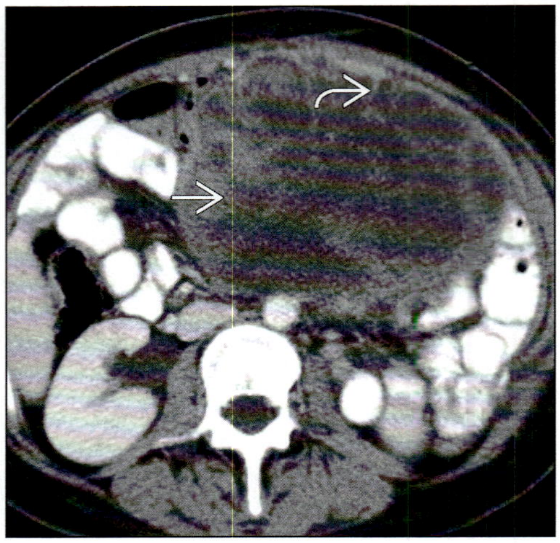

(Left) *Transverse transabdominal ultrasound shows an extremely large, slightly heterogeneously echogenic mass → filling most of the abdominopelvic cavity in this patient complaining of abdominal pain and weight gain.* ***(Right)*** *Axial CECT in the same patient shows a large heterogeneous mass → with extensive enhancing septations ↪ and areas of necrosis, worrisome for carcinoma. Subsequent hysterectomy showed uterine leiomyosarcoma.*

Stage IV, Recurrent Uterine Sarcoma

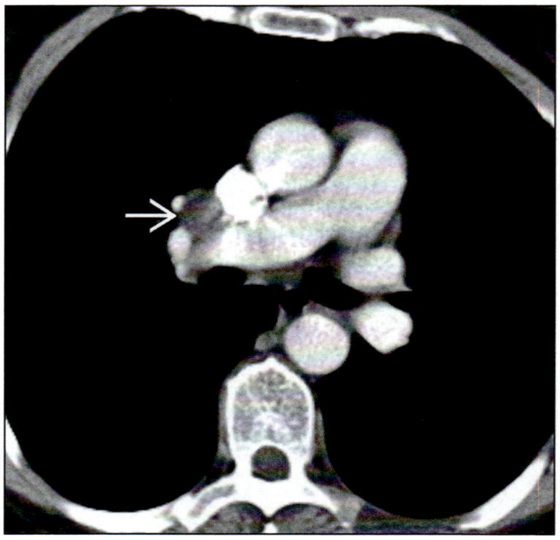

Stage IV, Recurrent Uterine Sarcoma

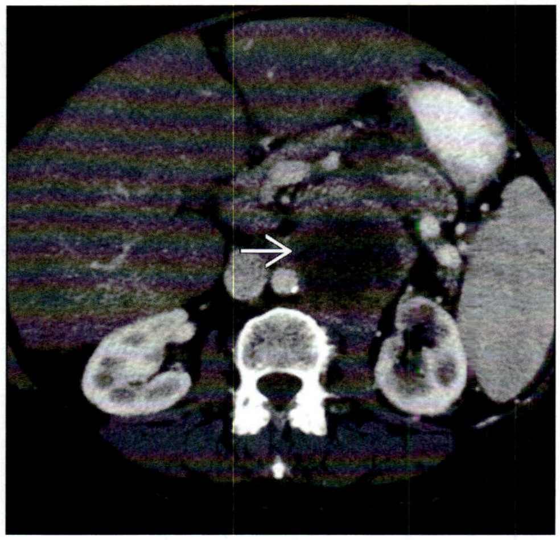

(Left) *Axial CECT in a patient with a history of uterine leiomyosarcoma shows a new enlarged lymph node → in the mediastinum just anterior to the right main pulmonary artery and lateral to the superior vena cava, worrisome for a metastatic lesion. Subsequent resection showed metastatic disease.* ***(Right)*** *Axial CECT shows a large necrotic left paraaortic mass → in this patient with a history of uterine leiomyosarcoma, compatible with recurrence.*

Stage IV, Recurrent Uterine Sarcoma

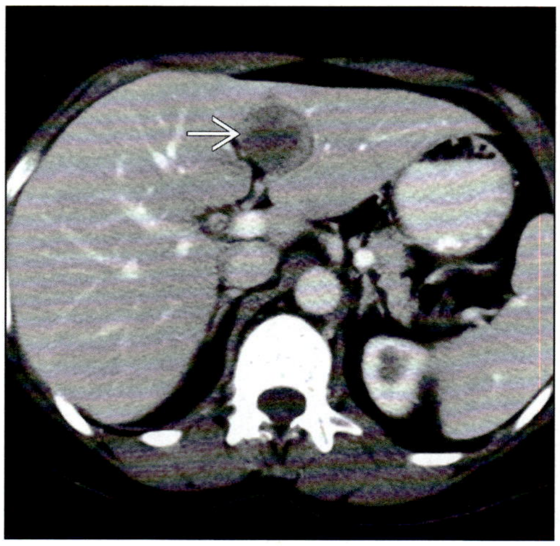

Stage IV, Recurrent Uterine Sarcoma

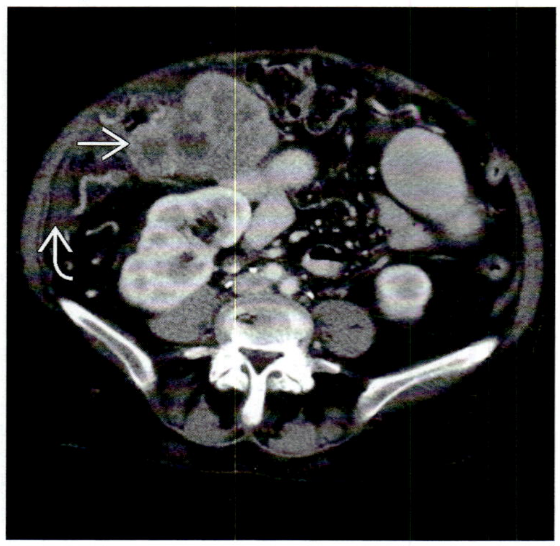

(Left) *Axial CECT in a patient with a history of uterine leiomyosarcoma shows a low-attenuation hepatic lesion → with mild enhancing wall and central necrosis, compatible with recurrent disease.* ***(Right)*** *Axial CECT shows recurrent tumor → within the small bowel mesentery in this patient with a history of uterine leiomyosarcoma. Also note early nodular carcinomatosis ↪ along the right side of the omentum.*

Stage IV, Recurrent Uterine Sarcoma

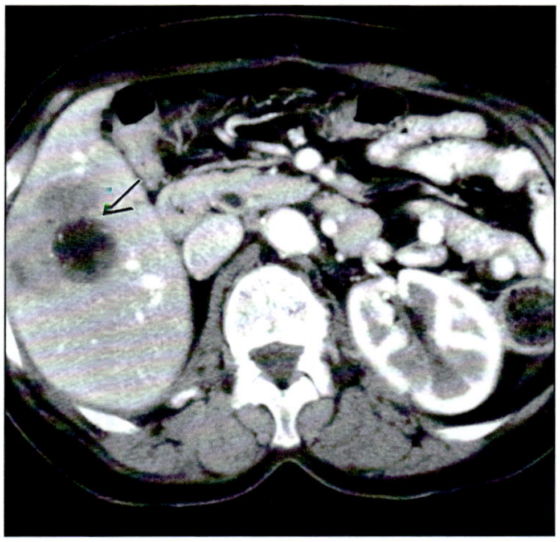

Stage IV, Recurrent Uterine Sarcoma

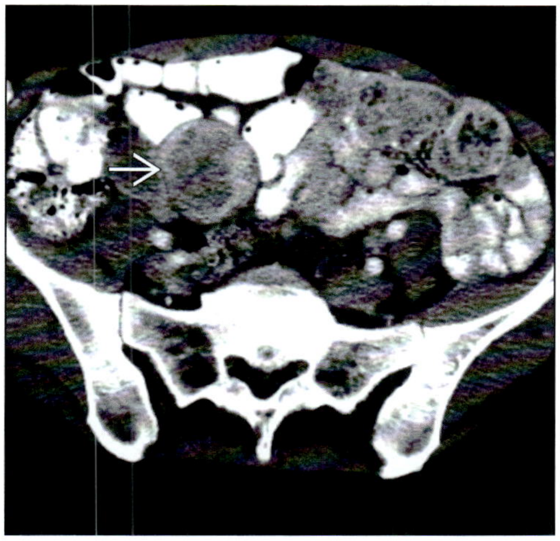

(Left) Axial CECT in a patient with uterine leiomyosarcoma shows a complex lesion → with a more solid anterolateral component and a more necrotic posteromedial portion, compatible with recurrent disease. ***(Right)*** Axial CECT in the same patient also shows a rounded metastatic lesion → in the small bowel mesentery that is very easy to identify with the well-opacified small bowel adjacent to it.

Stage IV, Recurrent Uterine Sarcoma

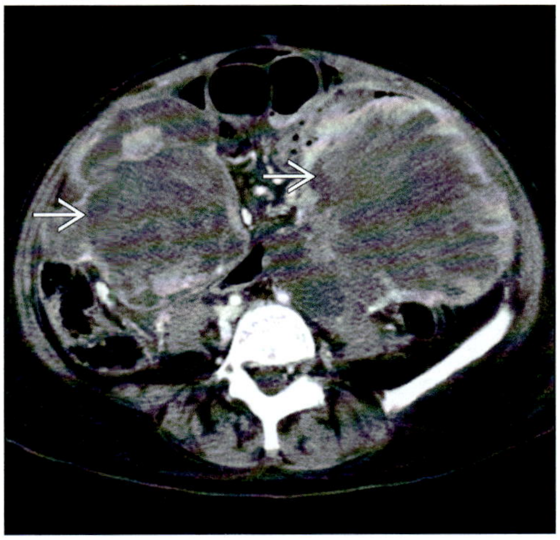

Stage IV, Recurrent Uterine Sarcoma

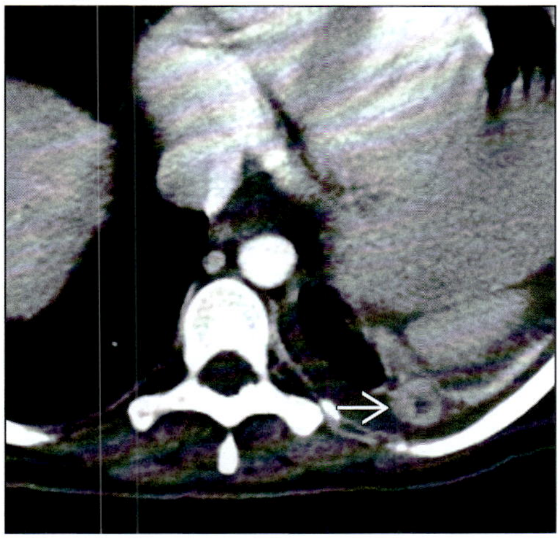

(Left) Axial CECT shows multiple characteristic large necrotic masses → with enhancing septa, compatible with recurrent uterine leiomyosarcoma. ***(Right)*** Axial CECT shows a trace left-sided pleural effusion and an enhancing pleural-based lesion →, subsequently biopsied under CT guidance showing recurrent uterine leiomyosarcoma.

Stage IV, Recurrent Uterine Sarcoma

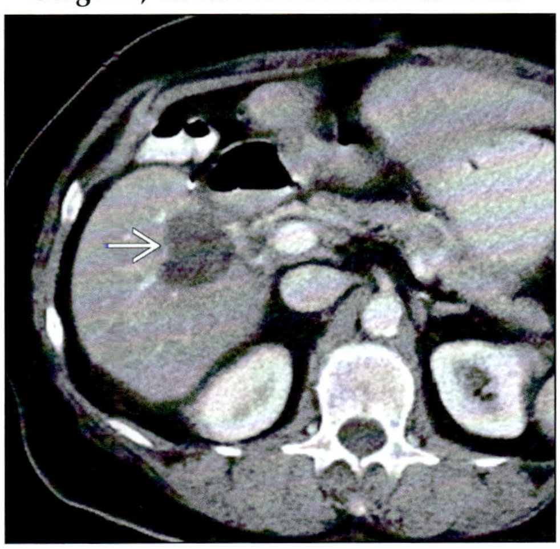

Stage IV, Recurrent Uterine Sarcoma

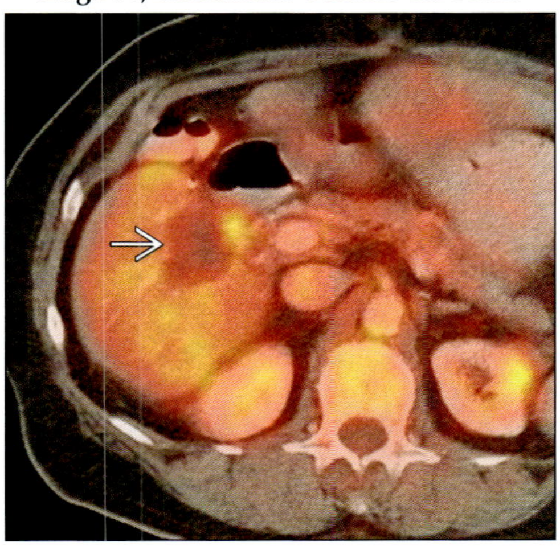

(Left) Axial CECT shows a new low-attenuation lesion → in the liver status post resection of a prior lesion, worrisome for metastatic disease. ***(Right)*** Axial PET/CT in the same patient shows no increased FDG activity →, which could be misinterpreted as benign. However, sarcomas may have variable FDG activity. Subsequent ultrasound-guided biopsy in this patient showed recurrent uterine leiomyosarcoma.

CORPUS UTERI CARCINOMA

*(**Left**) Axial CECT shows a low-attenuation lesion → in the liver of a patient with a history of uterine leiomyosarcoma. The lesion is nonspecific but did measure above water attenuation. (**Right**) Axial PET/CT in the same patient shows no increased FDG activity in the hepatic lesion →. With a history of sarcoma, a negative PET study should be interpreted cautiously, as sarcomas similar to this case may be non-FDG avid.*

Stage IV, Recurrent Uterine Sarcoma

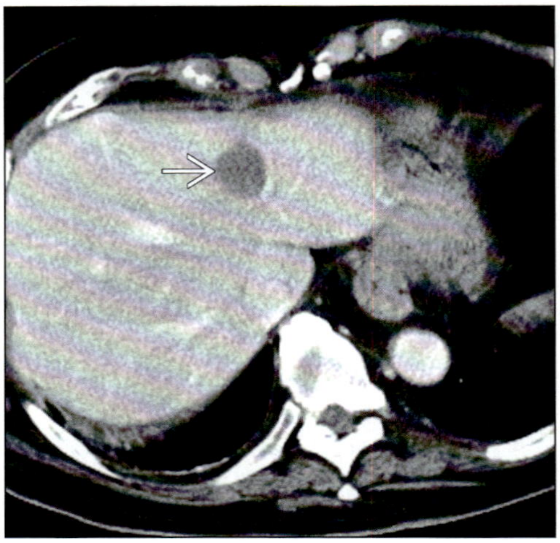

Stage IV, Recurrent Uterine Sarcoma

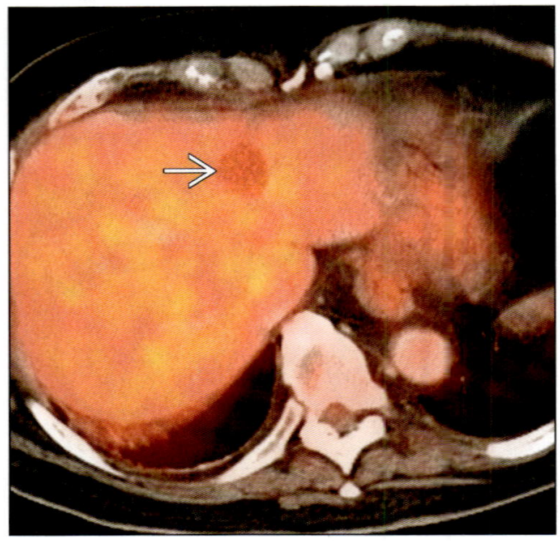

*(**Left**) Axial CECT during the hepatic arterial phase shows extensive vascularity → within this recurrent uterine leiomyosarcoma of the liver. Sarcomas often outgrow their blood supply and become necrotic centrally. (**Right**) Gross pathology specimen shows the large resected hepatic lesion → against the minimal amount of normal hepatic tissue seen along the right upper border ↪.*

Stage IV, Recurrent Uterine Sarcoma

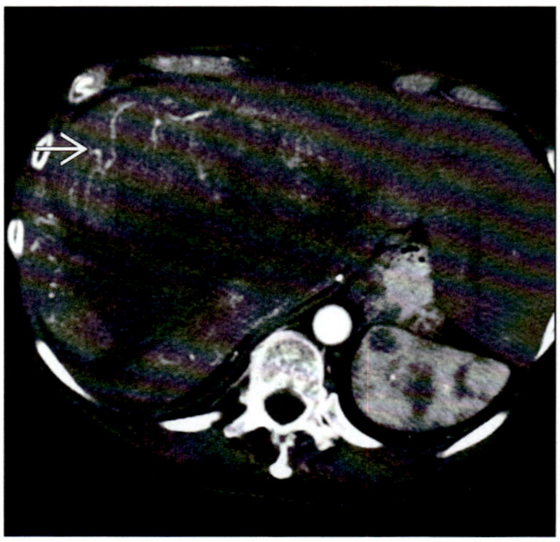

Stage IV, Recurrent Uterine Sarcoma

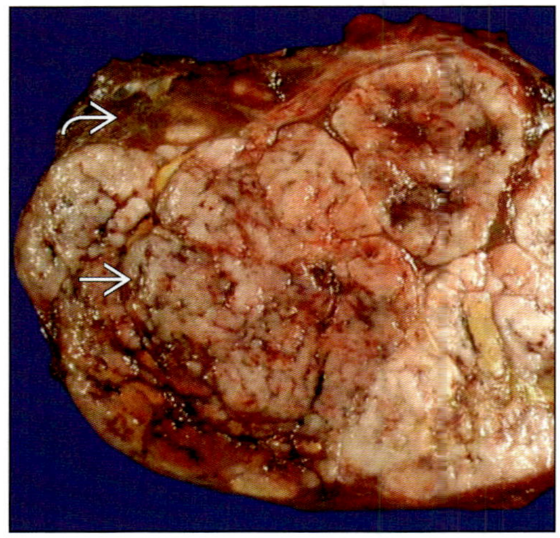

*(**Left**) Axial CECT shows bilateral well-circumscribed large lesions → in a patient with a history of uterine leiomyosarcoma, very worrisome for metastatic disease. (**Right**) Axial fused PET/CT from the same patient shows no increased FDG activity in the lesions → above background lung. Subsequent CT-guided biopsy revealed metastatic uterine leiomyosarcoma.*

Stage IV, Recurrent Uterine Sarcoma

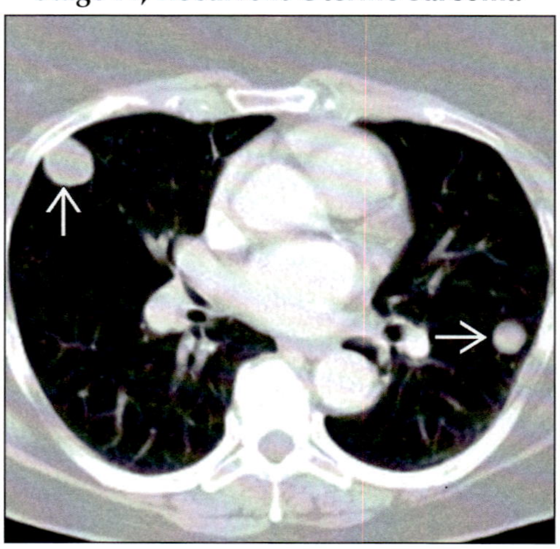

Stage IV, Recurrent Uterine Sarcoma

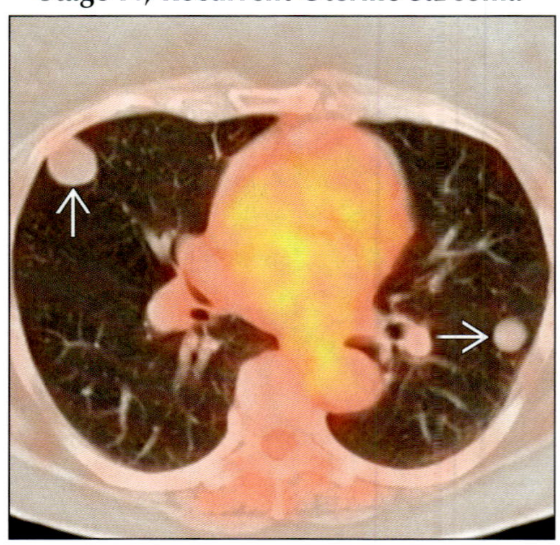

Stage IV, Recurrent Uterine Sarcoma

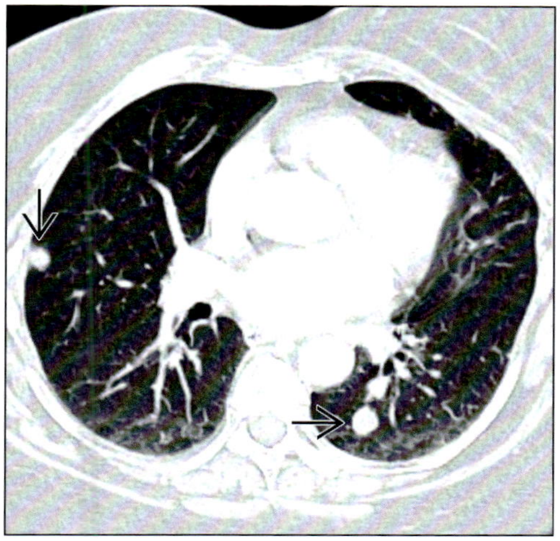

Stage IV, Recurrent Uterine Sarcoma

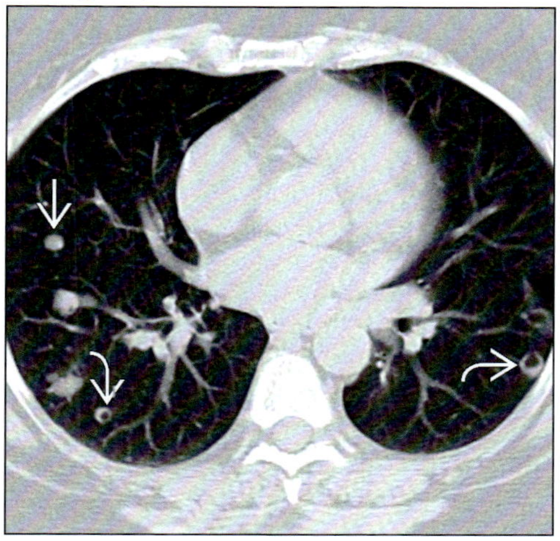

(Left) *Axial CECT shows typical well-circumscribed bilateral lung metastases* → *from uterine leiomyosarcoma. With this appearance, FDG PET could be performed, but biopsy should be considered, as sarcomas may not be FDG avid.* ***(Right)*** *Axial CECT shows bilateral metastases from uterine leiomyosarcoma* ➡*. Note that there is cavitation in some of the lesions* ➦*, a finding that may be seen with uterine leiomyosarcoma, among other malignancies.*

Stage IV, Recurrent Uterine Sarcoma

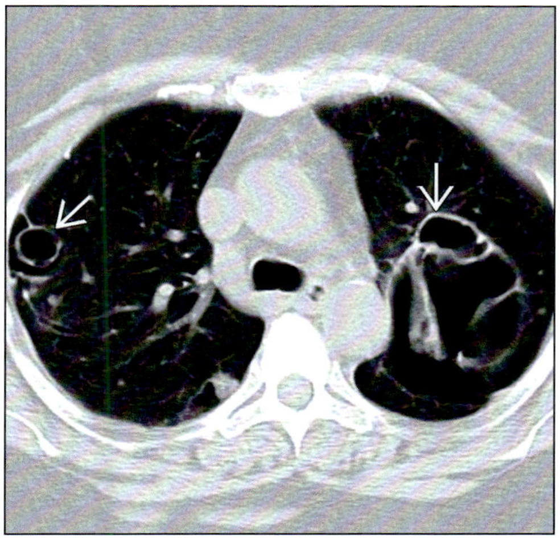

Stage IV, Recurrent Uterine Sarcoma

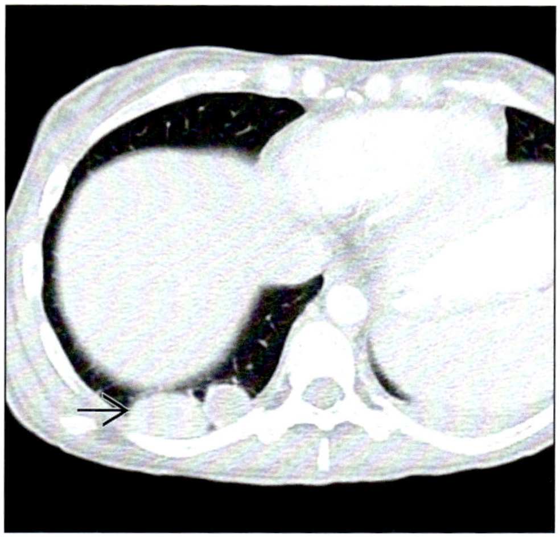

(Left) *Axial CECT shows bilateral pulmonary metastases from uterine leiomyosarcoma* ➡*. Note the extensive cavitation in some of the lesions, a finding that may be seen with uterine leiomyosarcoma, among other malignancies.* ***(Right)*** *Axial CECT shows 2 well-circumscribed lesions* → *in the right lower lobe, biopsy proven to be recurrent uterine leiomyosarcoma. Lower lobe lesions, particularly when new, should be biopsied.*

Stage IV, Recurrent Endometrial

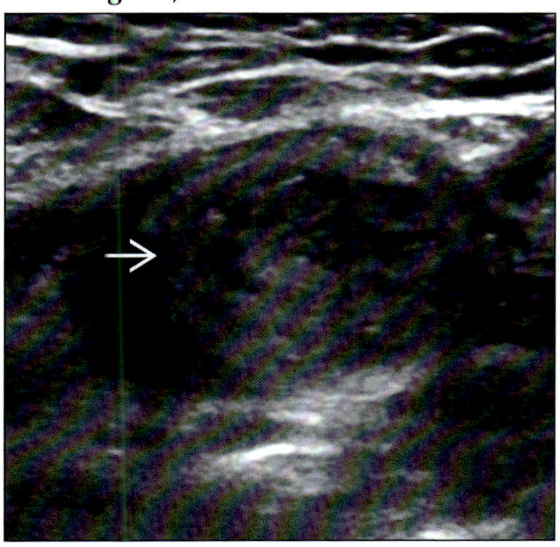

Stage IV, Recurrent Endometrial

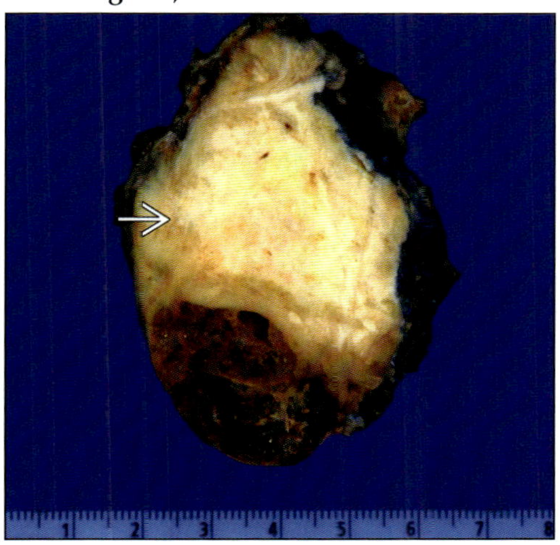

(Left) *Transverse grayscale ultrasound shows a nodule* ➡ *in the thyroid isthmus with slightly heterogeneous echotexture in this patient with a history of metastatic endometrial carcinoma. Although very atypical, pathology revealed metastatic endometrial carcinoma.* ***(Right)*** *Gross pathology image from the same patient shows a solid yellowish lesion* ➡ *in the resected thyroid isthmus, shown to be metastatic endometrial carcinoma.*

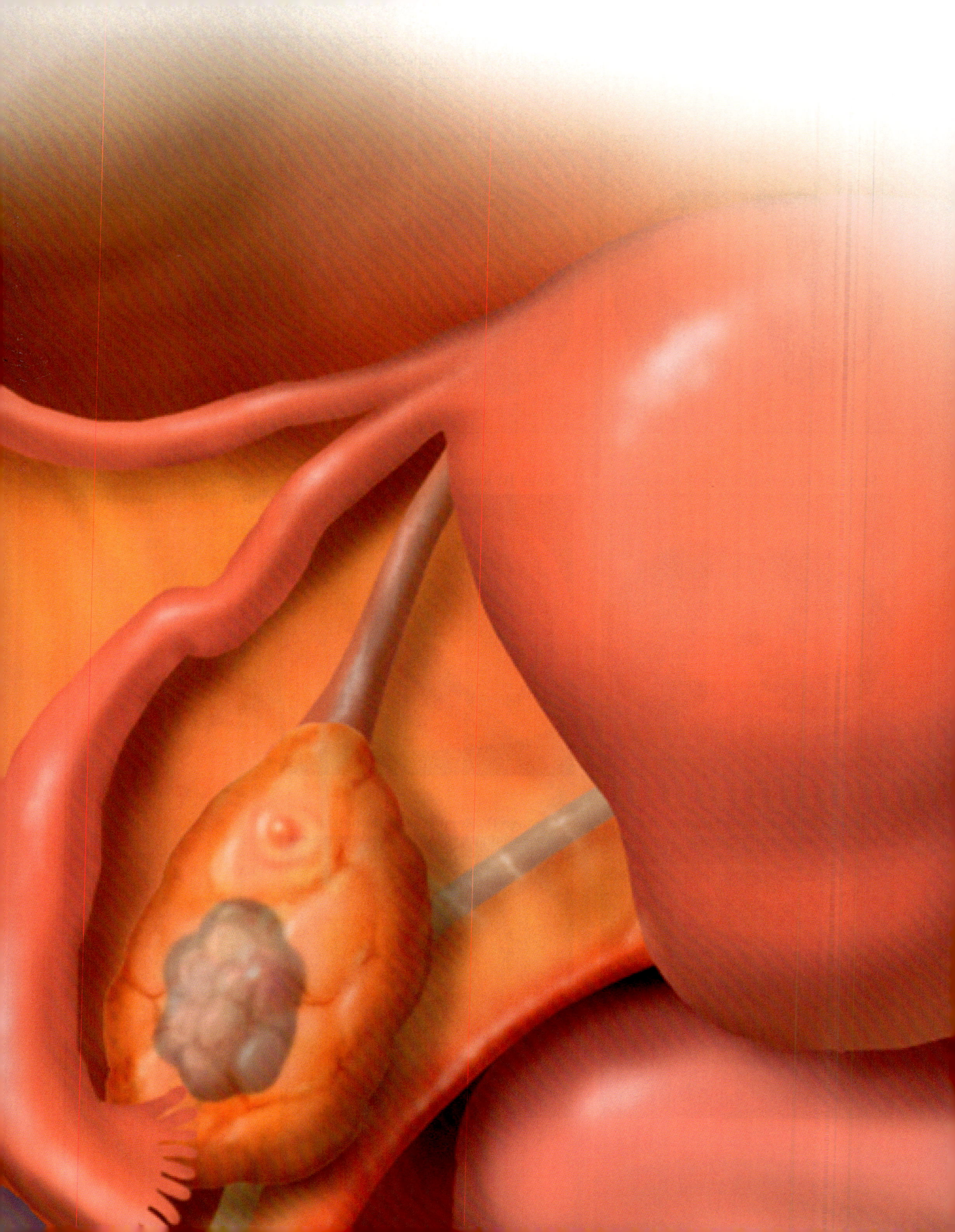

Ovarian Carcinoma

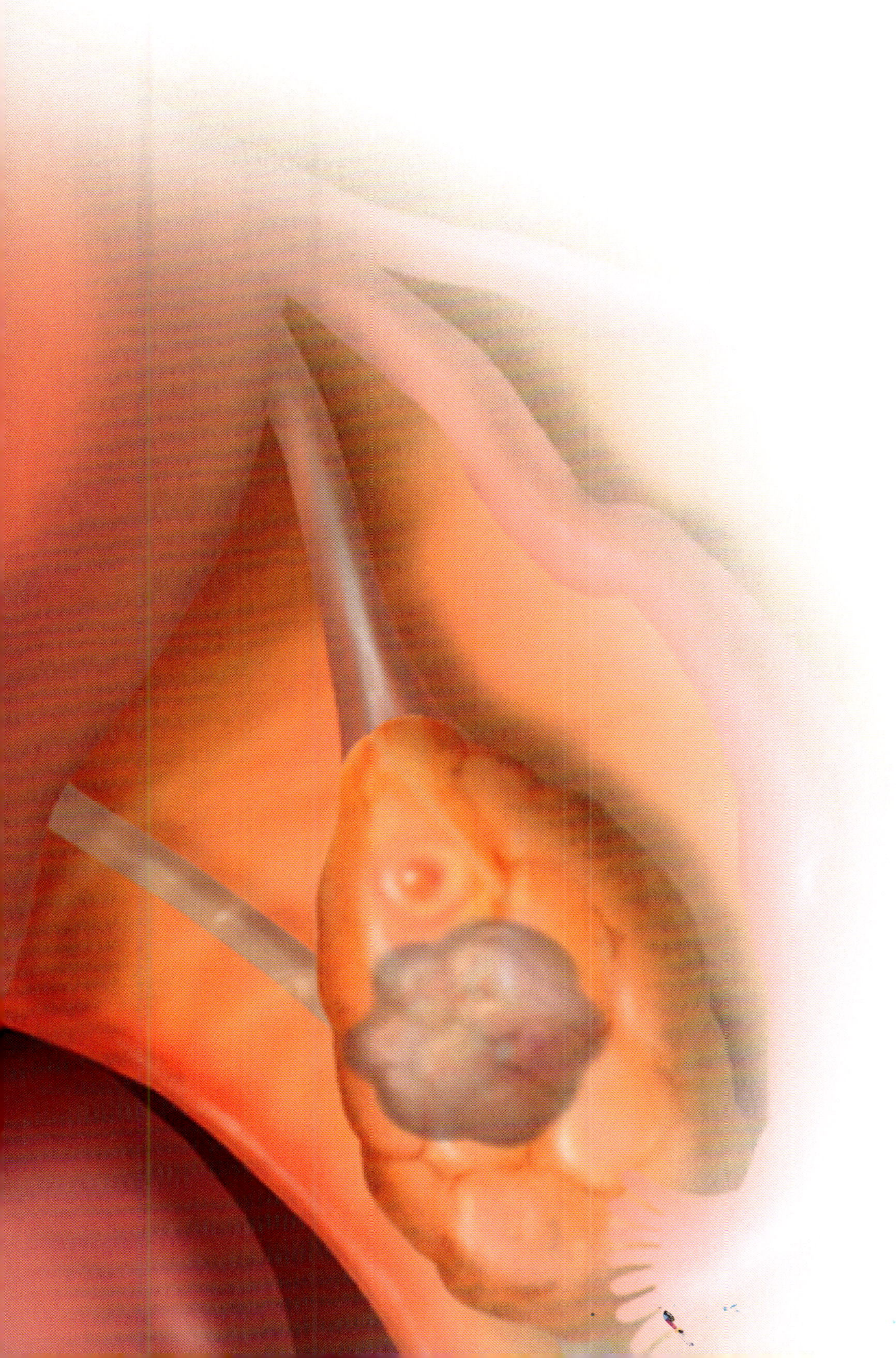

OVARIAN CARCINOMA

(T) Primary Tumor

Adapted from 7th edition AJCC Staging Forms.

TNM	*FIGO*	*Definitions*
TX		Primary tumor cannot be assessed
T0		No evidence of primary tumor
T1	I	Tumor limited to ovaries (1 or both)
T1a	IA	Tumor limited to 1 ovary; capsule intact, no tumor on ovarian surface; no malignant cells in ascites or peritoneal washing
T1b	IB	Tumor limited to both ovaries; capsules intact, no tumor on ovarian surface; no malignant cells in ascites or peritoneal washings
T1c	IC	Tumor limited to 1 or both ovaries with any of the following: Capsule ruptured, tumor on ovarian surface, malignant cells in ascites or peritoneal washings
T2	II	Tumor involves 1 or both ovaries with pelvic extension
T2a	IIA	Extension &/or implants on uterus &/or tube(s); no malignant cells in ascites or peritoneal washings
T2b	IIB	Extension to &/or implants on other pelvic tissues; no malignant cells in ascites or peritoneal washings
T2c	IIC	Pelvic extension &/or implants with malignant cells in ascites or peritoneal washings
T3	III	Tumor involves 1 or both ovaries with peritoneal metastasis outside the pelvis
T3a	IIIA	Microscopic peritoneal metastasis beyond pelvis (no macroscopic tumor)
T3b	IIIB	Macroscopic peritoneal metastasis beyond pelvis ≤ 2 cm in greatest dimension
T3c	IIIC	Peritoneal metastasis beyond pelvis > 2 cm in greatest dimension &/or regional lymph node metastasis

(N) Regional Lymph Nodes

NX		Regional lymph nodes cannot be assessed
N0		No regional lymph node metastasis
N1	IIIC	Regional lymph node metastasis

(M) Distant Metastasis

M0		No distant metastasis
M1	IV	Distant metastasis (excludes peritoneal metastasis)

AJCC Stages/Prognostic Groups

Adapted from 7th edition AJCC Staging Forms.

Stage	*T*	*N*	*M*
I	T1	N0	M0
IA	T1a	N0	M0
IB	T1b	N0	M0
IC	T1c	N0	M0
II	T2	N0	M0
IIA	T2a	N0	M0
IIB	T2b	N0	M0
IIC	T2c	N0	M0
III	T3	N0	M0
IIIA	T3a	N0	M0
IIIB	T3b	N0	M0
IIIC	T3c	N0	M0
	Any T	N1	M0
IV	Any T	Any N	M1

OVARIAN CARCINOMA

T1a

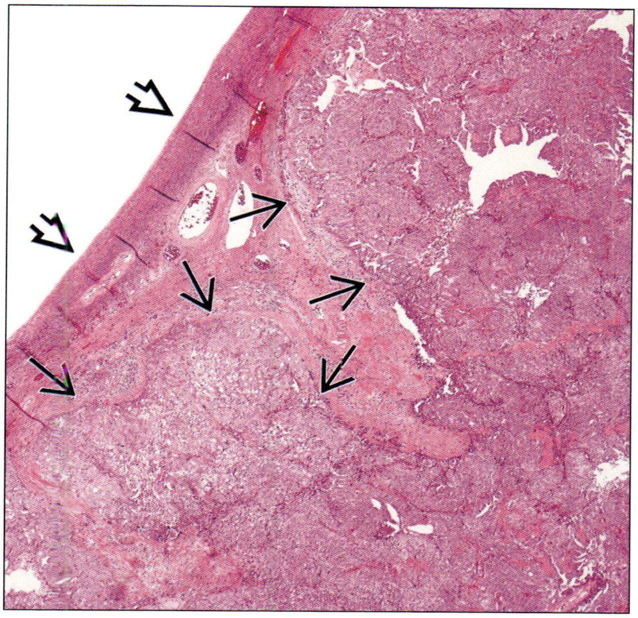

Low-power magnification of H&E shows ovarian carcinoma that is limited to 1 ovary with intact capsule (T1a). Sheets of tumor cells ➙ are seen with intact capsule ⇨. (Original magnification 20x.)

T1a

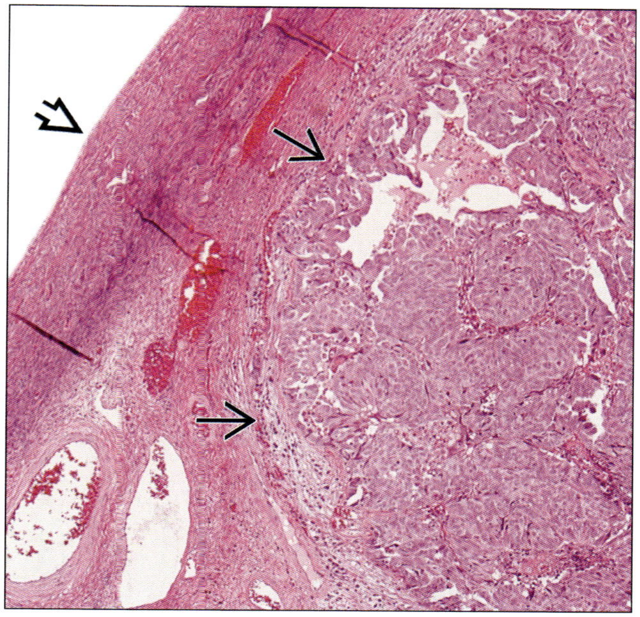

High-power magnification shows sheets of serous carcinoma cells ➙ and an intact capsule ⇨ overlying ovarian stroma. (Original magnification 100x.)

T1c

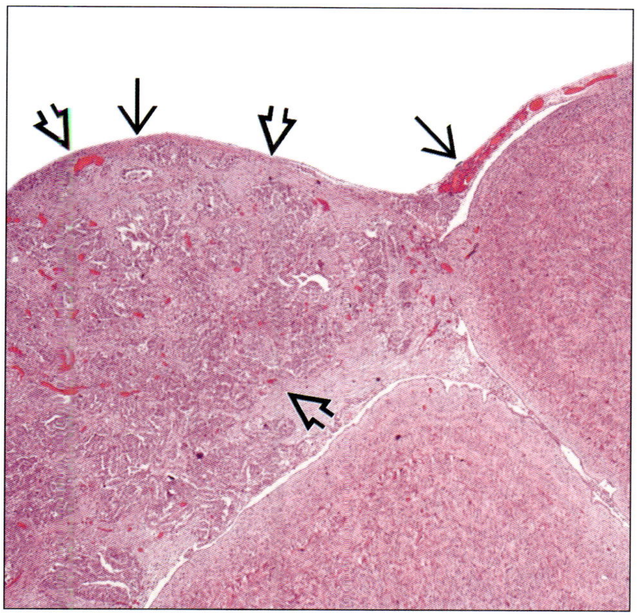

Low-power magnification shows ovarian tumor extending through the capsule to the ovarian surface (T1c). The H&E stain shows ovarian tumor ⇨ extending to the ovarian surface ➙. Note normal ovarian tissue on the right side of the photomicrograph. (Original magnification 20x.)

T1c

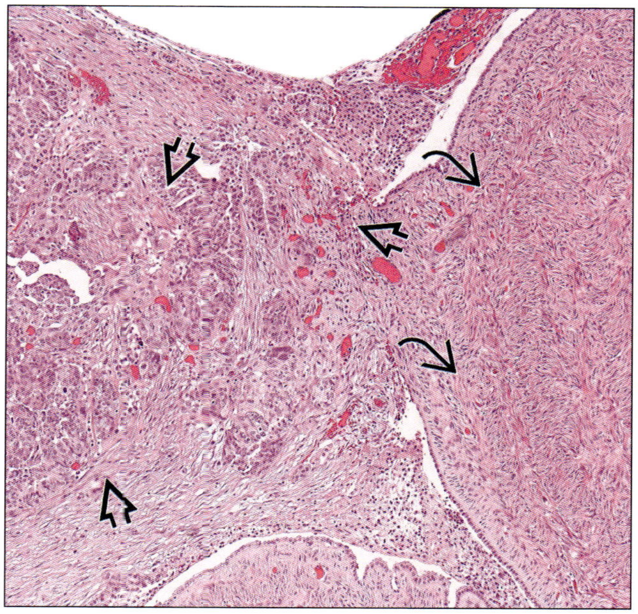

Higher magnification shows a close-up of the cords and nests of tumor cells ⇨ and ovarian plump spindle stromal cells ↷. (Original magnification 100x.)

OVARIAN CARCINOMA

T2a

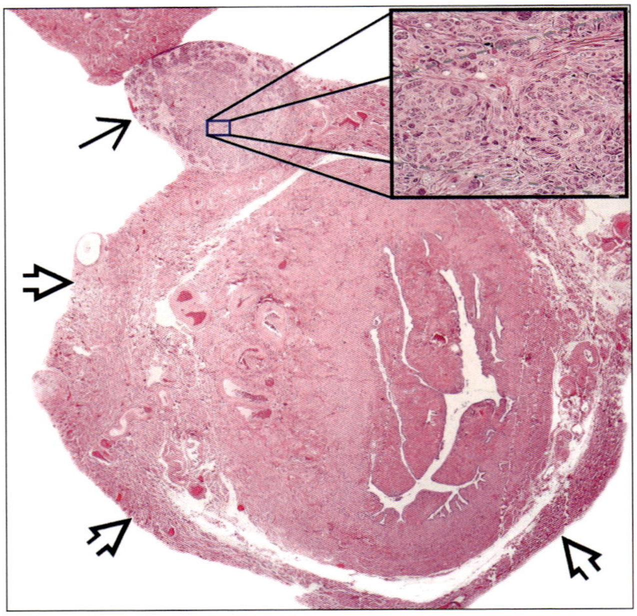

Low-power magnification of H&E stain shows a cross section of a fallopian tube ⇨ with ovarian tumor nodule ⇨ implanted on the serosal aspect. The inset shows a high magnification view of the neoplastic malignant cells of the nodule.

T2b

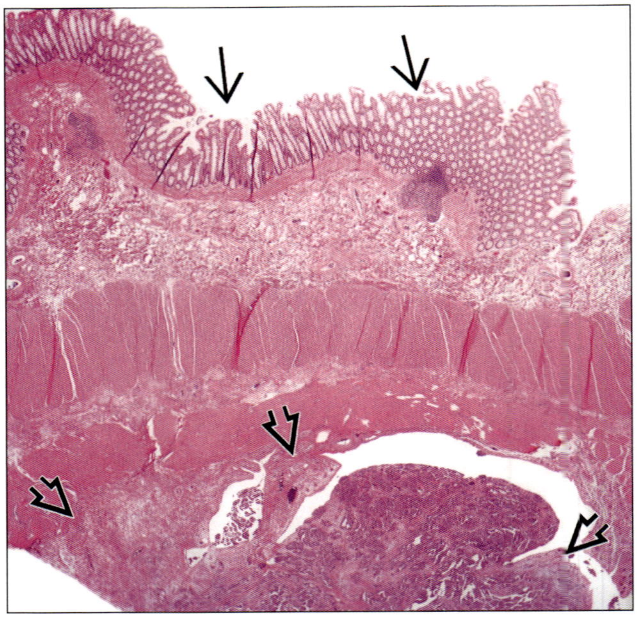

Low-power magnification of H&E stain shows an implanted ovarian nodule to the serosal surface of the recto-sigmoid colon (T2b). The mucosal side of the rectosigmoid is highlighted ⇨, as well as the tumor nodule ⇨. (Original magnification 40x.)

T3

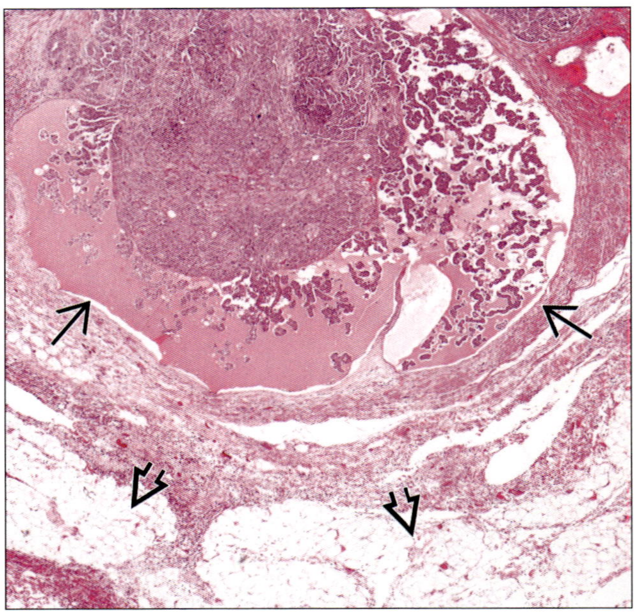

H&E section shows peritoneal metastasis of ovarian papillary serous carcinoma outside the pelvis (T3). The nodule in the upper part of the slide ⇨ represents the metastatic tumor and is implanted in the fibro-fatty tissue ⇨ of the peritoneum (lower aspect of the slide). (Original magnification 20x.)

T3c

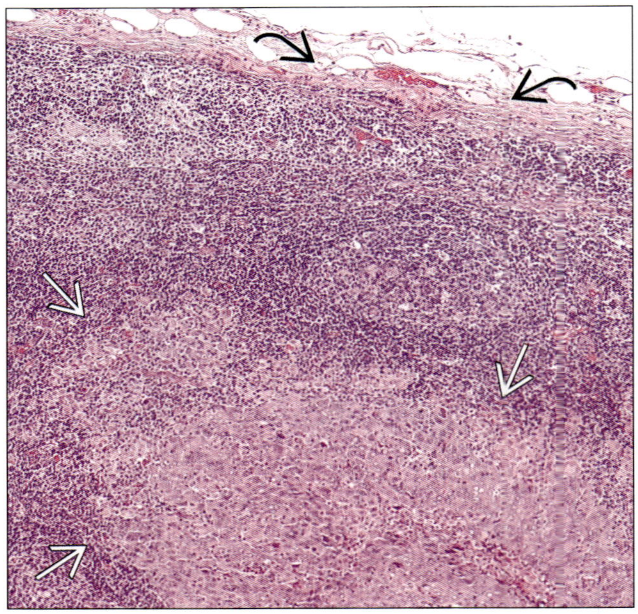

Low-power magnification of H&E stain shows a metastatic ovarian carcinoma to a regional lymph node (T3c). The lymph node capsule is highlighted ⇨; tumor nest ➡ is present within the lymph node. (Original magnification 40x.)

T1a (FIGO IA)

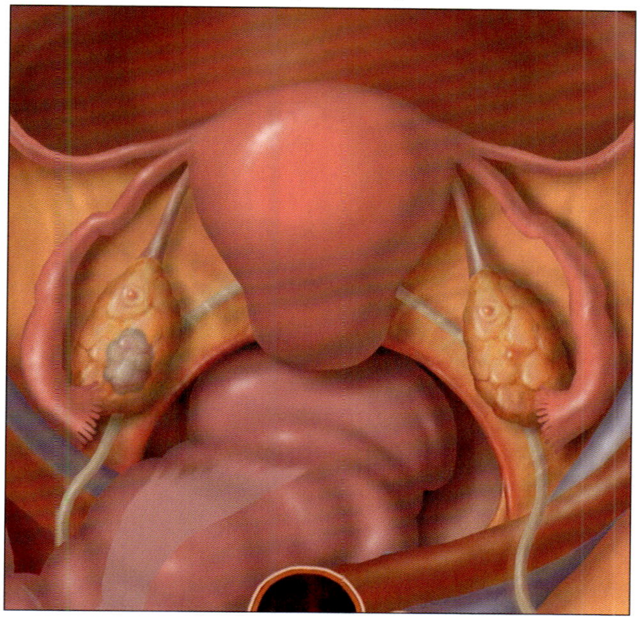

T1a tumors are limited to 1 ovary with intact capsule, no tumor on the ovarian surface, and no malignant cells in ascites or peritoneal washings.

T1b (FIGO IB)

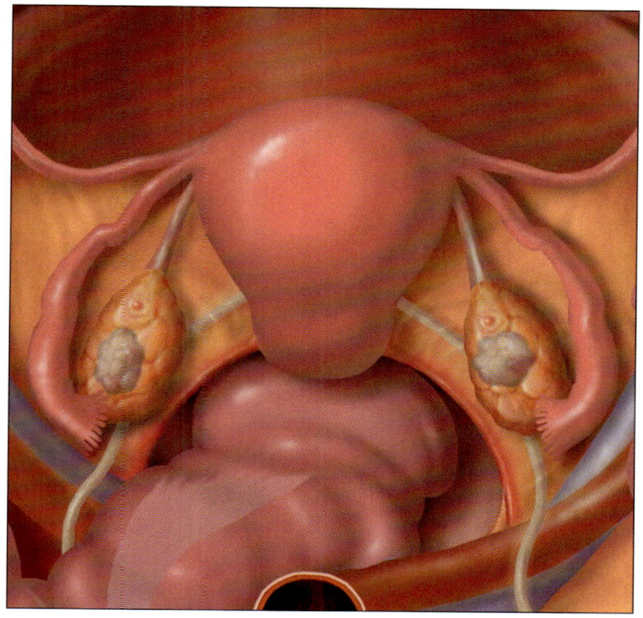

T1b tumors are limited to both ovaries with intact capsules, no tumor on the ovarian surface, and no malignant cells in ascites or peritoneal washings.

T1c (FIGO IC)

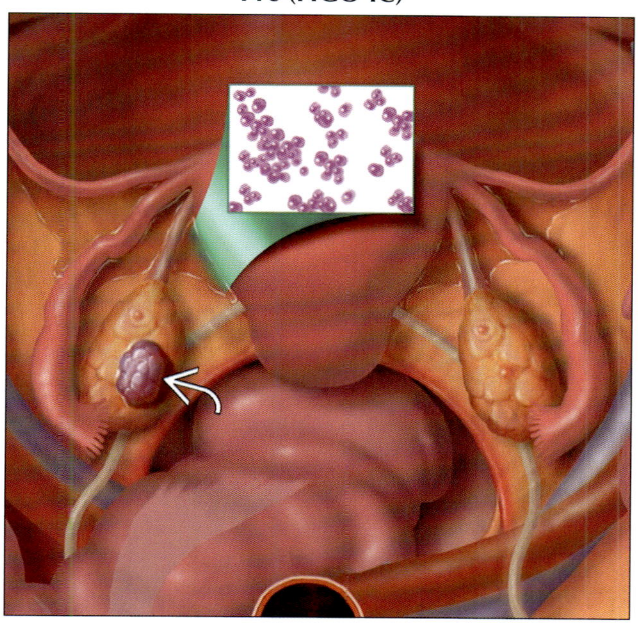

T1c tumors are limited to 1 or both ovaries with capsule rupture, tumor on the ovarian surface ➔, or malignant cells in ascites or peritoneal washings.

T2a (FIGO IIA)

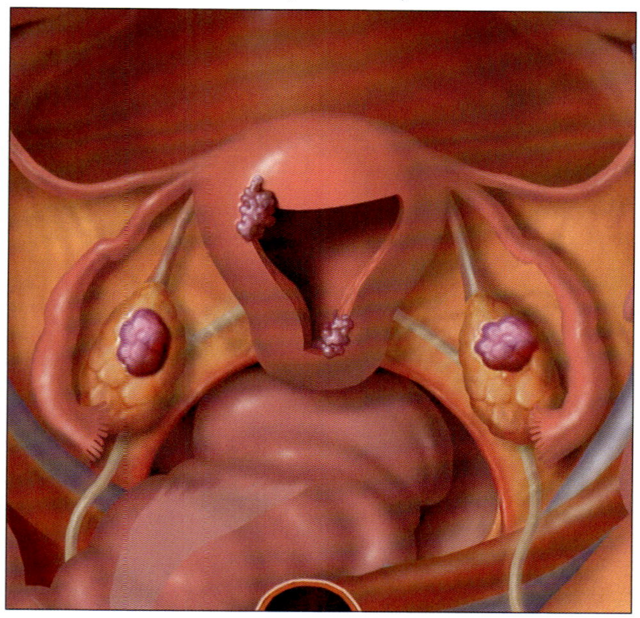

T2a tumors involve 1 or both ovaries with pelvic extension to the uterus or fallopian tube. No malignant cells are found in ascites or peritoneal washings.

OVARIAN CARCINOMA

T2b (FIGO IIB)

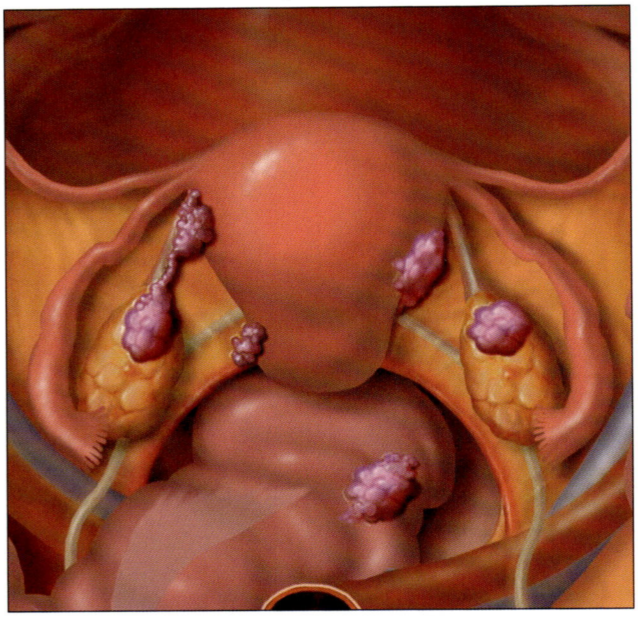

T2b tumors involve 1 or both ovaries with pelvic extension &/or implants to other pelvic organs. No malignant cells in ascites or peritoneal washings are found.

T2c (FIGO IIC)

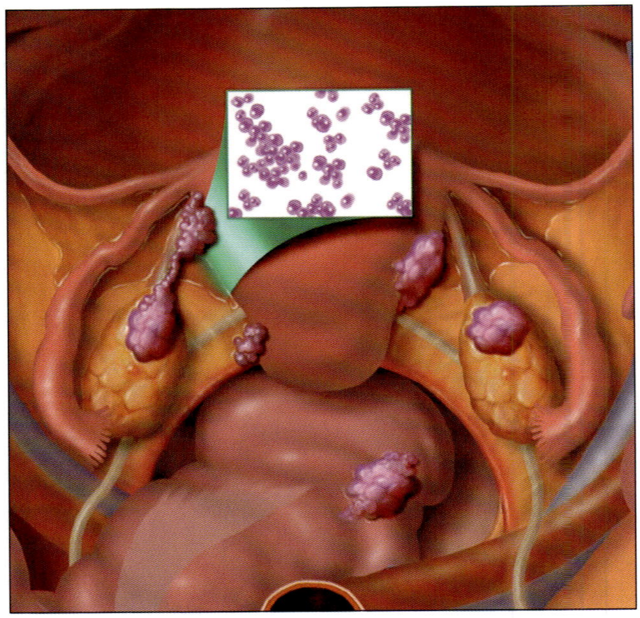

T2c tumors involve 1 or both ovaries with pelvic extension &/or implants, with malignant cells in ascites or peritoneal washings.

T3a (FIGO IIIA)

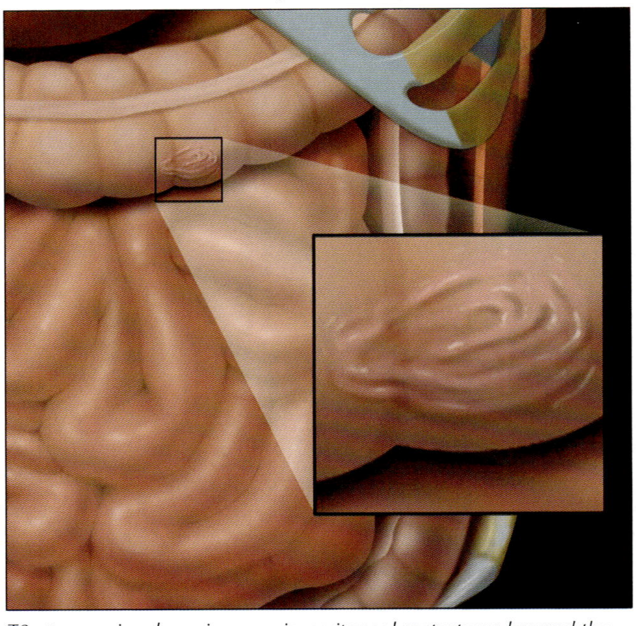

T3a tumors involve microscopic peritoneal metastases beyond the pelvis. This cannot be visualized by imaging; rather, it is found through peritoneal biopsy at staging laparotomy.

T3b (FIGO IIIB)

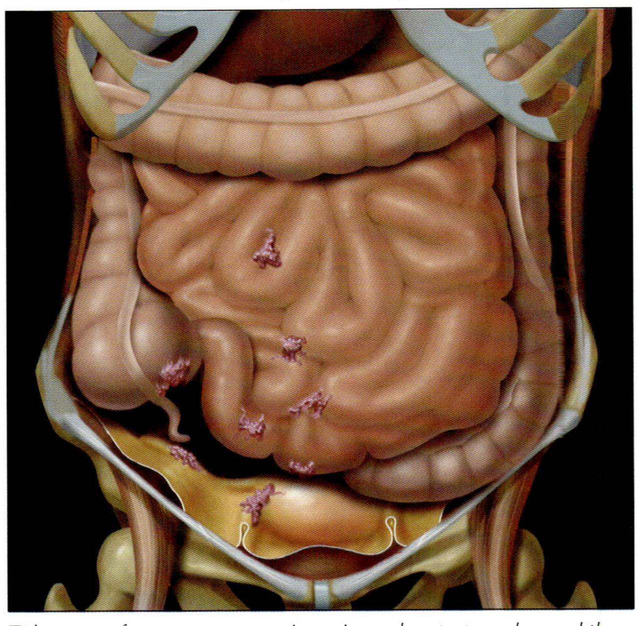

T3b tumors feature macroscopic peritoneal metastases beyond the pelvis that are less than or equal to 2 cm in greatest dimension.

T3c (FIGO IIIC)

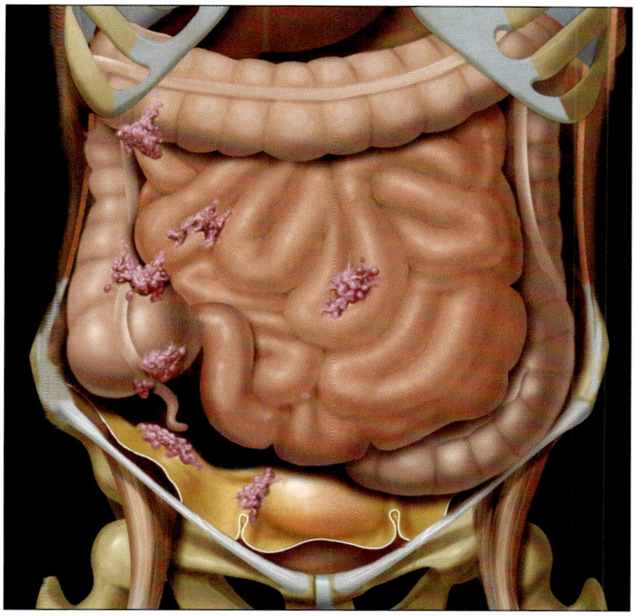

T3c tumors involve macroscopic peritoneal metastases beyond the pelvis greater than 2 cm in greatest dimension.

Nodal Drainage of the Ovary

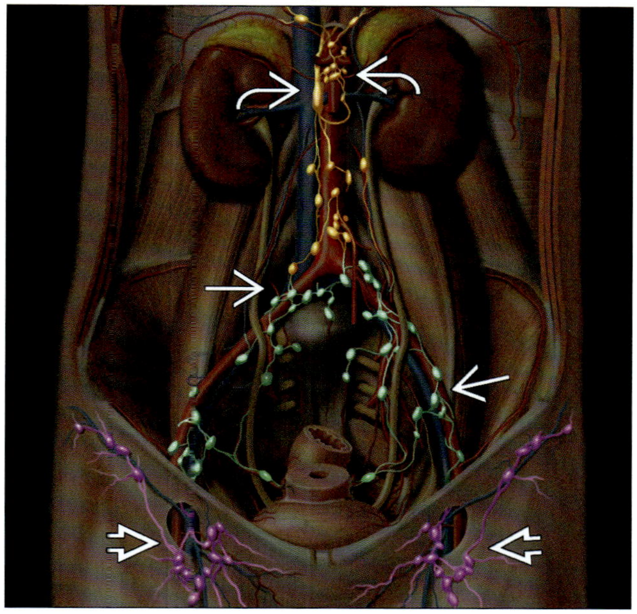

The main ovarian lymphatics follow the ovarian veins to the paraaortic lymph nodes ➭. Lymphatic spread may also occur through the broad ligament to the pelvic lymph nodes ➡ and along the round ligament to the inguinal lymph nodes ⇨.

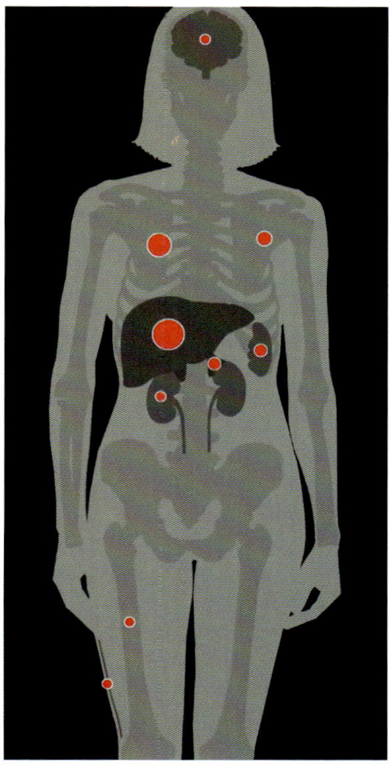

METASTASES, ORGAN FREQUENCY

Liver	45-48%
Lung	34-39%
Pleura	25%
Adrenal gland	15-21%
Spleen	15-20%
Bone	11%
Kidney	7-10%
Skin and subcutaneous tissue	5%
Brain	3-6%

OVARIAN CARCINOMA

OVERVIEW

General Comments

- Primary peritoneal carcinoma (unusual tumor of similar histiogenic origin to primary ovarian carcinoma) included with ovarian carcinoma in 7th edition AJCC Staging Manual

Classification

- Primary ovarian carcinomas are differentiated by cell origin
  - Epithelial ovarian tumors (EOT): 90% of ovarian carcinomas
    - Serous cystadenocarcinoma (60%)
    - Endometrioid carcinoma (10%)
    - Clear cell carcinoma (10%)
    - Carcinosarcoma (10%)
    - Mixed (5%)
    - Mucinous cystadenocarcinoma (3%)
      - Less common than initially thought
      - Many mucinous tumors of ovaries are actually metastatic from gastrointestinal primary
    - Undifferentiated carcinoma (1%)
    - Brenner tumor (< 1%)
  - Nonepithelial ovarian tumors: 10% of ovarian carcinomas
    - Germ cell tumors
      - Dysgerminoma
      - Embryonal carcinoma
      - Immature teratoma
      - Olyembryoma
      - Choriocarcinoma
      - Mixed tumors
    - Tumor of sex cord or stroma
      - Malignant granulosa cell tumor
- Nonepithelial primary ovarian cancers may be staged using TNM classification system

PATHOLOGY

Routes of Spread

- Understanding pattern of spread is crucial for adequate radiological and surgical staging
- **Local spread**
  - Direct extension to surrounding pelvic structures
    - Commonly fallopian tubes, uterus, and contralateral adnexa
    - Less commonly rectum, bladder, and pelvic sidewall
  - Uterine involvement
    - Independent primary tumors of low histologic grade, usually of endometrioid type, with involvement limited to endometrium and ovary
      - Favorable prognosis; often no additional treatment
    - Tumors metastasizing from uterus to ovary or from ovary to uterus
      - Worse prognosis; adjuvant therapy is generally indicated
    - Distinction between primary vs. secondary involvement relies on histological examination
- **Peritoneal seeding**
  - Most common mode of tumor spread
  - Malignant cells shedding from tumor surface into peritoneal cavity
  - Malignant cells are distributed by gravity into cul-de-sac or follow normal routes of peritoneal fluid circulation
    - Preferential flow and seeding along right paracolic gutter, liver capsule, and right hemidiaphragm
  - Peritoneal fluid normally drains through rich lymphatic capillary network of diaphragm to supradiaphragmatic lymph nodes
    - Occlusion of these lymphatics by tumor cells blocks absorption of peritoneal fluid
    - Contributes to accumulation of malignant ascites
  - Most common sites of peritoneal metastases
    - Cul-de-sac
    - Greater omentum
    - Paracolic gutters
    - Small and large bowel surface
    - Liver surface
    - Subphrenic spaces
  - Other potential sites of metastases
    - Porta hepatis
    - Fissure for ligamentum teres
    - Lesser sac
    - Gastrosplenic and gastrohepatic ligaments
    - Splenic hilum
  - Primary peritoneal carcinoma
    - Unusual tumor of similar histiogenic origin to primary ovarian carcinoma
    - Primary tumor of peritoneum that diffusely involves peritoneal surface but spares or only superficially involves ovaries
    - Generally diagnosed in state of peritoneal carcinomatosis
    - Poor prognosis
    - Biopsy important to differentiate primary peritoneal carcinoma from peritoneal carcinomatosis (due to other cancers, mesothelioma, lymphomatosis, or tuberculous peritonitis)
  - Pseudomyxoma peritonei
    - Growing body of immunohistochemical and molecular genetic studies suggest that majority are actually secondary to appendiceal tumors in both men and women
    - Those that are ovarian in origin probably originated from mucinous tumors arising in teratomas
- **Lymphatic spread**
  - 3 primary pathways for lymphatic drainage
    - Main lymphatics follow ovarian veins → paraaortic and aortocaval lymph nodes at level of renal veins
    - Through broad ligament → pelvic lymph nodes, including external iliac, hypogastric, and obturator nodes
    - Along round ligament → inguinal lymph nodes
- **Hematogenous spread**
  - Least common mode of spread
  - Usually not present at initial diagnosis, can be found at restaging
    - In up to 50% of patients at autopsy

General Features

- Genetics

- Lifetime risk of ovarian cancer: 15-30% in women carrying genes responsible for most hereditary ovarian cancers (*BRCA1*, *BRCA2*)
- Hereditary nonpolyposis colon cancer (Lynch syndrome) has also been associated with endometrial and ovarian cancers
- Etiology
  - No known causative factor in development of ovarian carcinoma
  - Factors known to increase risk of developing ovarian cancer include
    - Family history is strongest known risk factor
      - ~ 10% of cases are thought to have hereditary basis
      - Women who have had breast cancer or who have family history of breast or ovarian cancer are at increased risk
    - Nulliparity, early menarche, and late menopause
    - Estrogen use alone as postmenopausal hormone therapy
    - Obesity may be associated with increased risk
  - Pregnancy and long-term use of oral contraceptives reduce risk of developing ovarian cancer
- Epidemiology & cancer incidence
  - Approximately 3% of all cancers among women
  - 2nd most common gynecological malignancy after endometrial carcinoma
    - Estimated 21,550 new cases in USA in 2009
  - Leading cause of death from gynecological cancers and 9th leading cause of cancer death in women
    - Estimated 14,600 deaths in USA in 2009

Gross Pathology & Surgical Features

- General features
  - 2/3 of cases involve both ovaries
  - Range from microscopic to about 20 cm in diameter
  - Typically multilocular and cystic, with intracystic, soft, friable papillae
    - Cysts contain serous, turbid, or bloody fluid
  - External surfaces may be smooth or bosselated and may display grossly exophytic papillary tumor on surface (at least T1c)
  - Solid areas and intracystic nodules are more common in carcinomas than in cystadenomas
  - Hemorrhage and necrosis are often present
- Endometrioid carcinoma arising in endometrioma
  - Gross findings of endometriotic cyst containing chocolate-colored fluid
  - 1 or more solid mural nodules reflecting foci of malignant transformation

Microscopic Pathology

- Major histologic types
  - **Serous cystadenocarcinoma**
    - Most common type of ovarian cancer
      - Accounts for > 50% of malignant ovarian neoplasms
    - Complex papillary and solid patterns with marked nuclear atypia, qualify as high-grade carcinomas
    - Characteristic pattern is lace-like or labyrinthine pattern
      - May be focal but often diffuse
      - Characterized by extensive bridging and coalescence of papillae resulting in solid sheets of tumor cells with interspersed slit-like spaces
    - Serous carcinomas that display extensive solid areas usually are composed of uniform sheets of cells with high-grade nuclear atypia
      - Usually there are focal areas with papillary architecture that permit diagnosis of serous carcinoma as opposed to undifferentiated carcinoma
    - Psammoma bodies are present in 25% of cases
  - **Endometrioid carcinoma**
    - Well-differentiated endometrioid adenocarcinoma accounts for most cases
    - Confluent or cribriform proliferation of glands lined by tall stratified columnar epithelium with sharp luminal margins
    - Villoglandular growth pattern also occurs
    - Squamous differentiation is present in 50% of cases
  - **Mucinous adenocarcinoma**
    - Stromal invasion measuring > 5 mm
    - Stromal invasion in primary ovarian mucinous neoplasms is characterized by 3 different patterns
      - Confluent glandular growth with crowded glands without intervening stroma
      - Clusters of single cells with abundant eosinophilic cytoplasm surrounded by clear spaces
      - Glands of varying sizes infiltrating stroma in haphazard pattern
    - Cytoplasm is scant and eosinophilic with irregular borders and occasional mucin droplets
  - **Brenner tumor**
    - Rounded nests of transitional or squamous cells like epithelium and glandular structures of cylindrical cells within abundant fibrous nonepithelial tissue
    - Microscopically resembles urothelial transitional cell carcinoma
  - **Clear cell adenocarcinoma**
    - Ovarian epithelial tumor in which most cells have clear cytoplasm
    - High association with pelvic endometriosis

IMAGING FINDINGS

Detection

- Primary goal of radiologic assessment is differentiation of malignant from benign tumors
- CA-125 is glycoprotein that is assessed by monoclonal antibody OC-125
  - ↑ CA-125 serum level ≥ 30 U/mL indicates presence of malignancy
  - False-positive results
    - In women with conditions affecting peritoneal surface, such as endometriosis
  - False-negative results
    - In women with early-stage invasive disease and borderline ovarian tumors
- **General imaging findings suggestive of malignancy**
  - Most predictive imaging findings for malignancy are
    - Solid mass, especially when necrosis is present
    - Presence of nonfat nodular components in cystic lesion
  - Other findings suggestive of malignancy

OVARIAN CARCINOMA

- Irregular, thick wall or septa (> 3 mm)
- Vascularity in solid mass or papillary projections
  - Doppler demonstration of blood flow
  - Enhancement on CT and MR
- Ancillary findings that are strong indicators of malignancy
  - Ascites
  - Peritoneal metastases
  - Lymphadenopathy
  - Pelvic organ or sidewall invasion
- **Special tumor features** may be present and can suggest specific type
  - Calcification in cystic or partially cystic tumor
    - Serous epithelial tumor
  - Associated endometrial hyperplasia or carcinoma
    - Endometrioid epithelial tumor (20-30% of patients)
  - Variable density (echogenicity) within loculi of multilocular tumor
    - Mucinous epithelial tumor
  - Pseudomyxoma peritonei virtually never occurs in association with primary ovarian mucinous tumors
- **Ultrasound**
  - Low cost and wide availability
  - Modality of choice to evaluate suspected or palpable adnexal mass
    - Adnexal masses are found on US in about 10% of premenopausal women
    - US seems to be similar with CT and MR in differentiation of malignant from benign ovarian tumors
      - Pattern recognition on US correctly classified 93% of lesions as benign or malignant (in experienced hands)
  - Transvaginal ultrasound (TVU) and transabdominal ultrasound (TAU) should be used together
    - TVU allows best evaluation of pelvic masses but limited field of view
    - TAU is better for large mass or if ovaries are displaced by enlarged leiomyomatous uterus
  - Ovarian volumes
    - Premenopausal women: Up to 20 cm^3
    - Postmenopausal women: Up to 8-10 cm^3
    - Ovarian volumes progressively decrease with age and years since menopause
    - Enlarged ovary for age, or ovary > 2x volume of other ovary, may be early indication of ovarian neoplasm
  - Spectral Doppler findings suggestive of malignancy
    - Low-resistance waveforms due to tumor neovascularity and arteriovenous shunting
    - Resistance index < 0.4 and pulsatility index < 1
    - Considerable overlap with benign physiological lesions
    - More suspicious in postmenopausal women, in whom benign lesions are less frequent
    - Color Doppler flow imaging alone is significantly inferior to combined US techniques, morphologic assessment alone, and contrast-enhanced US in diagnosis of ovarian cancer
  - Hemorrhagic cysts may appear similar to neoplasm
    - Repeat scanning 4-6 weeks following initial detection of indeterminate ovarian mass
  - Mixed results reported for use of US ± CA-125 in screening for ovarian cancer
    - Routine US screening of asymptomatic women → ↑ false-positive results → unnecessary laparoscopy or laparotomy
    - Positive predictive value for invasive cancer is 3.7% for abnormal CA-125, 1% for abnormal TVU, and 23.5% if both tests are abnormal
- **CT**
  - Increased number of incidental ovarian lesions discovered due to widespread use of CT
  - Recent advances in CT technology and availability of multidetector CT (MDCT) allow better detection and improved characterization of adnexal masses
  - MDCT: Sensitivity (90%), specificity (89%), positive predictive value (78%), negative predictive value (95%), and overall accuracy in diagnosing malignancy (89%)
- **MR**
  - Used mainly as problem-solving tool in setting of sonographically indeterminate or complex adnexal mass
  - Can provide tissue characterization based on signal properties
    - MR is superior to US and CT in differentiation of benign from malignant masses
  - Adequate evaluation of adnexal masses on MR imaging requires
    - T1WI and T2WI to delineate pelvic anatomy and tumor
    - Fat-saturated T1WI to distinguish between fat and hemorrhage
    - Gadolinium-enhanced T1WI to improve detection of solid components
  - Dynamic contrast-enhanced MR imaging has been used to analyze perfusion of solid components contained in ovarian tumors
    - Can differentiate among benign, borderline, and malignant tumors
    - Different parameters have been used
      - Include enhancement amplitude (EA), time of half rising (Tmax), and maximal slope (MS)
    - Invasive tumors tend to show early intense and persistent enhancement
- **FDG PET/CT**
  - May detect unexpected ovarian cancers during staging of other tumors
  - Low specificity since benign lesions, such as corpus luteum cyst in premenopausal women, can increase ovarian uptake
    - Increased ovarian FDG uptake in postmenopausal women, in whom benign lesions are less likely, is usually associated with malignancy
  - May detect ovarian carcinoma in so-called normal-sized ovary carcinoma syndrome (NOCS)
    - NOCS occurs when diffuse metastatic malignant disease with normal-sized ovaries is noted, but no origin is assigned by preoperative or intraoperative evaluation

Staging

- Staging is surgical, based on International Federation of Obstetrics and Gynecology (FIGO) system
  - Staging requires staging laparotomy, which includes
    - Total abdominal hysterectomy

- Bilateral salpingo-oophorectomy
- Omentectomy
- Retroperitoneal lymph node sampling
- Peritoneal and diaphragmatic biopsies
- Cytological evaluation of peritoneal washings

- Preoperative imaging staging of ovarian carcinoma
  - CT is primary imaging modality for preoperative staging of ovarian cancer
  - MR is at least as accurate as CT
    - Used when CT is contraindicated
      - e.g., in patients with poor renal function or allergy to iodinated contrast
    - 3.0T MR can achieve staging of ovarian cancer accuracy comparable to surgical staging
    - Adding DWI to routine MR improves sensitivity and specificity for depicting peritoneal metastases
      - Sensitivity and specificity of 90% and 95.5%, respectively
      - Peritoneal tumor showed restricted diffusion on DWI and ascites was of low signal intensity, increasing tumor conspicuity
  - FDG PET/CT
    - FDG PET is limited in resolution and not optimal for detecting lesions < 0.5 cm in size
  - CT and pelvic MR have replaced barium enema and intravenous pyelography (IVP) in preoperative staging of ovarian cancer
- Goals of preoperative imaging
  - Detection of metastatic lesions
    - Prevent understaging
    - Allow adequate intraoperative sampling of suspected lesions
  - Recognition of extensive, unresectable disease
- Factors generally indicating inoperable disease include
  - Invasion of pelvic sidewall, rectum, sigmoid colon, or bladder
  - Bulky peritoneal disease in
    - Porta hepatis
    - Intersegmental fissure of liver
    - Lesser sac
    - Gastrosplenic ligament
    - Gastrohepatic ligament
    - Subphrenic space
    - Small bowel mesentery
    - Supracolic omentum
    - Presacral space
  - Suprarenal and splenic adenopathy
  - Hepatic and splenic (parenchymal), pleural, or pulmonary metastases
- Preoperative CT and MR imaging are highly accurate in
  - Detection of inoperable tumor
  - Prediction of suboptimal debulking
- **Malignant ascites**
  - Ascites can result from increased production by tumor, peritoneal metastases, or decreased absorption
    - Ascites can result from diaphragmatic lymphatics blockage, indicating stage III disease
  - Any peritoneal fluid in postmenopausal women and more than small amount of fluid in premenopausal women is abnormal
  - Presence of ascites: Positive predictive value (75%) for presence of peritoneal metastases
- **Peritoneal disease**
  - Microscopic peritoneal disease is undetectable with imaging
  - Small peritoneal implants ≤ 2 cm are difficult to detect with imaging
  - Omentum is most common site of peritoneal spread of tumor
    - Early omental disease
      - Subtle, fine, reticular nodularity
    - Advanced omental disease
      - Mass-like omental thickening (omental cakes)
  - Common sites of involvement should be carefully evaluated, including subphrenic space, mesentery, and paracolic gutters
  - Presence of ascites or calcifications of peritoneal nodules make implants more conspicuous and easy to detect
  - Pseudomyxoma peritonei
    - Accumulation of mucinous ascites → hepatic, splenic, and mesenteric scalloping
    - When found, should raise possibility of primary appendiceal neoplasm with ovarian metastases rather than primary mucinous ovarian neoplasm
- **Local extension**
  - Local tumor extension involving surrounding pelvic organs is suggested by
    - Distortion or irregular interface between tumor and myometrium
    - Obscuration of tissue planes with either urinary bladder or colon
    - < 3 mm between tumor and pelvic sidewall
    - Displacement or encasement of iliac vessels
  - Local extension is easier to identify with MR than with either CT or US
    - Superior soft tissue contrast
- **Nodal disease**
  - Frequency of nodal metastases in T1 or T2 disease
    - Approximately 15%; increases to 65% in patients with M1 disease
  - Major limitation of CT and MR: Dependence on size of lymph node to determine nodal involvement
    - Enlarged lymph node is likely to be involved
    - Not possible to exclude metastatic disease in normal-sized node
  - Using short axis size threshold of ≥ 1 cm to define abnormal lymph nodes
    - Sensitivity of preoperative CT (50%), MR (83%)
    - Specificity of preoperative CT (92%), MR (95%)
  - Cardiophrenic nodes are detected in approximately 15% of patients with advanced disease
    - Often indicates poor prognosis; usually considered stage IV disease
    - Enlargement is defined as short axis diameter > 5 mm
  - Functional evaluation of lymph nodes
    - DWI MR is accurate in distinguishing malignant from benign pelvic lymph nodes
    - FDG PET
      - Detect metastases in normal-sized lymph nodes
      - Verify malignant tissue in enlarged nodes
- **Small bowel involvement**
  - Commonly occurs and is frequent cause of morbidity

OVARIAN CARCINOMA

- Either due to serosal implants or frank wall invasion
- **Liver involvement**
  - Important to distinguish implants on liver capsule (stage III) from true parenchymal metastases (stage IV)
    - Capsular implants are considered resectable, whereas parenchymal metastases generally are not
    - Capsular masses are usually smooth, well defined; have elliptic or biconvex appearance and sharp interface with liver parenchyma
    - Parenchymal metastases are less defined and surrounded by liver parenchyma
    - Capsular metastases may invade liver parenchyma
      - Fuzzy interface between mass and liver parenchyma
- **Pleural effusion**
  - Most common finding in stage IV disease
  - Presence of effusion is not sufficient for designation of stage IV disease
    - Cytologic evaluation is required
  - Pleural masses, nodularity, or thickening makes likelihood of pleural metastases extremely high

Restaging

- Imaging recommendations
  - Patients treated for ovarian cancer are followed-up with serial measurements of CA-125 and either CT scan or MR imaging of abdomen and pelvis
    - Serial serum CA-125 levels are accurate measure of disease burden for most women
  - PET/CT demonstrates greater accuracy and less interobserver variability than CT alone
  - Chest CT should not be performed routinely
    - Used if ↑ tumor markers and no sites of recurrence are detected on abdominal and pelvic CT
  - MR is more sensitive than PET/CT for detecting local pelvic recurrence and peritoneal lesions in recurrent ovarian carcinoma

CLINICAL ISSUES

Presentation

- Symptoms are usually nonspecific
- Common symptoms
  - Abdominal pressure, fullness, swelling, or bloating
  - Urinary urgency
  - Pelvic discomfort or pain
  - Women who experience such symptoms daily for more than a few weeks should seek medical evaluation
- Other signs and symptoms
  - Persistent indigestion, gas, or nausea
  - Unexplained changes in bowel habits, including diarrhea or constipation
  - Changes in bladder habits, including urinary frequency
  - Loss of appetite, unexplained weight loss or gain, increased abdominal girth
  - Dyspareunia
  - Low back pain
  - Abnormal vaginal bleeding is rarely symptom of ovarian cancer

Cancer Natural History & Prognosis

- Prognosis of ovarian cancer is generally poor, mainly due to late detection
  - Percentage of tumor stage at diagnosis
    - Stage I (34%)
    - Stage II (8%)
    - Stage III (43%)
    - Stage IV (11%)
- Staging is most important prognostic factor
  - 5-year survival rate depends on tumor stage
    - Stage IA (87.6%)
    - Stage IB (84.5%)
    - Stage IC (81.7%)
    - Stage IIA (69.3%)
    - Stage IIB (70.2%)
    - Stage IIC (64.1%)
    - Stage IIIA (52.2%)
    - Stage IIIB (45.3%)
    - Stage IIIC (32.1%)
    - Stage IV (15.3%)

Treatment Options

- Treatment options by stage
  - Stage I
    - Total abdominal hysterectomy + bilateral salpingo-oophorectomy + omentectomy
    - Undersurface of diaphragm should be visualized and biopsied; pelvic and abdominal peritoneal biopsies and pelvic and paraaortic lymph node biopsies are required
    - Peritoneal washings should be obtained routinely
    - Unilateral salpingo-oophorectomy
      - Alternative for selected patients who desire childbearing and have grade I tumors on histologic examination
      - May be associated with ↓ risk of recurrence
    - No further treatment if low-grade cancer; possible combination chemotherapy if high-grade cancer
  - Stage II
    - Total abdominal hysterectomy + bilateral salpingo-oophorectomy + debulking of as much tumor as possible + sampling of lymph nodes and other suspected tissues
    - Following surgery, combination chemotherapy ± radiation therapy
  - Stage III
    - Same as stage II
    - Possible follow-up surgery to remove any remaining tumor
  - Stage IV
    - Debulking surgery to remove as much tumor as possible, followed by combination chemotherapy

REPORTING CHECKLIST

T Staging

- Laterality
- Ascites
  - Carefully inspect peritoneal surfaces for soft tissue or calcified nodules
- Involvement of uterus, rectum, bladder, or pelvic sidewall
- Carefully check common sites of peritoneal implants

- DWI MR can be very useful in depicting peritoneal implants

N Staging

- Retroperitoneal lymph nodes, along ovarian veins
- Iliac lymph nodes, along broad ligament
- Inguinal lymph nodes, along round ligament

M Staging

- Liver is common site of metastatic disease
  - Capsular hepatic lesions are T3 disease
  - Hepatic parenchymal lesions are M1 disease
  - Capsular lesions can invade into liver parenchyma to become M1 disease
- Chest CT if CT of abdomen and pelvis is negative and tumor markers are high
  - Nodular pleural thickening strongly suggests pleural metastases
    - But positive pleural cytology is a requirement for M1 designation
  - Hilar, mediastinal, or supraclavicular adenopathy is considered M1 disease

SELECTED REFERENCES

1. American Joint Committee on Cancer: AJCC Cancer Staging Manual. 7th ed. New York: Springer, 2010
2. Low RN et al: Diffusion-weighted MRI of peritoneal tumors: comparison with conventional MRI and surgical and histopathologic findings--a feasibility study. AJR Am J Roentgenol. 193(2):461-70, 2009
3. Suga K et al: F-18 FDG PET-CT findings in a case of normal-sized ovarian cancer syndrome. Clin Nucl Med. 34(10):706-9, 2009
4. Booth SJ et al: The accurate staging of ovarian cancer using 3T magnetic resonance imaging--a realistic option. BJOG. 115(7):894-901, 2008
5. Ferreira CR et al: Mucinous ovarian tumors associated with pseudomyxoma peritonei of adenomucinosis type: immunohistochemical evidence that they are secondary tumors. Int J Gynecol Cancer. 18(1):59-65, 2008
6. Fujii S et al: Detection of peritoneal dissemination in gynecological malignancy: evaluation by diffusion-weighted MR imaging. Eur Radiol. 18(1):18-23, 2008
7. Sebastian S et al: PET-CT vs. CT alone in ovarian cancer recurrence. Abdom Imaging. 33(1):112-8, 2008
8. Thomassin-Naggara I et al: Dynamic contrast-enhanced magnetic resonance imaging: a useful tool for characterizing ovarian epithelial tumors. J Magn Reson Imaging. 28(1):111-20, 2008
9. Tsili AC et al: Adnexal masses: accuracy of detection and differentiation with multidetector computed tomography. Gynecol Oncol. 110(1):22-31, 2008
10. Kim CK et al: Detection of recurrent ovarian cancer at MRI: comparison with integrated PET/CT. J Comput Assist Tomogr. 31(6):868-75, 2007
11. Liu J et al: Ultrasonography, computed tomography and magnetic resonance imaging for diagnosis of ovarian carcinoma. Eur J Radiol. 62(3):328-34, 2007
12. Chen M et al: Differentiation between malignant and benign ovarian tumors by magnetic resonance imaging. Chin Med Sci J. 21(4):270-5, 2006
13. Woodward PJ et al: From the archives of the AFIP: radiologic staging of ovarian carcinoma with pathologic correlation. Radiographics. 24(1):225-46, 2004
14. Seidman JD et al: Pathology of ovarian carcinoma. Hematol Oncol Clin North Am. 17(4):909-25, vii, 2003
15. Coakley FV: Staging ovarian cancer: role of imaging. Radiol Clin North Am. 40(3):609-36, 2002

OVARIAN CARCINOMA

*(**Left**) Longitudinal color Doppler ultrasound shows a mixed solid-cystic left ovarian mass with a large solid component. There is blood flow within both the solid component and the wall. The other ovary was normal; there is no ascites. (**Right**) Longitudinal color Doppler ultrasound shows increased blood flow within a mixed solid-cystic right ovarian mass. The Doppler wave form shows low resistance flow of 0.2 due to tumor neovascularity and vascular shunting.*

Stage IA (T1a N0 M0)

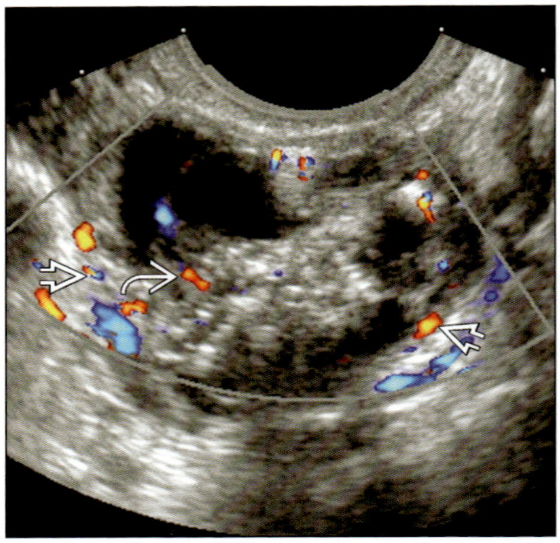

Stage IA (T1a N0 M0)

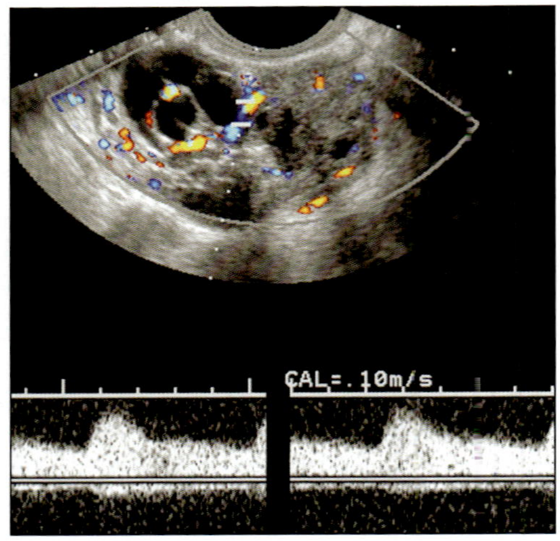

*(**Left**) Axial PET/CT in a 55-year-old patient with a history of breast cancer shows an incidental finding of a slightly enlarged left ovary with an area of increased metabolic activity. (**Right**) Coronal PET/CT in the same patient shows increased focal ovarian metabolic activity. This finding is not specific and can be seen in the setting of benign or malignant disease. However, such findings are more specific in postmenopausal women, in whom benign lesions are less likely.*

Stage IA (T1a N0 M0)

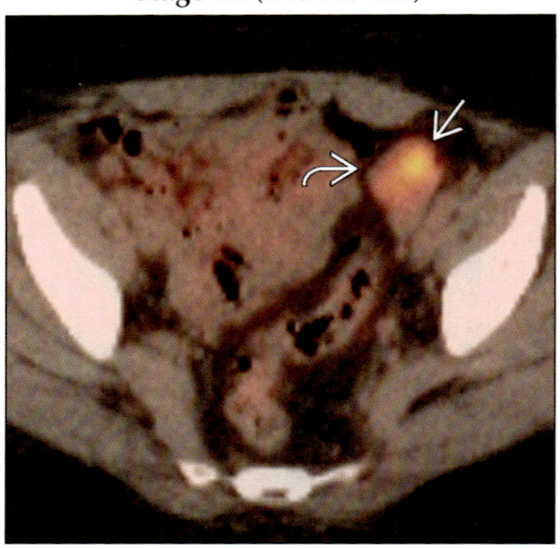

Stage IA (T1a N0 M0)

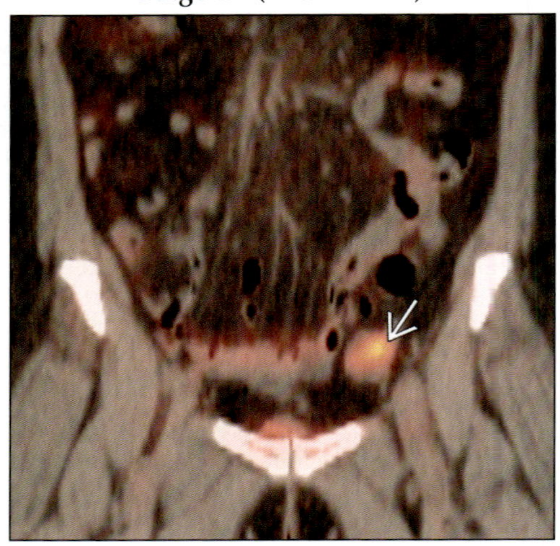

*(**Left**) Axial CECT shows a large cystic ovarian mass with thick septa and no evidence of peritoneal metastases. (**Right**) Axial CECT in the same patient shows a soft tissue mass filling the endometrial cavity. Histological examination showed low histological grade of both tumors, with associated atypical endometrial hyperplasia and ovarian endometriosis, findings that favor independent primary tumors. Streak artifacts result from metallic hip replacement.*

Stage IA (T1a N0 M0)

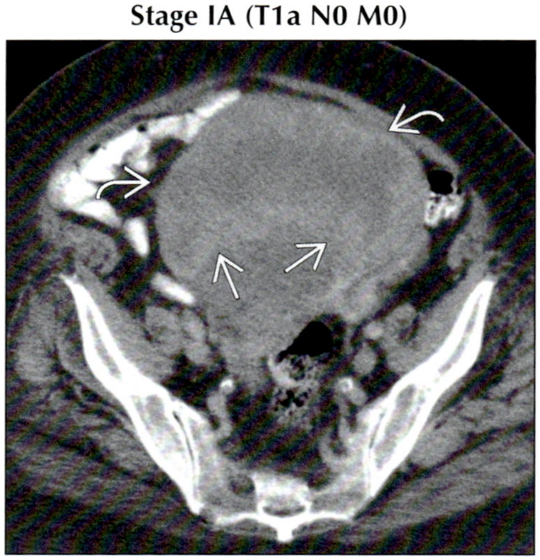

Stage IA (T1a N0 M0)

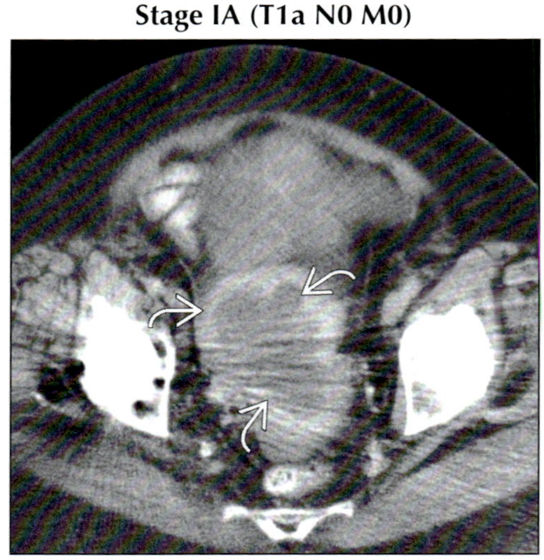

OVARIAN CARCINOMA

Stage IA (T1a N0 M0)

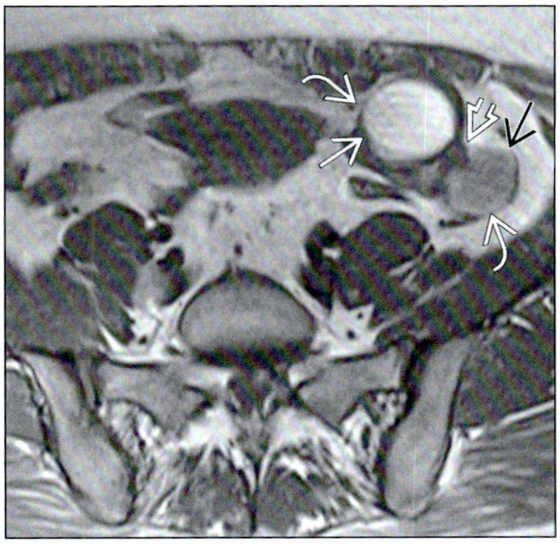

Stage IA (T1a N0 M0)

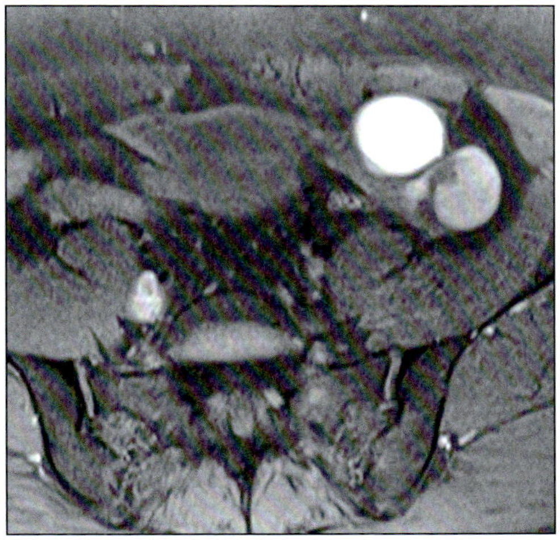

(Left) *Axial T1WI MR in a 40-year-old woman with long history of pelvic pain shows a complex left ovarian multilocular cystic lesion ➔. One of the cystic compartments ➔ is of very high signal intensity, while another compartment ➔ is slightly hyperintense relative to muscles. Note a small papillary projection ➔ within the 2nd compartment.* ***(Right)*** *Axial T1WI FS MR in the same patient shows 2 hyperintense cystic compartments due to endometriomas.*

Stage IA (T1a N0 M0)

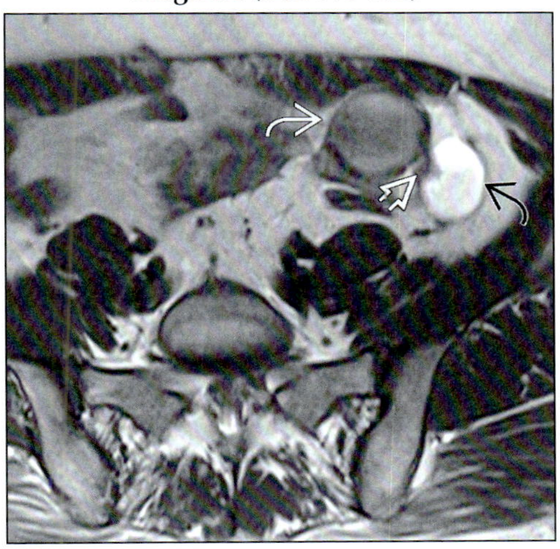

Stage IA (T1a N0 M0)

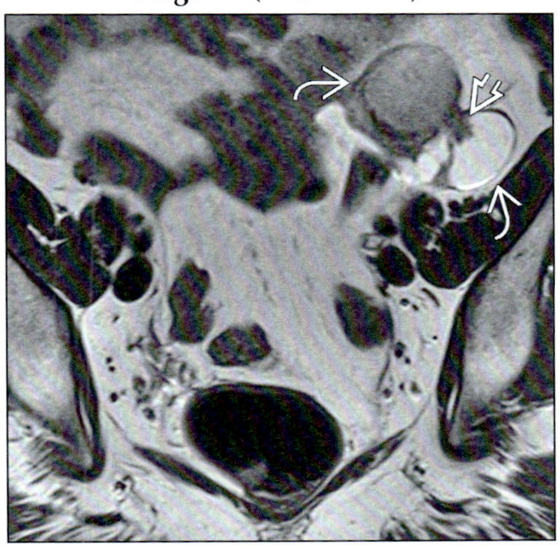

(Left) *Axial T2WI MR in the same patient shows low T2 signal intensity of the 1st compartment ➔ and high T2 signal intensity of the 2nd compartment ➔. The high T1 signal intensity and low T2 signal intensity (T2 shading) is characteristic of endometriomas. Note the small intracystic papillary lesion ➔.* ***(Right)*** *Coronal T2WI MR in the same patient shows the multilocular cystic mass ➔ and the intracystic papillary lesion ➔.*

Stage IA (T1a N0 M0)

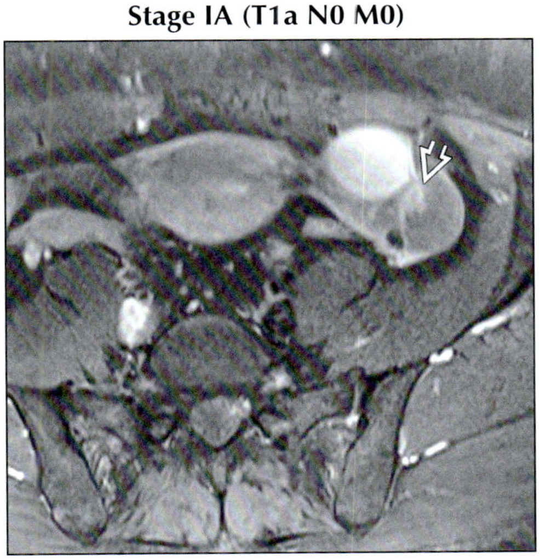

Stage IA (T1a N0 M0)

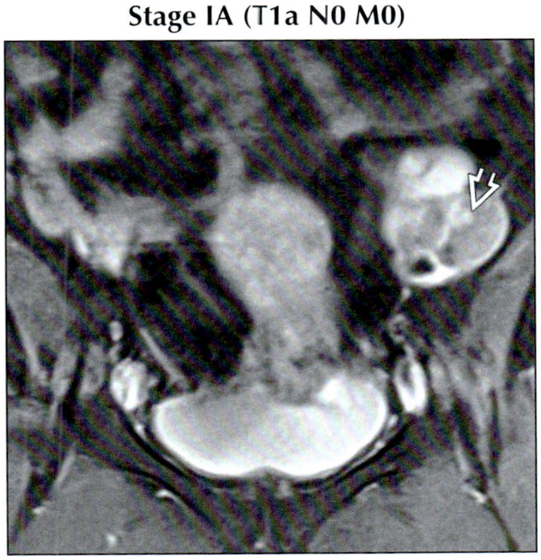

(Left) *Axial T1 C+ FS MR in the same patient shows enhancement of the small papillary lesion ➔ within the cyst.* ***(Right)*** *Coronal T1 C+ FS MR in the same patient shows enhancement of the intracystic papillary lesion ➔. This was proved at surgery to be clear cell carcinoma. Clear cell and endometrioid adenocarcinoma are the 2 histologic types developing within endometriomas.*

OVARIAN CARCINOMA

*(**Left**) Axial CECT shows bilateral, ovarian, multilocular, mainly cystic masses with loculi exhibiting different attenuation. The right ovary has 2 loculi; the more anterior loculus has higher attenuation than the more posterior loculus. (**Right**) Axial CECT in the same patient shows bilateral ovarian masses. The presence of multiple loculi of different attenuation in an ovarian mass is a feature of mucinous tumors.*

Stage IB (T1b N0 M0)

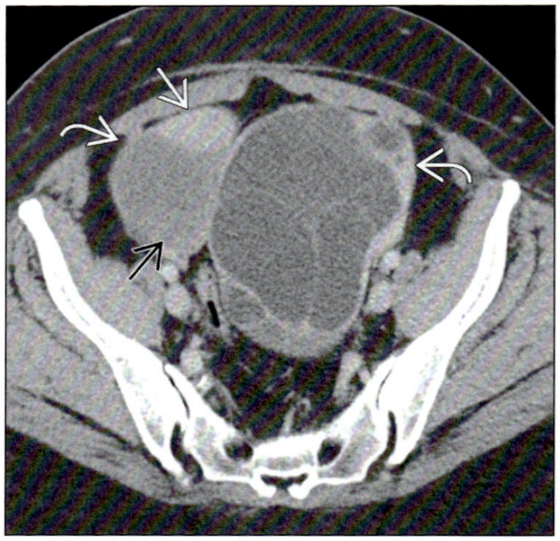

Stage IB (T1b N0 M0)

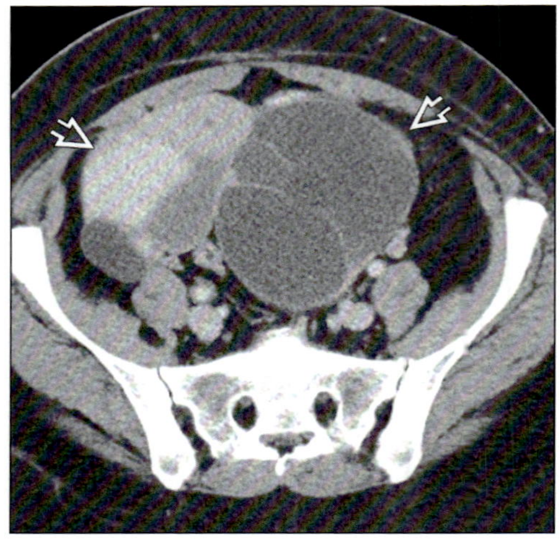

*(**Left**) Axial T2WI MR shows a large left ovarian mass that is partially solid and partially cystic. A small amount of ascitic fluid is seen in the cul-de-sac. (**Right**) Coronal T2WI MR in the same patient shows a mixed solid-cystic ovarian mass with mural nodules. At surgery malignant cells were found in the ascitic fluid. The size of an ovarian mass does not affect staging as long as the tumor is limited to the ovary and there is no capsular rupture.*

Stage IC (T1c N0 M0)

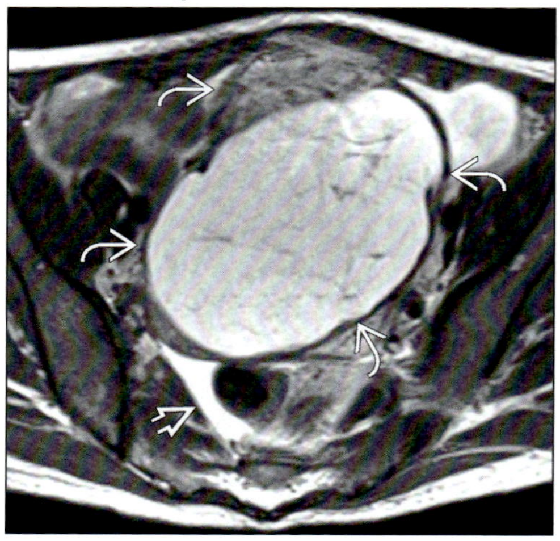

Stage IC (T1c N0 M0)

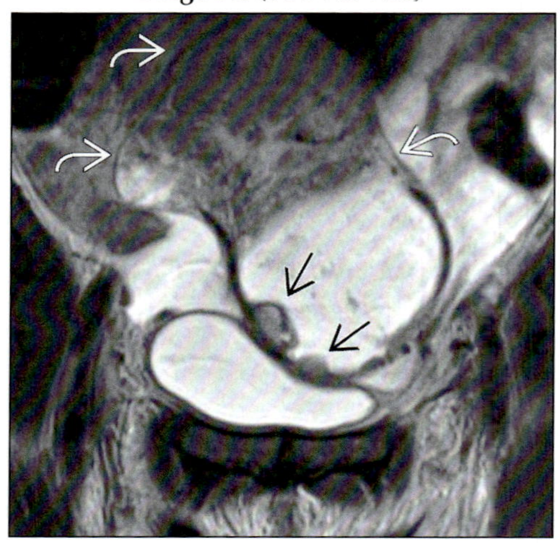

*(**Left**) Axial CECT shows a heterogeneous left ovarian mass and another heterogeneous mass that fills the uterine cavity. Histology revealed a primary ovarian tumor with metastasis to the uterus. (**Right**) Axial CECT in the same patient shows an omental mass confined to the pelvis. Uterine involvement alone would constitute T2a disease, but the presence of pelvic omental involvement makes this T2b disease.*

Stage IIB (T2b N0 M0)

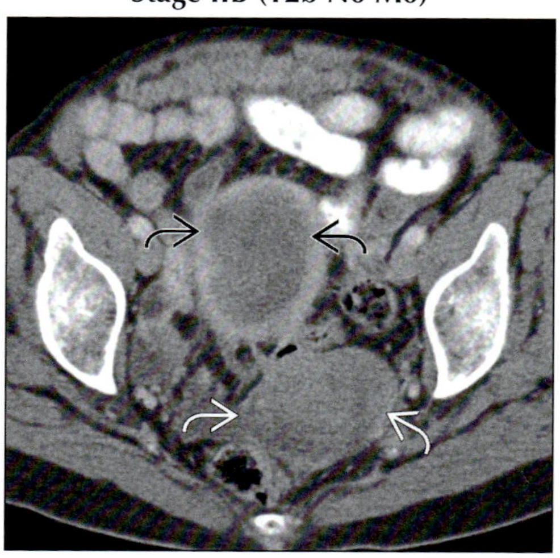

Stage IIB (T2b N0 M0)

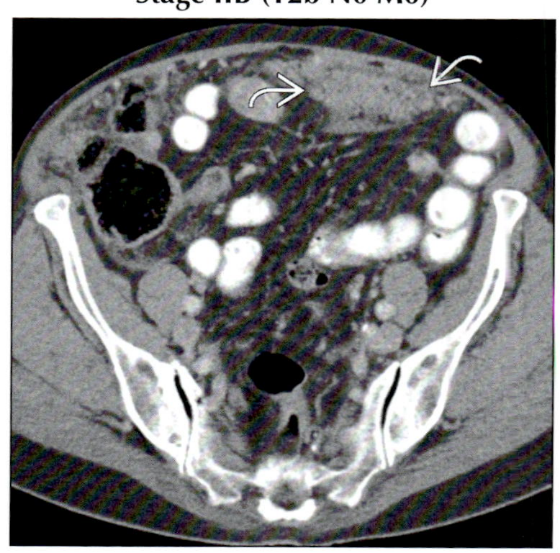

OVARIAN CARCINOMA

Stage IIB (T2b N0 M0)

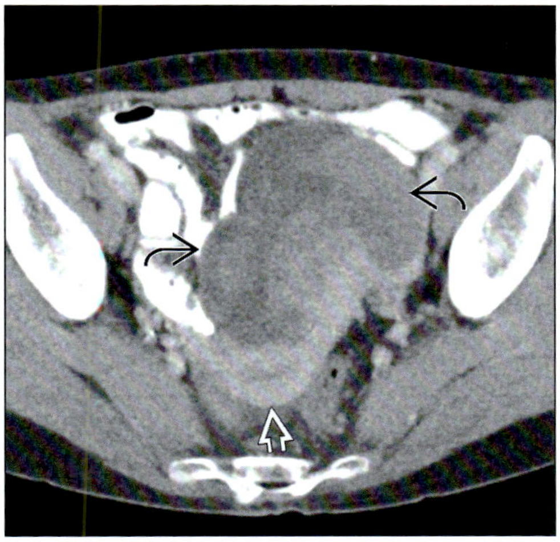

Stage IIB (T2b N0 M0)

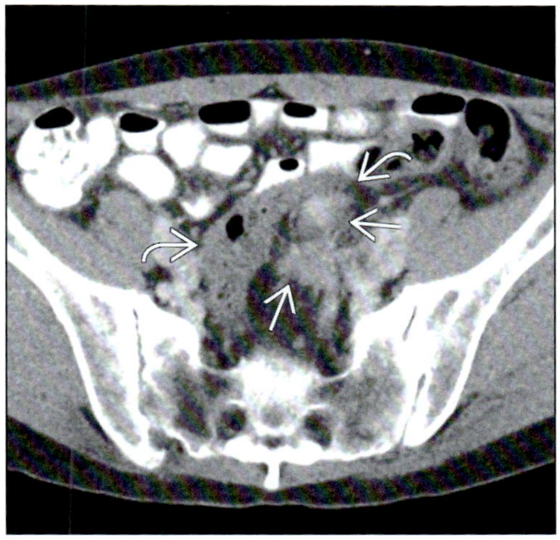

(Left) *Axial CECT shows a left heterogeneous ovarian mass separate from the uterus. There is no ascites.* ***(Right)*** *Axial CECT in the same patient shows an infiltrating mass involving the sigmoid mesocolon. The mass does not extend to the sigmoid colon.*

Stage IIIB (T3b N0 M0)

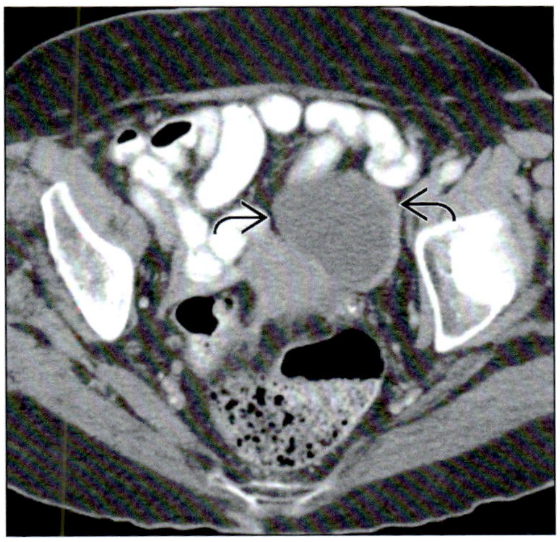

Stage IIIB (T3b N0 M0)

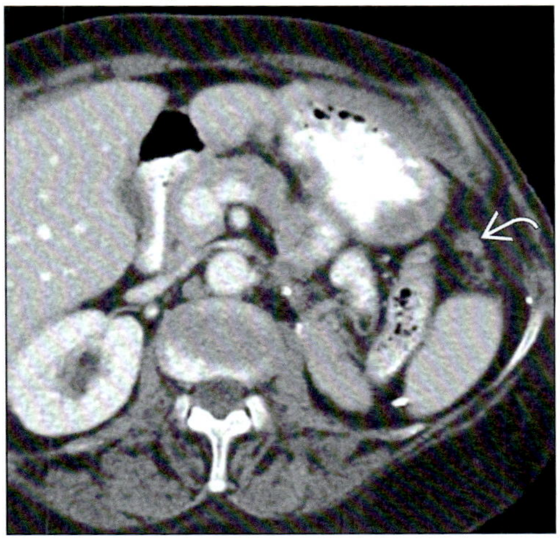

(Left) *Axial CECT shows a 5 cm, unilocular, cystic, left ovarian mass without obvious septa or mural nodules. This is a relatively benign appearance.* ***(Right)*** *Axial CECT in the same patient shows subtle omental nodules, indicating T3b disease. The presence of omental disease is surprising given the rather benign appearance of the ovarian cystic mass. Surgery confirmed a malignant clear cell ovarian carcinoma with peritoneal disease outside the pelvis.*

Stage IIIB (T3b N0 M0)

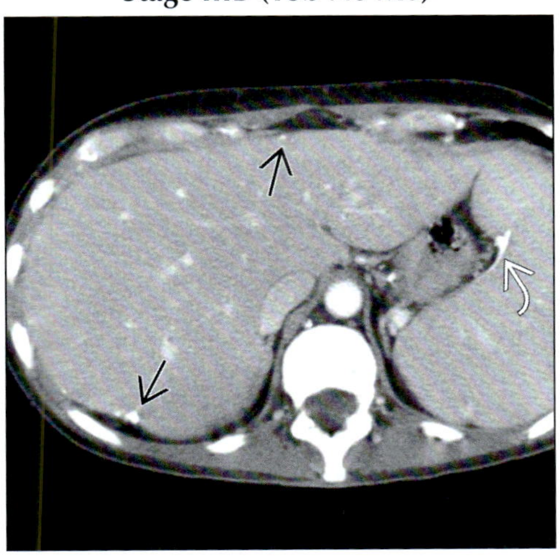

Stage IIIB (T3b N0 M0)

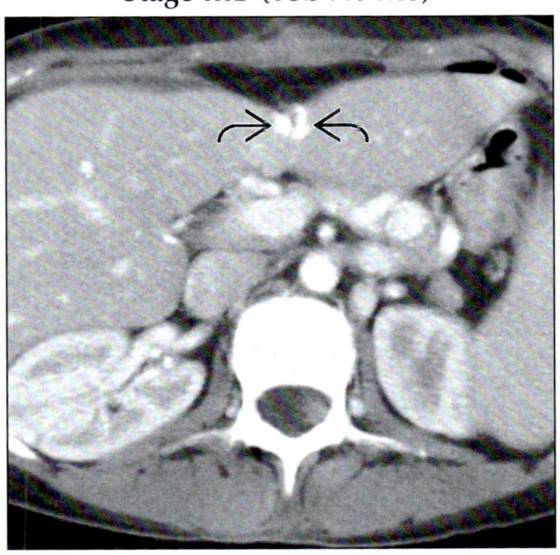

(Left) *Axial CECT shows small calcified peritoneal implants along the liver capsule and in the splenic hilum.* ***(Right)*** *Axial CECT in the same patient shows calcified small peritoneal metastases along the falciform ligament. The calcifications make otherwise small, undetectable peritoneal implants more conspicuous. The presence of calcified peritoneal implants is characteristic of metastatic serous cystadenocarcinoma.*

OVARIAN CARCINOMA

(Left) *Axial CECT shows nodular thickening of the omentum →.* **(Right)** *Axial CECT in the same patient shows ascites → with nodular peritoneal thickening → in a patient with primary peritoneal carcinoma, an unusual tumor of histiogenic origin similar to primary ovarian carcinoma. It diffusely involves the peritoneum but spares or only superficially involves ovaries. Generally diagnosed in the state of peritoneal carcinomatosis, it has a poor prognosis.*

Stage IIIB (T3b N0 M0)

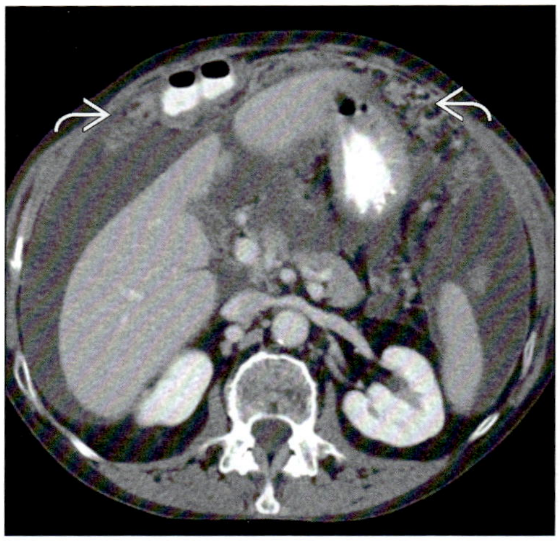

Stage IIIB (T3b N0 M0)

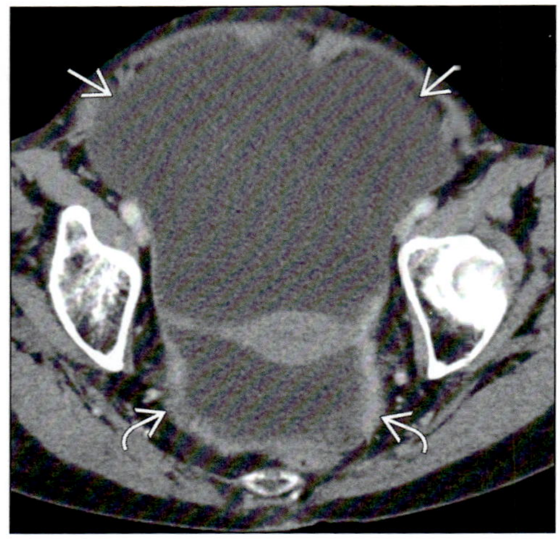

(Left) *Axial CECT in a 37-year-old woman who presented with abdominal distension and was found to have pelvic masses on vaginal exam shows a mixed solid and cystic right ovarian mass →. Ascites is present →. The mass displaces the colon → without obvious invasion.* **(Right)** *Axial CECT in the same patient shows another mass → superior to the right ovarian mass. The left ovarian vein → can be traced to this mass establishing its origin from the left ovary.*

Stage IIIC (T3c N0 M0)

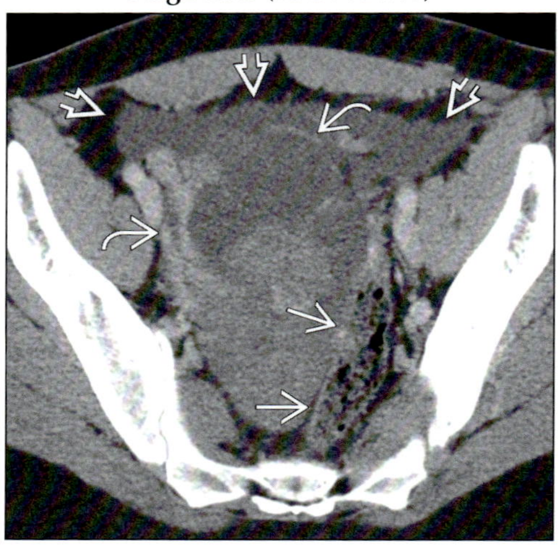

Stage IIIC (T3c N0 M0)

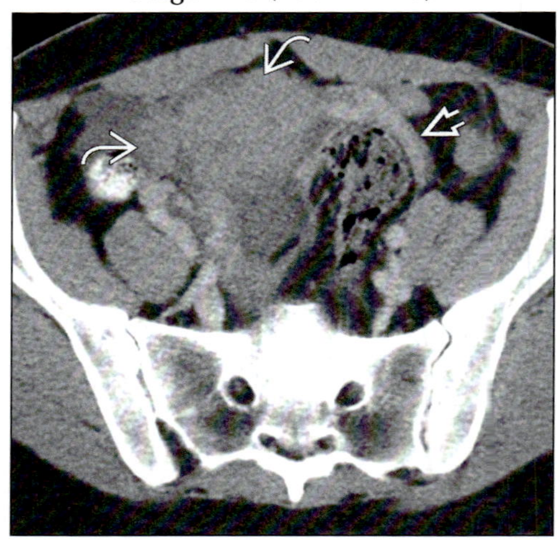

(Left) *Axial CECT in the same patient shows a 3rd mass → within the abdomen that represents an abdominal peritoneal metastasis larger than 2 cm. Subtle omental nodularity → is also present.* **(Right)** *Coronal CECT in the same patient shows the left ovarian mass → with a separate peritoneal metastatic lesion →.*

Stage IIIC (T3c N0 M0)

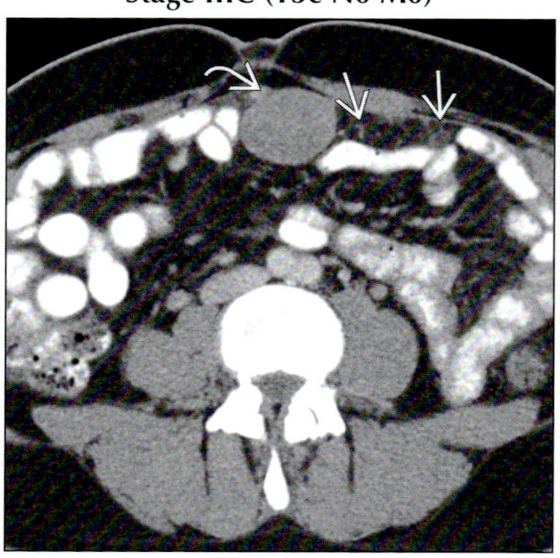

Stage IIIC (T3c N0 M0)

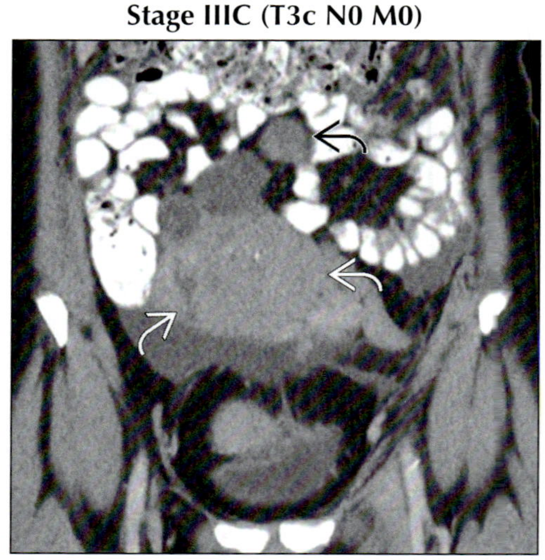

OVARIAN CARCINOMA

Stage IIIC (T3c N0 M0)

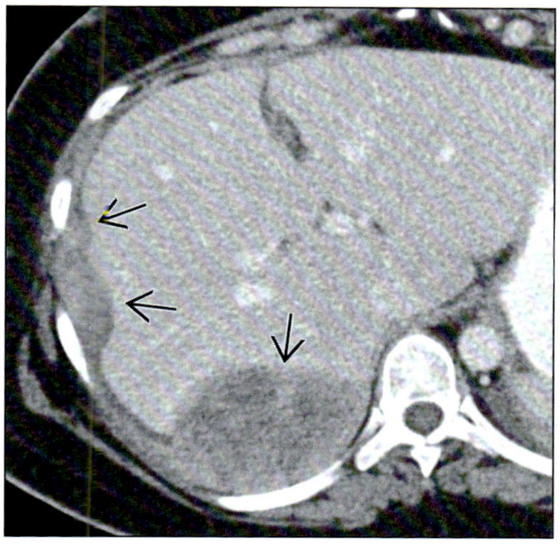

Stage IIIC (T3c N0 M0)

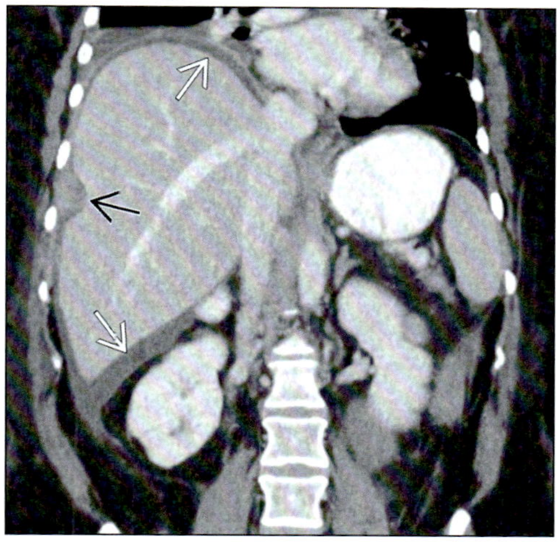

(Left) *Axial CECT shows large perihepatic peritoneal implants →. Note the sharp interface between the implants and the liver. Ascites is also present.* ***(Right)*** *Coronal reformat CECT in the same patient shows a perihepatic peritoneal implant → indenting the liver parenchyma but without parenchymal invasion. Perihepatic ascites is also seen →. Coronal reformat better delineates capsular implants and confirms the peritoneal, rather than pleural, location.*

Stage IIIC (T1a N1 M0)

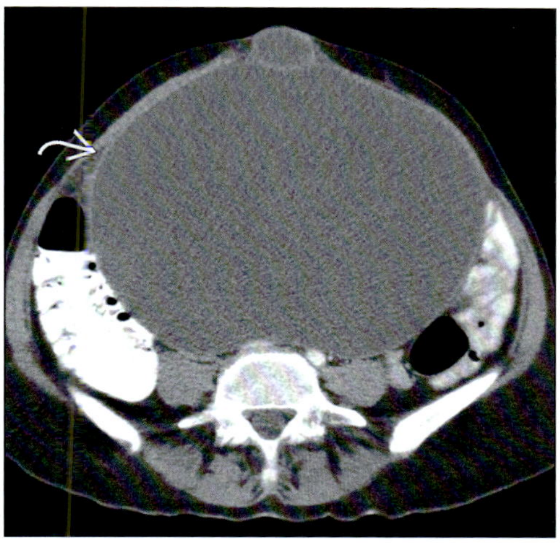

Stage IIIC (T1a N1 M0)

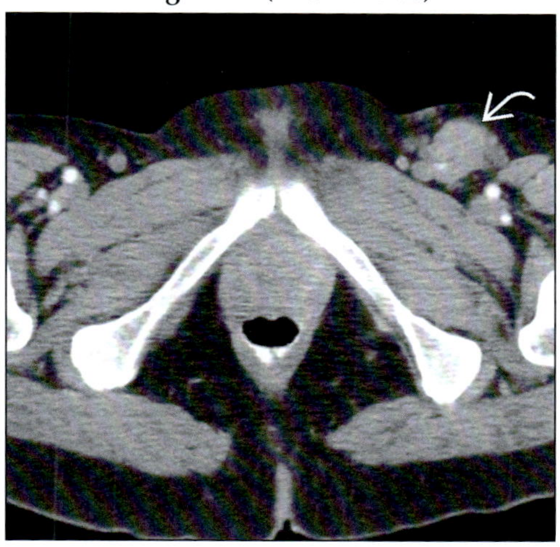

(Left) *Axial CECT shows a large, cystic left ovarian lesion → extending into the abdomen and displacing the bowel loops on both sides. There was no ascites or evidence of peritoneal metastases.* ***(Right)*** *Axial CECT in the same patient shows an enlarged left inguinal lymph node →. Metastases to inguinal nodes result from tumor spread through lymphatics along the round ligament.*

Stage IIIC (T2b N1 M0)

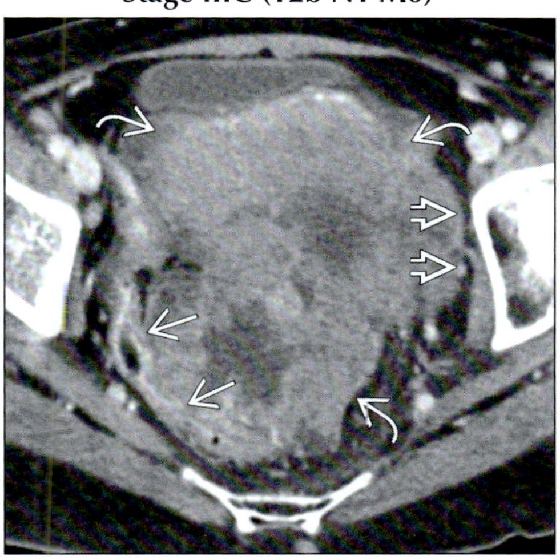

Stage IIIC (T2b N1 M0)

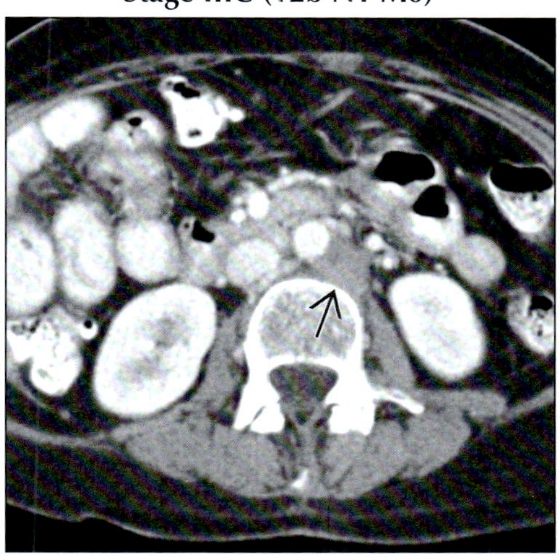

(Left) *Axial CECT shows a large solid mass arising from the left ovary →. The mass displaces the sigmoid colon → and is less than 3 mm from the left obturator internus muscle →. Involvement of the pelvic sidewall makes the tumor inoperable in most institutions. Extensive pelvic involvement constitutes T2b disease.* ***(Right)*** *Axial CECT in the same patient shows an enlarged left paraaortic lymph node →. Regional nodal metastases constitute N1 disease.*

OVARIAN CARCINOMA

*(**Left**) Axial T2WI MR in a 55-year-old woman shows a mixed solid and cystic right ovarian mass with thick septa within the cystic component. (**Right**) Axial T2WI MR in the same patient shows the large multilocular cystic component of the mass with solid tumor invading into the wall of the sigmoid colon. There is also an enlarged right internal iliac lymph node.*

Stage IIIC (T2b N1 M0)

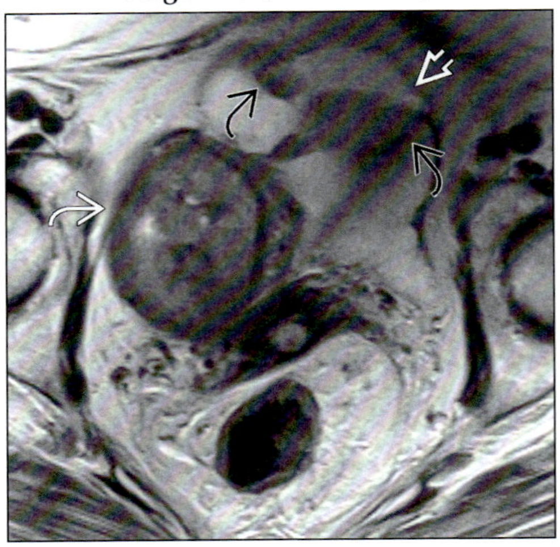

Stage IIIC (T2b N1 M0)

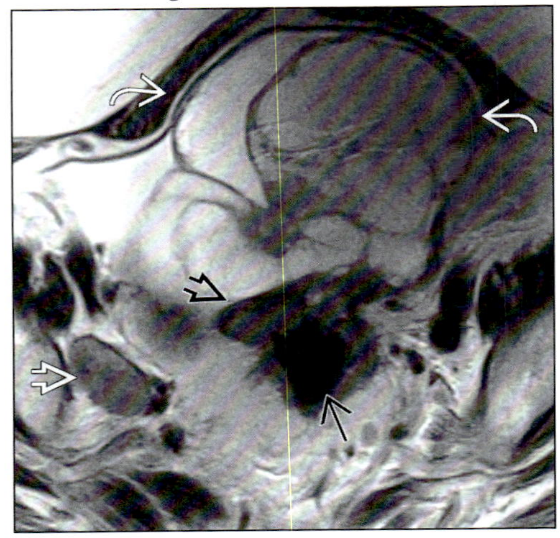

*(**Left**) Axial T2WI MR in a patient with advanced local disease shows invasion of the myometrium. The tumor is less than 3 mm from the pelvic side wall. The rectum is displaced but not invaded. Bilateral external iliac lymphadenopathy indicates N1 disease. (**Right**) Sagittal T2WI MR in the same patient shows invasion of the posterior wall of the uterus sparing the endometrium. The urinary bladder is not involved.*

Stage IIIC (T2b N1 M0)

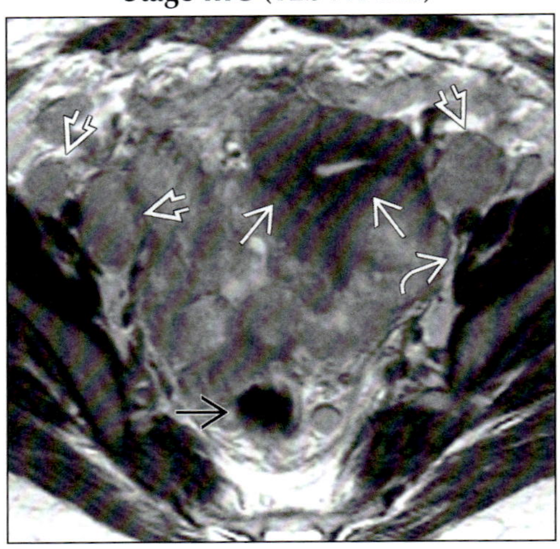

Stage IIIC (T2b N1 M0)

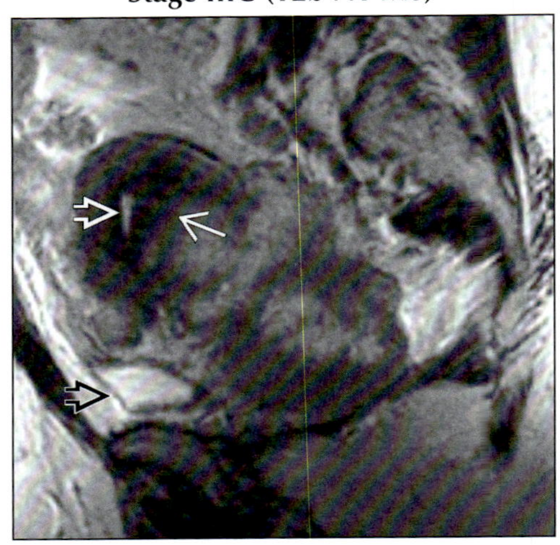

*(**Left**) Axial T1WI C+ FS MR in the same patient shows a large mass occupying almost the entire pelvis. There is an irregular interface between the tumor and the uterus due to uterine invasion. The tumor comes within 3 mm of the pelvic sidewall. Bilateral external iliac nodes are also seen. (**Right**) Axial T1WI C+ FS MR in the same patient shows enhancing tumor invading and wrapping around the rectum to involve the uterosacral ligament.*

Stage IIIC (T2b N1 M0)

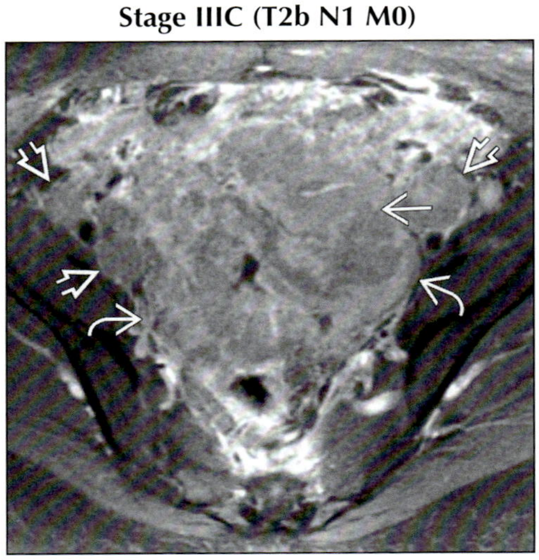

Stage IIIC (T2b N1 M0)

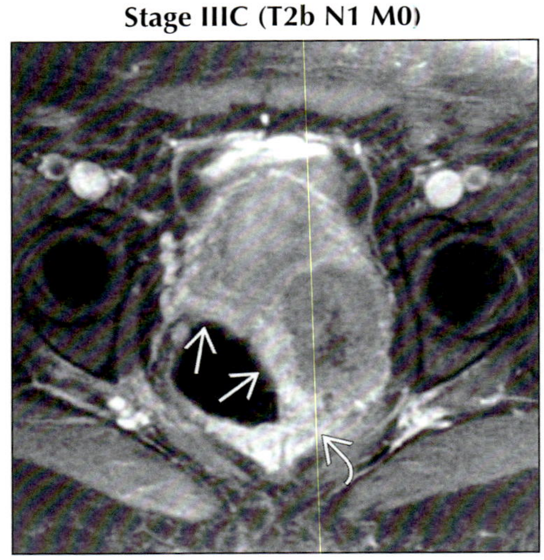

Stage IIIC (T3c N1 M0)

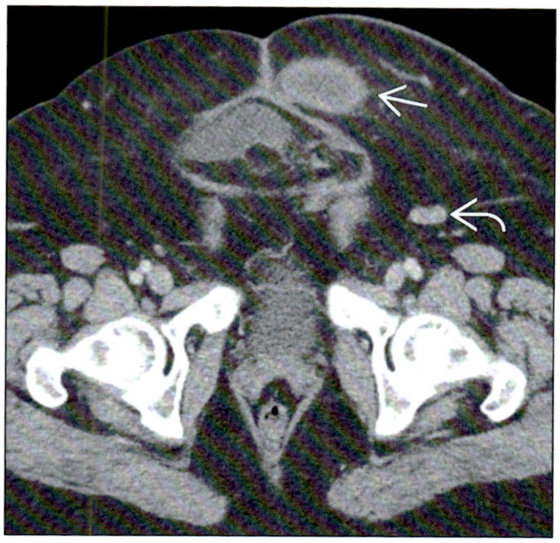

Stage IIIC (T3b N1 M0)

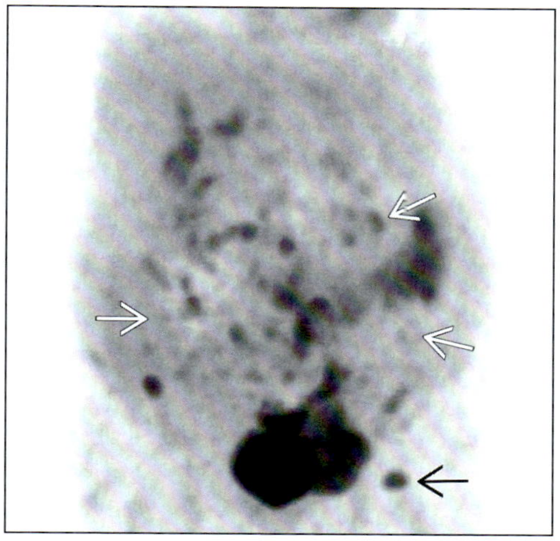

(Left) *Axial CECT in a patient with advanced ovarian carcinoma demonstrates a 10 mm left inguinal lymph node ➔. This node is not pathologic by any size criterion. Note the small anterior abdominal wall postoperative subcutaneous seroma ➔.* ***(Right)*** *Coronal PET in the same patient shows extensive peritoneal metastatic disease ➔. Peritoneal lesions are less than 2 cm in greatest dimension. The left inguinal node ⇨ shows increased metabolic activity.*

Stage IV (T3c N0 M1)

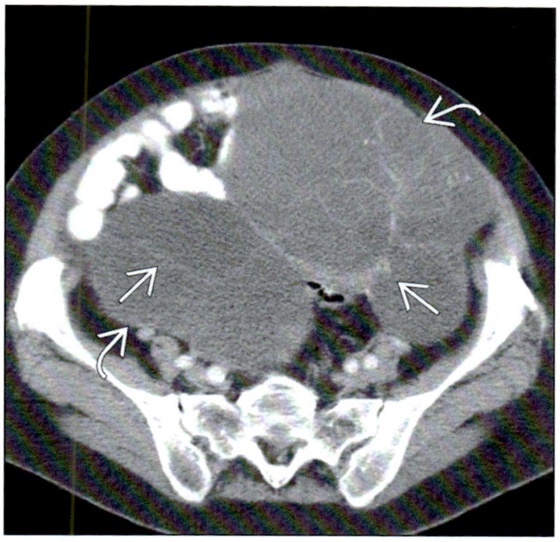

Stage IV (T3c N0 M1)

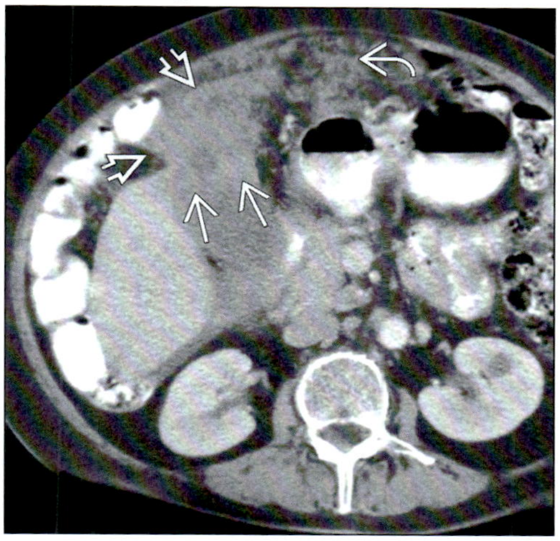

(Left) *Axial CECT shows large bilateral multilocular ovarian masses ➔ with internal septations ➔.* ***(Right)*** *Axial CECT in the same patient shows omental metastases ➔ with a large omental mass ➔ invading the fundus of the gallbladder ➔. Large peritoneal metastases (> 2 cm) within the abdomen constitute T3c disease, and invasion of the gallbladder constitutes M1 disease.*

Stage IV (T3c N0 M1)

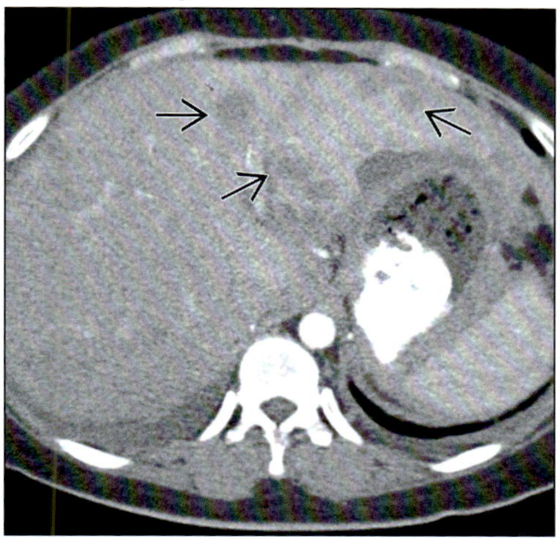

Stage IV (T3c N0 M1)

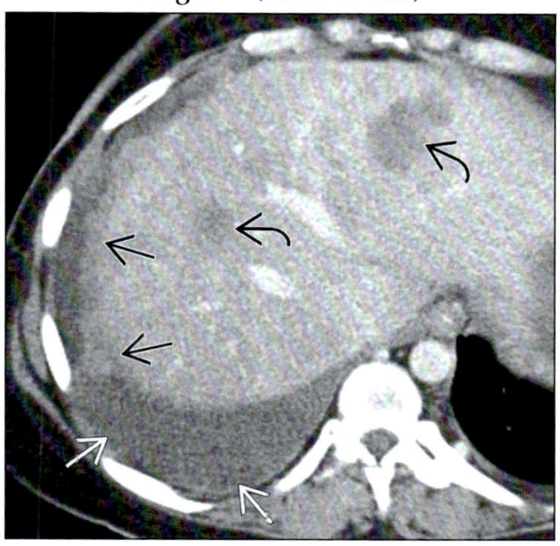

(Left) *Axial CECT in a patient with advanced local disease shows multiple, poorly enhancing parenchymal liver lesions ⇨. Intraparenchymal liver lesions constitute M1 disease.* ***(Right)*** *Axial CECT in the same patient shows multiple parenchymal hepatic lesions ⇨. Note the right-sided pleural effusion ➔ and pleural nodules ⇨. The presence of malignant pleural effusion constitutes M1 disease. Pleural nodularity is highly suggestive of pleural metastases.*

OVARIAN CARCINOMA

(Left) *Axial CECT in a patient with recurrent ovarian carcinoma and multiple large peritoneal implants shows that 1 lesion → invades the posterior wall of the stomach. Another lesion → involves the omentum, and 2 lesions → involve the gastrohepatic ligament. Also note the dilated common bile duct →.* ***(Right)*** *Axial CECT in the same patient shows that the common bile duct dilatation is due to a subtle parenchymal pancreatic head mass →.*

Stage IV (T3c N0 M1)

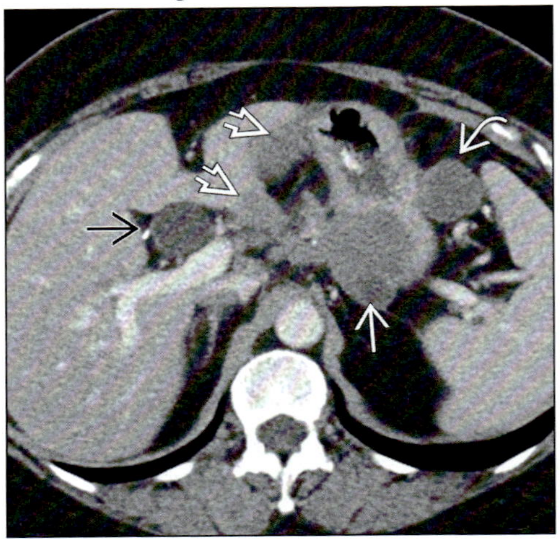

Stage IV (T3c N0 M1)

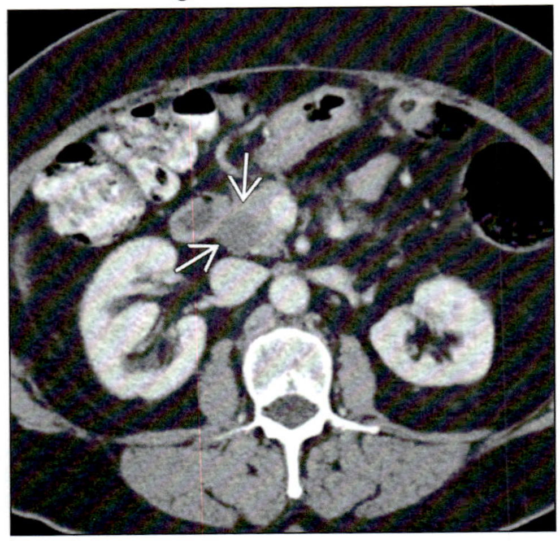

(Left) *Axial T2WI MR in the same patient shows a relatively hyperintense peritoneal implant → invading the posterior wall of the stomach →. The common bile duct is markedly dilated →.* ***(Right)*** *Axial T2WI MR in the same patient shows a hyperintense intraparenchymal pancreatic head mass →.*

Stage IV (T3c N0 M1)

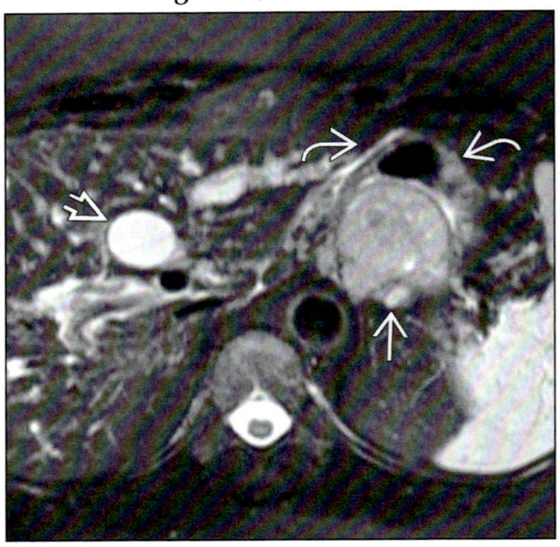

Stage IV (T3c N0 M1)

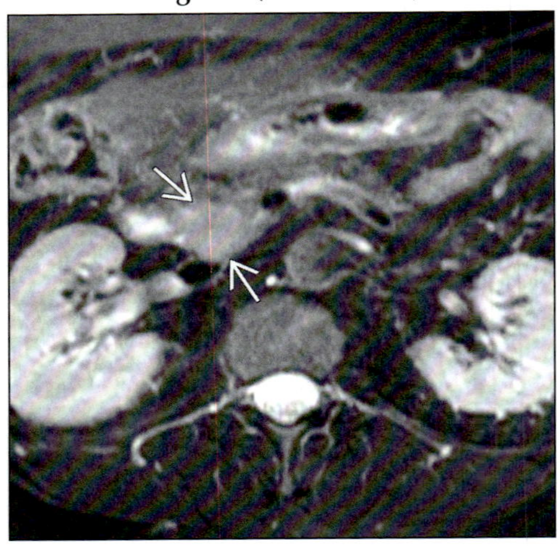

(Left) *Axial T1WI C+ FS MR in the same patient shows multiple peritoneal implants involving the posterior wall of the stomach →, omentum →, and gastrohepatic ligament →. Note that the lesions are poorly enhancing after contrast administration.* ***(Right)*** *Axial T1WI C+ FS MR in the same patient shows a similarly poorly enhancing intraparenchymal pancreatic head mass →, causing common bile duct obstruction.*

Stage IV (T3c N0 M1)

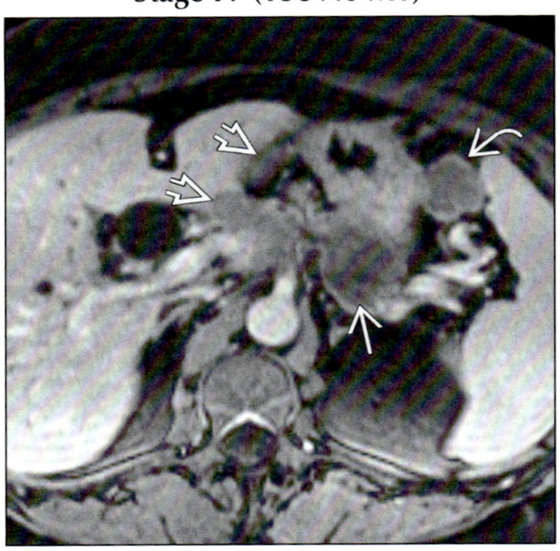

Stage IV (T3c N0 M1)

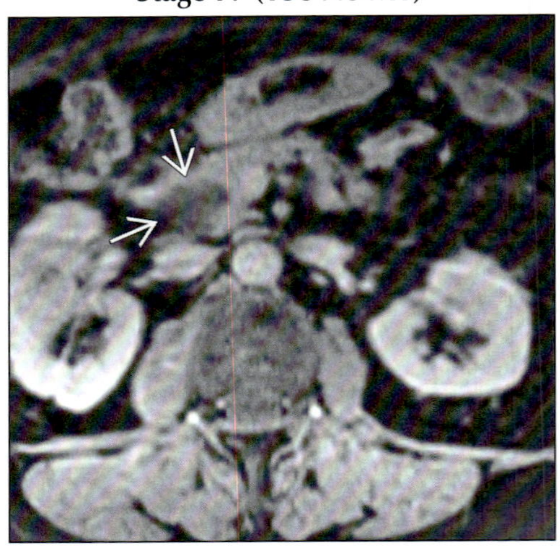

OVARIAN CARCINOMA

Stage IV (T3a N1 M1)

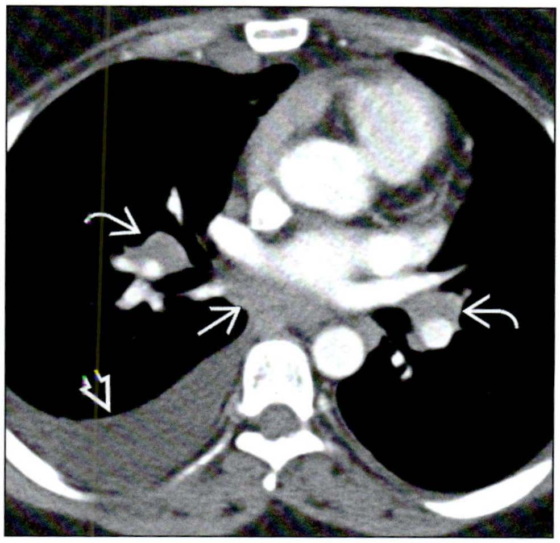

Stage IV (T3a N1 M1)

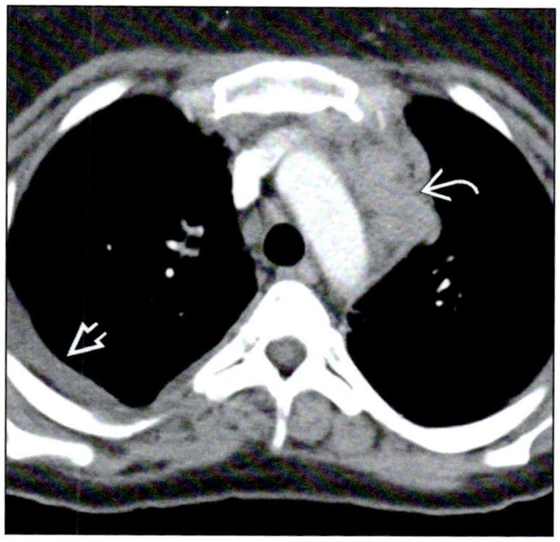

(Left) *Axial CECT in a patient with advanced local disease (not shown) demonstrates bilateral hilar and subcarinal lymphadenopathy. Note also the right-sided pleural effusion.* ***(Right)*** *Axial CECT in the same patient shows prevascular mediastinal lymphadenopathy. Right-sided pleural effusion is seen. The presence of mediastinal metastatic disease constitutes M1 disease.*

Stage IV (T3b N1 M1)

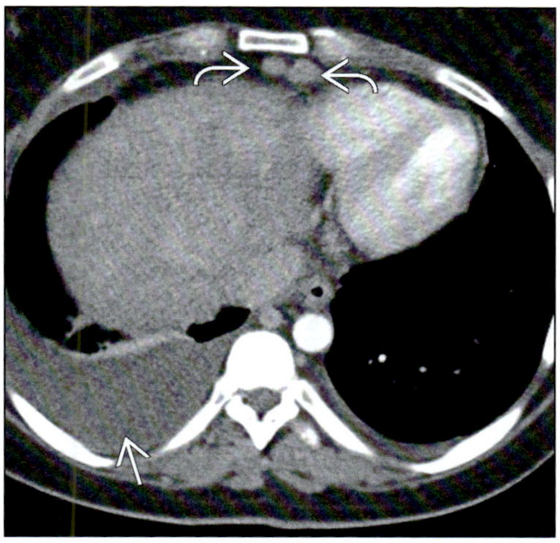

Stage IV (T3c N1 M1)

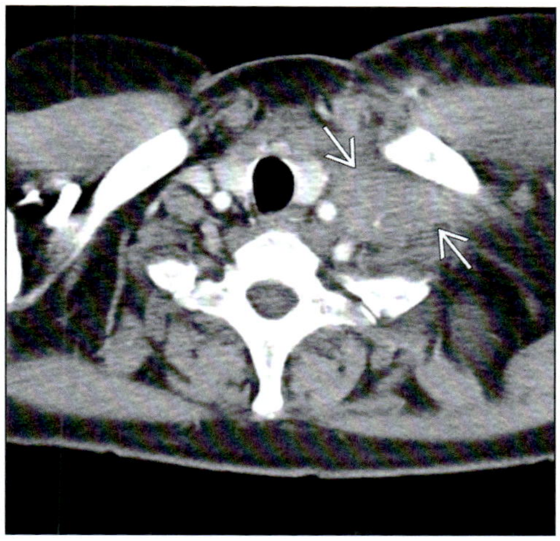

(Left) *Axial CECT shows enlarged cardiophrenic lymph nodes. A cardiophrenic node > 5 mm is suspicious for metastatic disease. Right-sided pleural effusion is also seen. Many consider metastatic disease to the cardiophrenic node to be M1 disease.* ***(Right)*** *Axial CECT in a patient with advanced local disease shows an enlarged left supraclavicular lymph node. Metastatic disease to supraclavicular nodes constitutes M1 disease.*

Stage IV (T3c N0 M1)

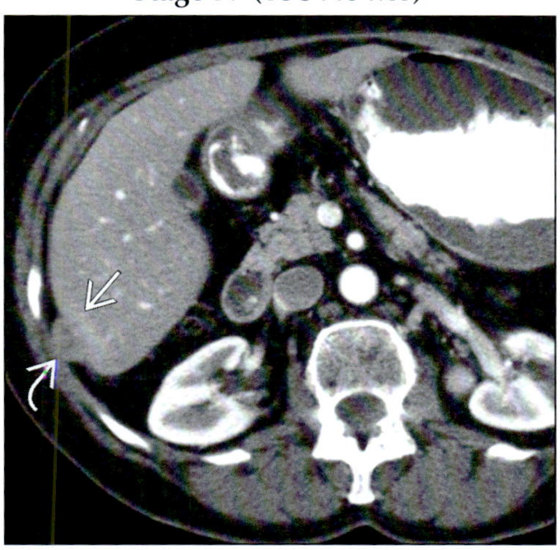

Stage IV (T3c N0 M1)

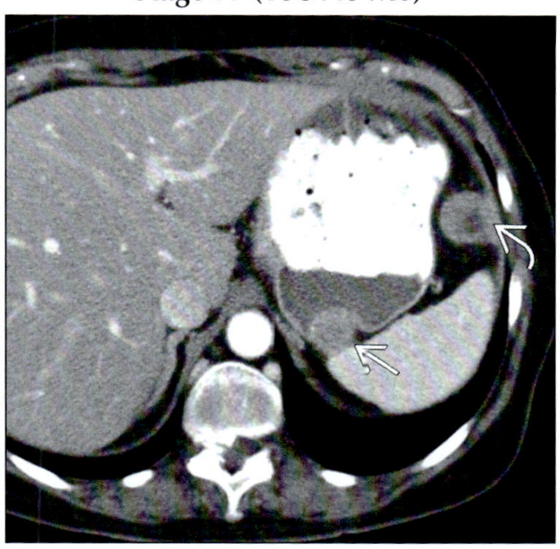

(Left) *Axial CECT shows a liver capsular implant invading into the liver parenchyma. An ill-defined interface between the capsular implant and the underlying liver parenchyma indicates liver invasion and stage IV disease.* ***(Right)*** *Axial CECT in the same patient shows 2 peritoneal implants. The 1st invades the right diaphragm, and the 2nd involves the gastrosplenic ligament. Gastrosplenic ligament implants indicate inoperable disease.*

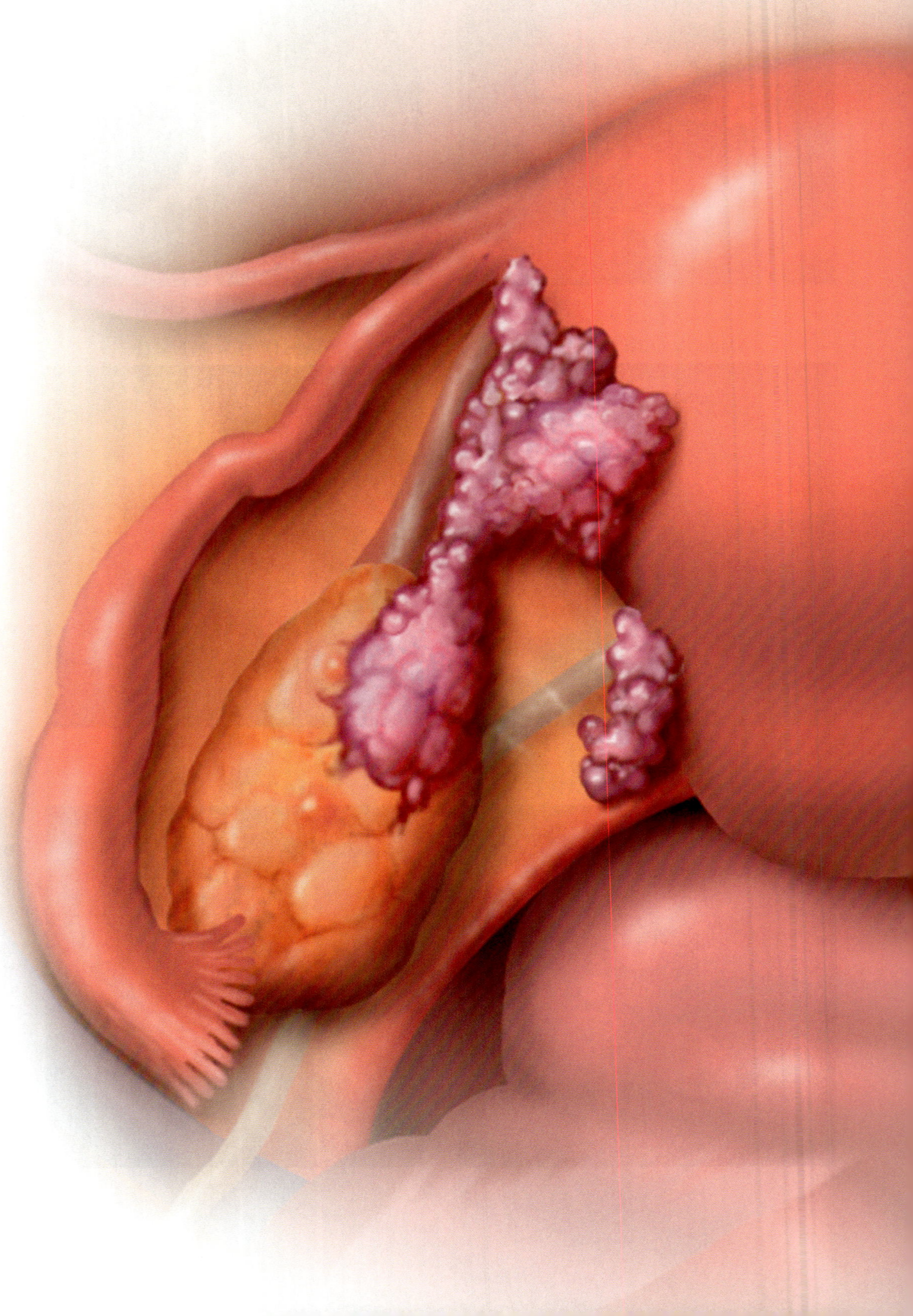

Fallopian Tube Carcinoma

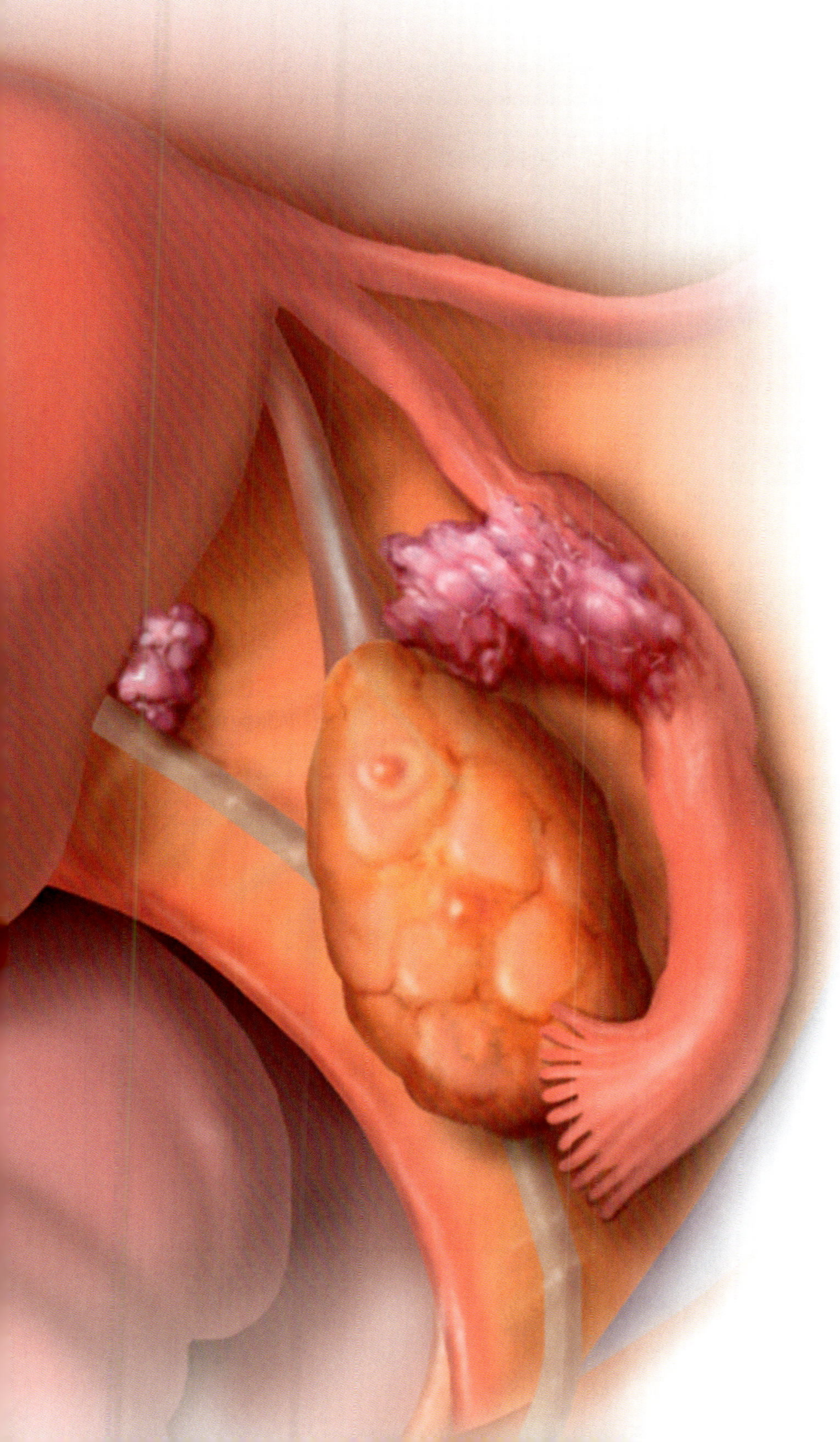

FALLOPIAN TUBE CARCINOMA

(T) Primary Tumor

Adapted from 7th edition AJCC Staging Forms.

TNM	*FIGO*	*Definitions*
TX		Primary tumor cannot be assessed
T0		No evidence of primary tumor
Tis[1]	0	Carcinoma in situ (limited to tubal mucosa)
T1	I	Tumor limited to the fallopian tube(s)
T1a	IA	Tumor limited to 1 tube, without penetrating the serosal surface; no ascites
T1b	IB	Tumor limited to both tubes, without penetrating the serosal surface; no ascites
T1c	IC	Tumor limited to 1 or both tubes with extension onto or through the tubal serosa or with malignant cells in ascites or peritoneal washings
T2	II	Tumor involves 1 or both fallopian tubes with pelvic extension
T2a	IIA	Extension &/or metastasis of uterus &/or ovaries
T2b	IIB	Extension to other pelvic structures
T2c	IIC	Pelvic extension with malignant cells in ascites or peritoneal washings
T3	III	Tumor involves 1 or both fallopian tubes, with peritoneal implants outside the pelvis
T3a	IIIA	Microscopic peritoneal metastasis outside the pelvis
T3b	IIIB	Macroscopic peritoneal metastasis outside the pelvis ≤ 2 cm in greatest dimension
T3c	IIIC	Peritoneal metastasis > 2 cm in diameter

(N) Regional Lymph Nodes

NX		Regional lymph nodes cannot be assessed
N0		No regional lymph node metastasis
N1	IIIC	Regional lymph node metastasis

(M) Distant Metastasis

M0		No distant metastasis
M1	IV	Distant metastasis

[1]*FIGO no longer includes stage 0 (Tis). Note: Liver capsule metastasis is T3/stage III; liver parenchymal metastasis is M1/stage IV; pleural effusion must have positive cytology for M1/stage IV.*

AJCC Stages/Prognostic Groups

Adapted from 7th edition AJCC Staging Forms.

Stage	*T*	*N*	*M*
0	Tis	N0	M0
IA	T1a	N0	M0
IB	T1b	N0	M0
IC	T1c	N0	M0
IIA	T2a	N0	M0
IIB	T2b	N0	M0
IIC	T2c	N0	M0
IIIA	T3a	N0	M0
IIIB	T3b	N0	M0
IIIC	T3c	N0	M0
	Any T	N1	M0
IV	Any T	Any N	M1

FALLOPIAN TUBE CARCINOMA

Tis

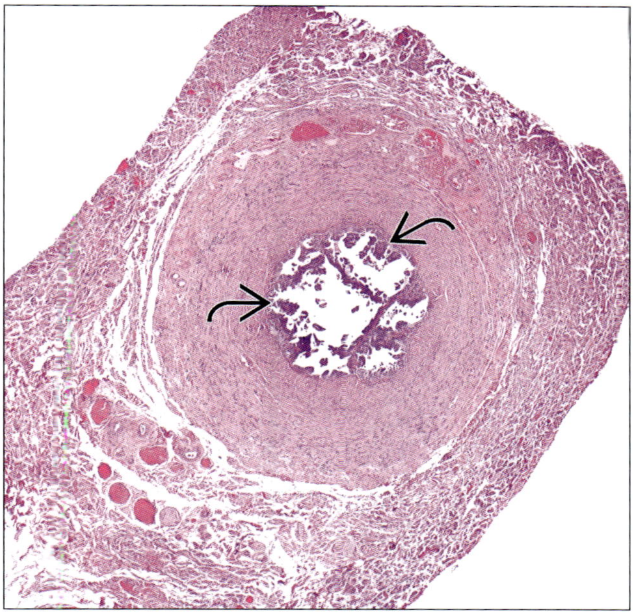

Low-power magnification of H&E stained full section of carcinoma in situ and fallopian tube shows the lumen lined by endosalpingeal epithelial cells forming papillae. (Original magnification 20x.)

Tis

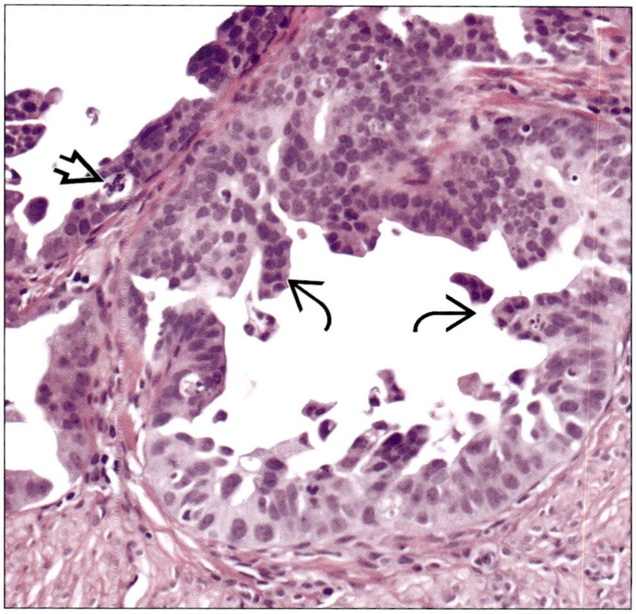

High-power magnification of the epithelial cells with carcinoma in situ shows loss of polarity with papillary formation that lack stromal cores. Note the cellular atypia of the lining cells and the mitotic figure. The basement membrane is intact. (Original magnification 400x.)

T1a (FIGO IA)

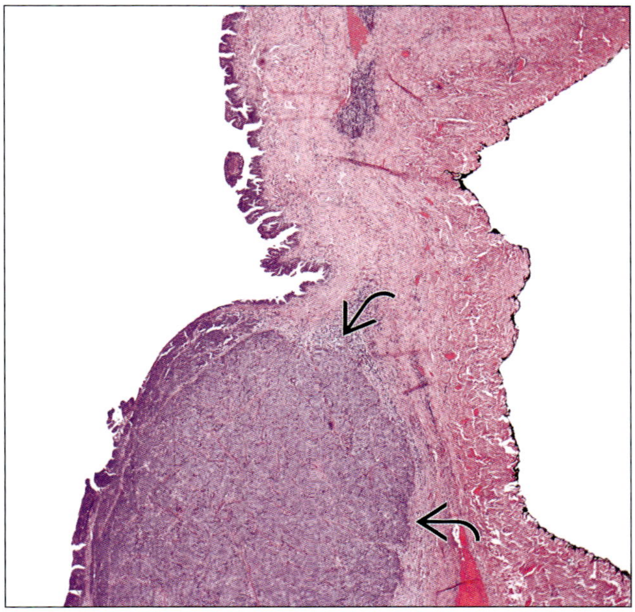

Low-power magnification shows tumor limited to the fallopian tube (T1a). H&E stain shows tumor cells within the wall of the fallopian tube. The left side clear space represents the luminal aspect of the fallopian tube with the lining epithelium. The tumor is limited to the wall of the fallopian tube. (Original magnification 40x.)

T1a (FIGO IA)

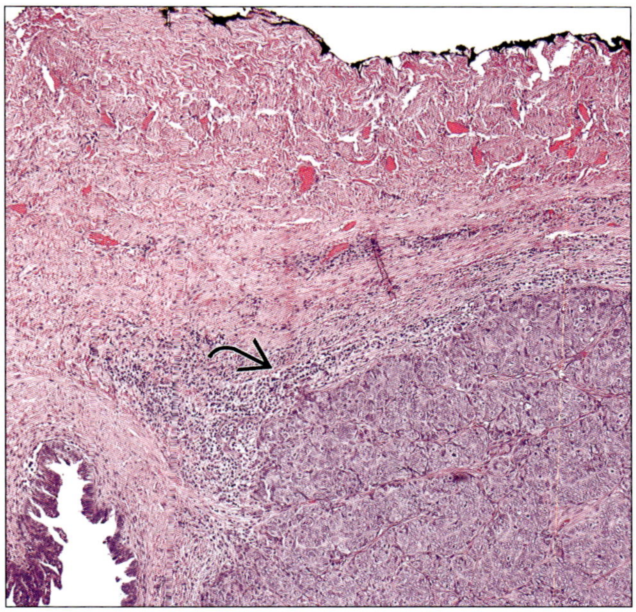

Intermediate-power magnification depicts a close-up on the sheets of tumor cells that do not extend to the serosal aspect (inked black, top) of the tube. (Original magnification 100x.)

FALLOPIAN TUBE CARCINOMA

T1c (FIGO IC)

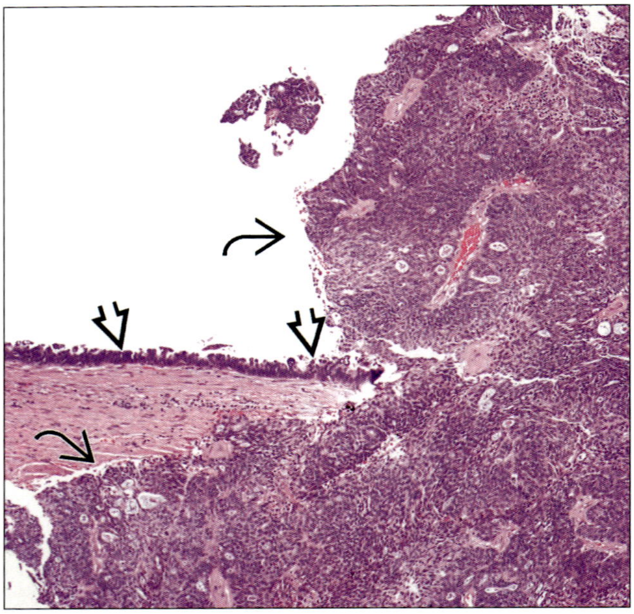

H&E stain from the wall of a fallopian tube demonstrates tumor invading through the wall of the tube. Note the surface epithelium on the luminal side. (Original magnification 100x.)

T2a (FIGO IIA)

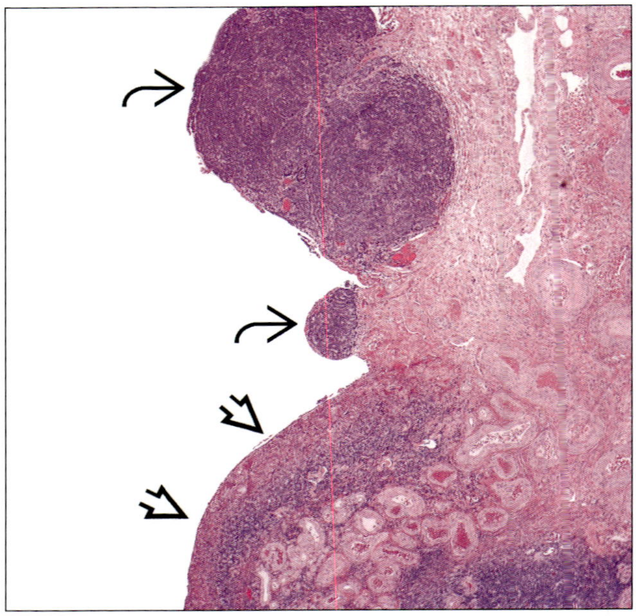

H&E section of tumor with pelvic extension to the surface of the ovary (T2a) displays tumor nodules visible on the surface of the ovary. (Original magnification 40x.)

T2a (FIGO IIA)

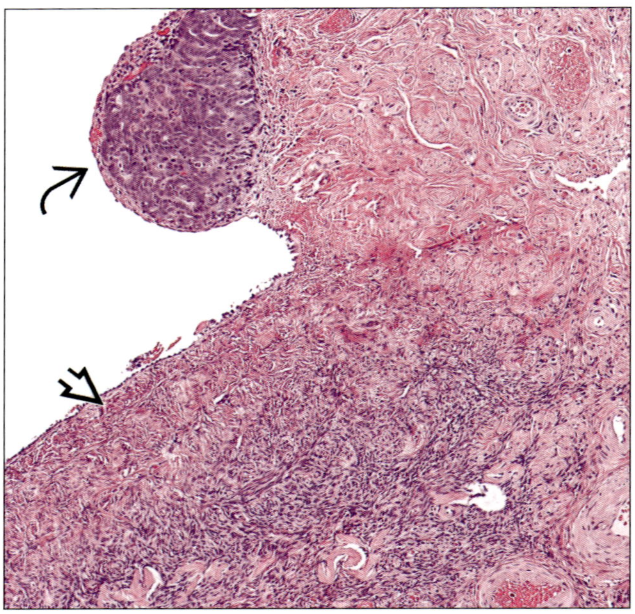

Intermediate-power magnification shows tumor nodule on the surface of the ovary. Note the stroma composed of whorls of plump spindle cells of fibroblastic type that is characteristic of the ovary. (Original magnification 100x.)

T3 (FIGO III)

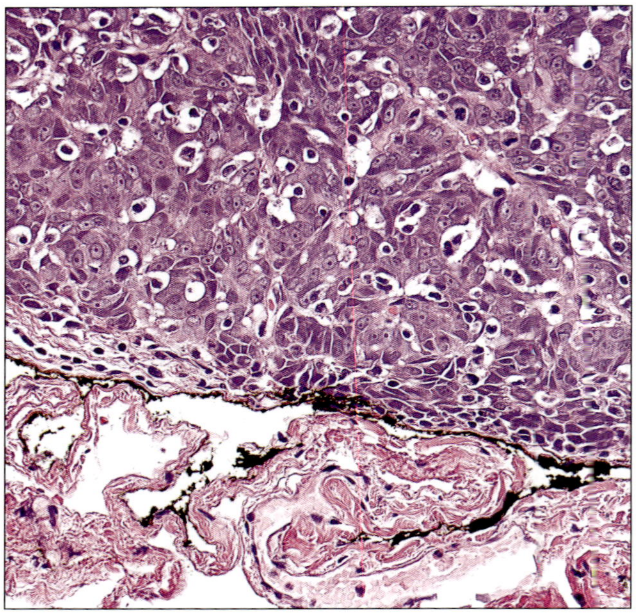

H&E stain demonstrates peritoneal tumor implants outside the pelvis (T3). (Original magnification 400x.)

FALLOPIAN TUBE CARCINOMA

T1a (FIGO IA)

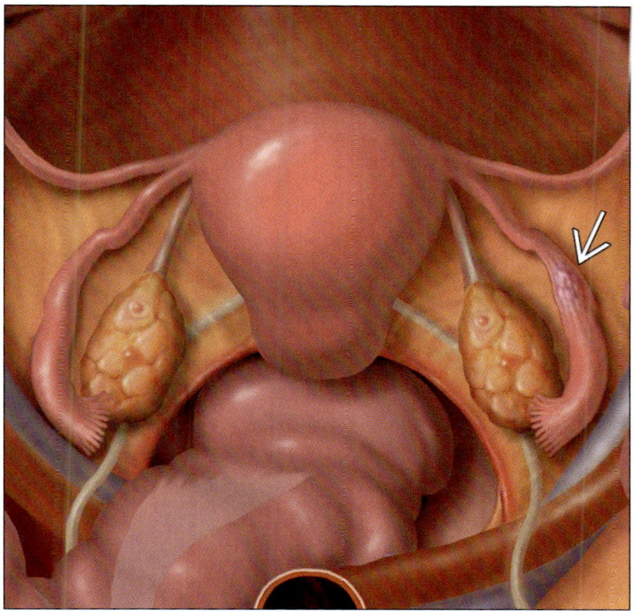

Graphic of the uterus as viewed from above shows T1a disease: Tumor is limited to 1 fallopian tube →, without penetrating the serosal surface, and there is no ascites.

T1b (FIGO IB)

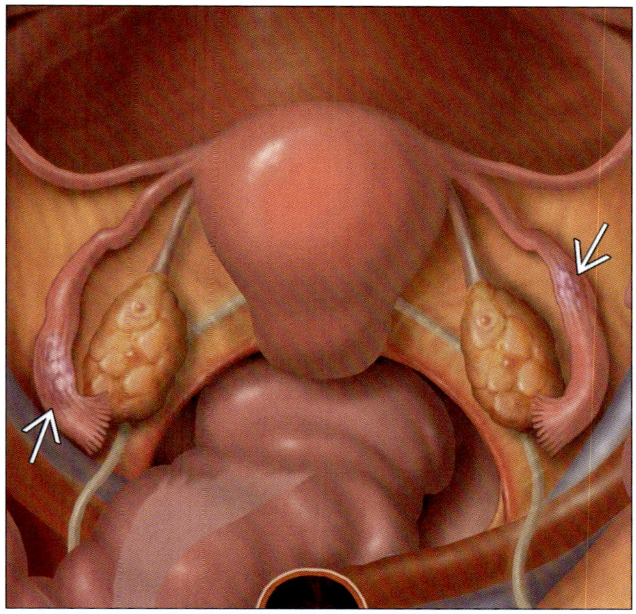

Graphic of the uterus as viewed from above shows T1b disease: Tumor is limited to both fallopian tubes →, without penetrating the serosal surface, and there is no ascites.

T1c (FIGO IC)

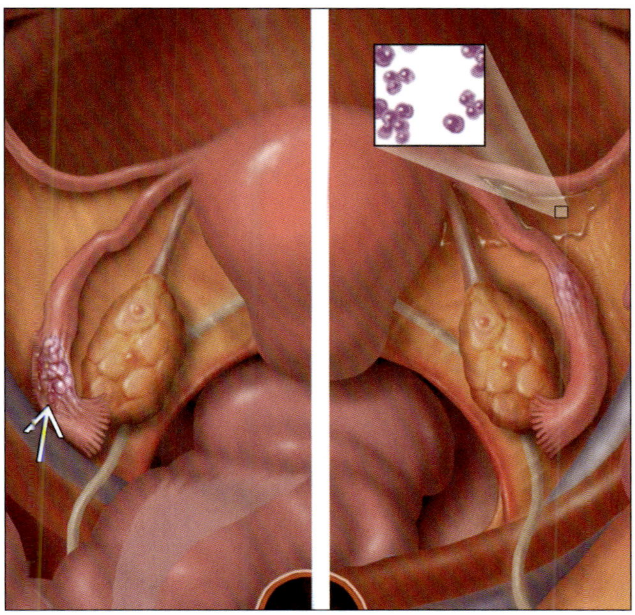

Two graphics of the uterus as viewed from above show T1c disease: Tumor is limited to 1 or both fallopian tubes, with extension onto or through the tubal serosa →, shown on the left, and with malignant cells in ascites or peritoneal washings on the right.

T2a (FIGO IIA)

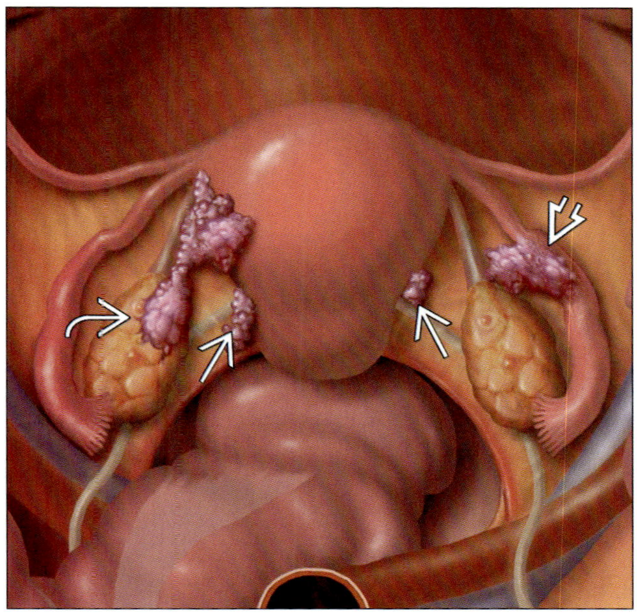

Graphic of the uterus as viewed from above shows T2a disease: Tumor involving 1 or both fallopian tubes →, with pelvic extension to the uterus → &/or ovaries →.

FALLOPIAN TUBE CARCINOMA

T2b (FIGO IIB)

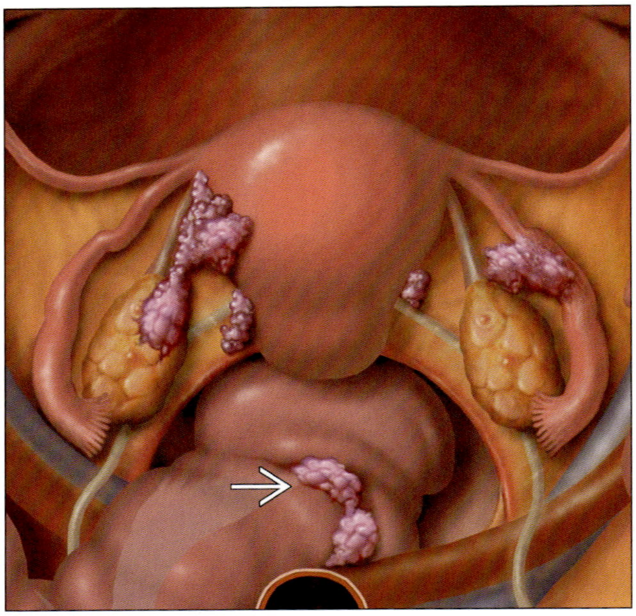

Graphic of the uterus as viewed from above shows T2b disease: Tumor involving 1 or both fallopian tubes with extension to pelvic organs other than the uterus and ovaries. Shown here is extension to the rectum ➔.

T2c (FIGO IIC)

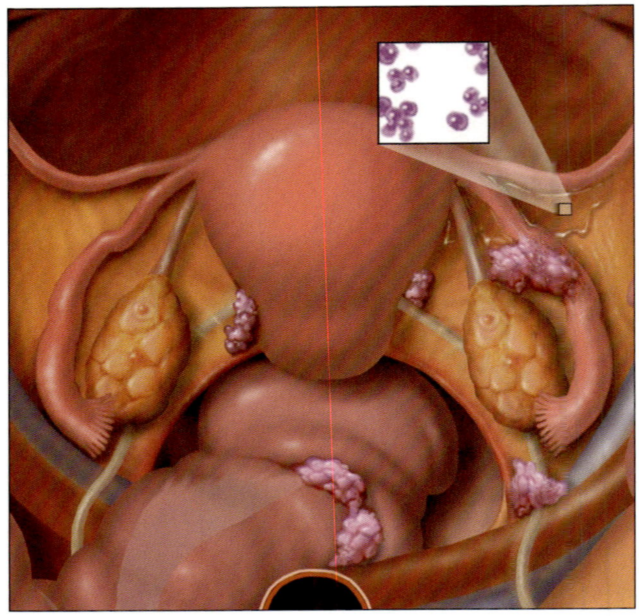

Graphic of the uterus as viewed from above shows T2c disease: Pelvic extension with malignant cells in ascites or peritoneal washings.

T3a (FIGO IIIA)

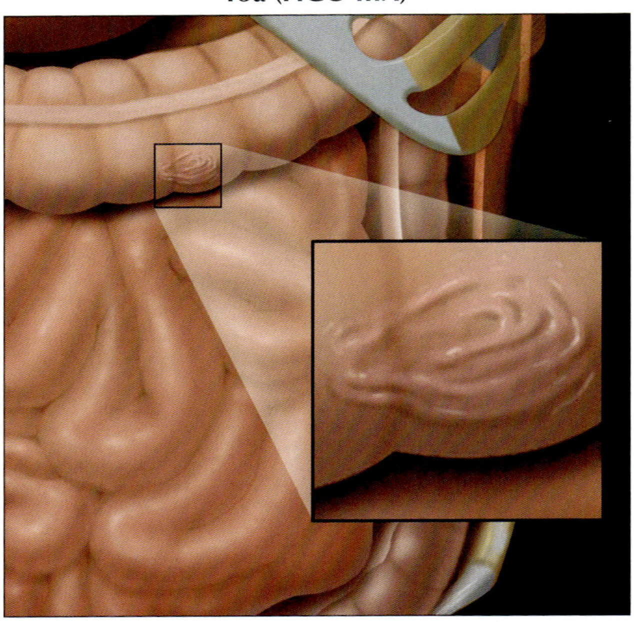

T3a tumors involve microscopic peritoneal metastases beyond the pelvis. These cannot be visualized by imaging; rather, they are found through peritoneal biopsy at staging laparotomy.

T3b (FIGO IIIB)

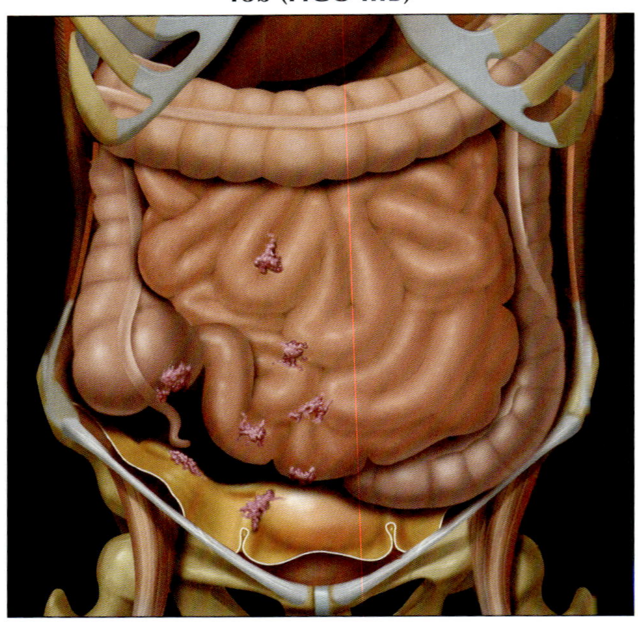

T3b tumors feature macroscopic peritoneal metastases beyond the pelvis that are less than or equal to 2 cm in greatest dimension.

FALLOPIAN TUBE CARCINOMA

T3c (FIGO IIIC)

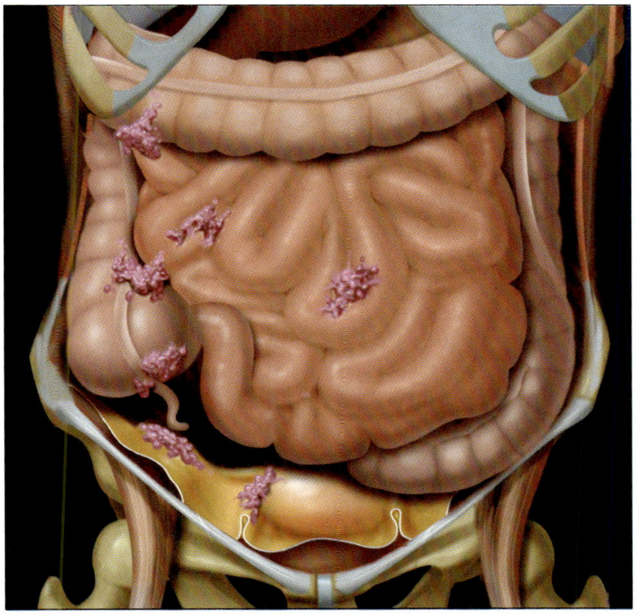

T3c tumors involve macroscopic peritoneal metastases beyond the pelvis larger than 2 cm in greatest dimension.

Nodal Drainage of the Fallopian Tubes

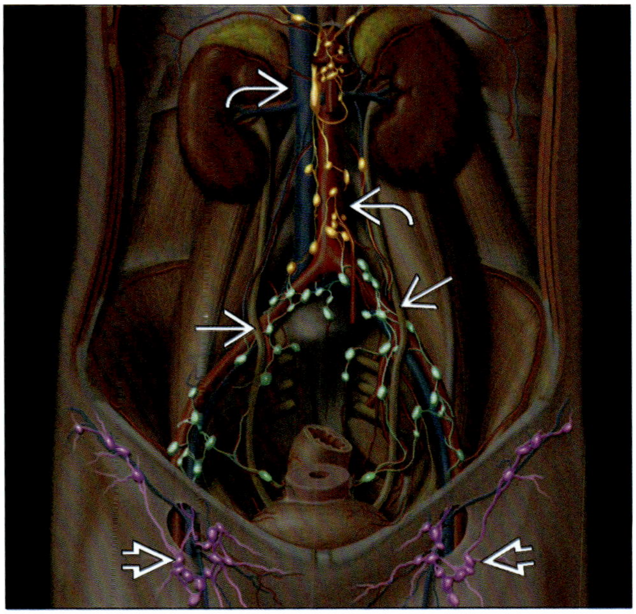

Fallopian tube lymphatics follow the ovarian veins to the paraaortic lymph nodes. Lymphatic spread may also occur through the broad ligament to the pelvic lymph nodes and along the round ligament to the inguinal lymph nodes.

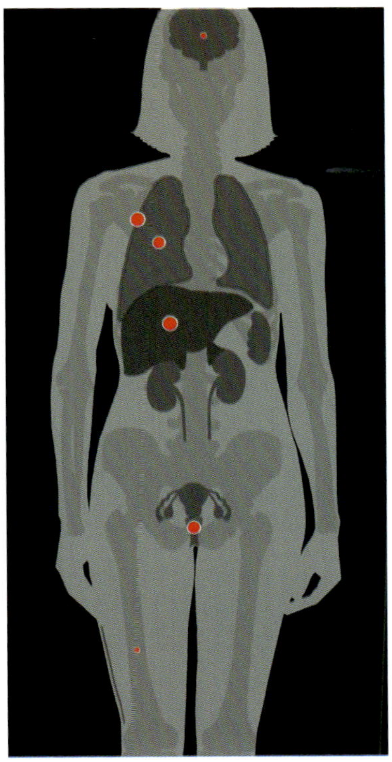

METASTASES, ORGAN FREQUENCY	
Liver	20.5%
Pleura	18%
Vagina	15.5%
Lung	13%
Bones	2.6%
Brain	2.6%

FALLOPIAN TUBE CARCINOMA

OVERVIEW

Classification

- Histological types of primary fallopian tube carcinoma (PFTC) include
  - Papillary serous carcinoma (49.5-83.3%)
  - Endometrioid (8.3-50%)
  - Mixed (3.9-16.7%)
  - Clear cell (1.9%)
  - Transitional (11.7%)

PATHOLOGY

Routes of Spread

- Pattern of spread is similar to ovarian carcinoma
- Peritoneal spread
  - In approximately 80% of patients with advanced disease, metastases are confined to peritoneal cavity
- Lymphatic spread
  - Lymphatic drainage of PFTC mirrors that of uterine fundus and ovaries
    - Along ovarian vessels → paraaortic nodes
    - Along broad ligament → pelvic nodes
    - Along round ligament of uterus → superficial inguinal nodes
  - Early lymphatic metastases are common
    - Incidence of positive nodes is 40–60% when there is extratubal tumor spread
- Hematogenous spread
  - Can occur to liver, pleura, vagina, lungs, and brain
- Transluminal spread
  - Spread to proximal part of fallopian tube and uterus

General Features

- Genetics
  - PFTC has been described in high-risk breast-ovarian cancer families with germ-line *BRCA1* and *BRCA2* mutations
    - *BRCA* mutations were noted in 16% of invasive PFTC patients
    - Occult PFTC found in 5.6% of *BRCA* patients who underwent prophylactic risk-reducing salpingo-oophorectomy
    - 44% of occult malignancies found in prophylactic oophorectomy specimens are of tubal origin
    - Increasing evidence that tubal fimbriae may be preferred site of origin of adnexal cancer in carriers of *BRCA* gene mutations
- Etiology
  - Etiology of PFTC is unknown
    - Hormonal, reproductive, and possibly genetic factors thought to ↑ epithelial ovarian tumors risk might also ↑ PFTC risk
    - 25-30% of cases in nulliparous women
    - 5x higher bilateral occurrence in infertile patients than in fertile patients
    - No statistically significant correlation between PFTC and age, race, weight, education level, pelvic inflammatory disease, infertility, previous hysterectomy, endometriosis, lactose intolerance, or smoking
    - Better prognosis in nulliparous women
    - High parity may be protective
    - Pregnancy and use of oral contraceptives ↓ risk significantly
- Epidemiology & cancer incidence
  - Least common of gynecological malignancies
    - Accounts for approximately 0.3–1.8% of female genital malignancies
    - Annual incidence is 3.6-4.1 per 1,000,000 women
    - True incidence may be underestimated because of difficulty in differentiating PFTC from epithelial ovarian carcinoma, especially in advanced cases
  - In 1 series, 35% of women with PFTC had history of breast cancer
  - Most frequently occurs between 4th and 6th decades of life
    - Median age of occurrence of 55 years (range: 17–88 years)
  - Bilateral tumors reported in 10-27% of cases
- Associated diseases, abnormalities
  - CA-125 is useful tumor marker for diagnosis, assessment of response to treatment, and detection of tumor recurrence during follow-up
    - > 80% of patients have elevated pretreatment serum CA-125 levels
    - Pretreatment serum CA-125 level is independent prognostic factor of disease-free survival and overall survival
    - Lead time (↑ CA-125 levels prior to clinical or radiological diagnosis of recurrence) is 3 months (range: 0.5–7 months)

Gross Pathology & Surgical Features

- Most arise in ampulla and project into tubal lumen, often causing occlusion
- Pattern of growth can be nodular, papillary, infiltrative, or massive
- Criteria for diagnosis of PFTC
  - Main tumor in tube and arises from endosalpinx
  - Histological pattern reproduces epithelium of tubal mucosa (papillary pattern)
  - If wall is involved, transition from benign to malignant tubal epithelium should be demonstrated
  - Ovaries and endometrium are normal or have much smaller tumor volume than that of tube

Microscopic Pathology

- H&E
  - Most common histologic type is papillary serous carcinoma
    - Histologically identical to ovarian serous adenocarcinoma
    - Produces large amount of serous fluid → tubal distension and hydrosalpinx
  - Serous tumors show papillary patterns, cords or sheets of pleomorphic cells

IMAGING FINDINGS

Detection

- **Ultrasound**
  - Sonographic appearance of PFTC is nonspecific, mimicking other pelvic diseases, such as tubo-ovarian abscess, ovarian tumor, and ectopic pregnancy

FALLOPIAN TUBE CARCINOMA

- Presence of partially solid/cystic mass separate from ovary is highly suggestive of PFTC
- Sonographic features include
  - Sausage-shaped solid mass
  - Cystic anechoic tubular structure with mural nodules
  - Multilocular mass with "cog and wheel" appearance
  - Color Doppler US: Low impedance vascular flow within solid components

- CT
  - When associated with hydrosalpinx
    - Mixed solid cystic adnexal mass or tubular cystic structure with papillary projections
    - Solid components have attenuation equal to that of other soft tissue masses and enhance less than myometrium
  - When not associated with hydrosalpinx
    - Sausage-shaped solid adnexal mass has attenuation equal to that of other soft tissue masses and enhances less than myometrium
  - Attempt should be made to identify ovaries separate from adnexal tubal mass
    - Ovaries can be identified by following ovarian vein &/or round ligament
  - Associated findings include
    - Peritumoral ascites resulting from tubal decompression through fimbrial end
    - Intrauterine fluid collection
    - Peritoneal implants
- MR
  - When associated with hydrosalpinx
    - Mixed solid cystic adnexal mass or tubular cystic structure with papillary projections
    - Cystic component of low signal intensity on T1W images and high signal intensity on T2W images
      - Cystic component may have high T1 signal intensity due to hemorrhage
    - Solid components show enhancement after administration of IV gadolinium
  - When not associated with hydrosalpinx
    - Solid adnexal mass with predominantly low signal intensity on T1WI and high signal intensity on T2WI
    - Heterogeneous enhancement after administration of IV gadolinium
  - Change in appearance on serial imaging due to tube decompression and passage of fluid from distended tube into uterus
  - Associated findings include
    - Peritumoral ascites
    - Intrauterine fluid collection
    - Peritoneal implants
- PET/CT
  - Can help identify site of primary tumor as PFTC in patients with metastatic disease of unknown origin
  - May detect unsuspected PFTC during staging of other tumors, particularly breast carcinoma

Staging

- PFTC is staged surgically, based on International Federation of Obstetrics and Gynecology (FIGO) system
- Staging and operability mirror that of epithelial ovarian cancer (EOC)
- Staging requires staging laparotomy, which includes
  - Total abdominal hysterectomy
  - Bilateral salpingo-oophorectomy
  - Omentectomy
  - Systematic pelvic and paraaortic nodal dissection
  - Peritoneal and diaphragmatic biopsies
  - Cytological evaluation of peritoneal washings
- CT
  - Primary imaging modality for preoperative staging PFTC
  - In many cases, preoperative diagnosis is that of EOC
  - Goals of preoperative imaging, as with EOC, are
    - Recognition of extensive disease that is unresectable
    - Detection of metastatic disease to prevent understaging and allow adequate intraoperative sampling of suspected lesions
  - Factors that generally indicate inoperable disease include
    - Invasion of pelvic sidewall, rectum, sigmoid colon, or bladder
    - Bulky peritoneal disease
      - Porta hepatis
      - Intersegmental fissure of liver
      - Lesser sac
      - Gastrosplenic ligament
      - Gastrohepatic ligament
      - Subphrenic space
      - Small bowel mesentery
      - Supracolic omentum
      - Presacral space
    - Suprarenal and splenic adenopathy
    - Hepatic and splenic (parenchymal), pleural, or pulmonary metastases
- MR
  - MR can be used as alternative to CT for local staging

Restaging

- CT
  - Modality of choice for restaging and detection of recurrent disease
- PET/CT
  - Useful in identifying patients with recurrent PFTC

CLINICAL ISSUES

Presentation

- Abdominal pain is frequent complaint (30-49%)
  - May lead to earlier presentation
  - Pain is colicky and lower abdominal
  - Pain is caused by distension of partially blocked fallopian tube by fluid, which is then relieved by passage of blood or discharge
- Latzko classical triad of symptoms reported in 15% of cases
  - Intermittent profuse serosanguineous vaginal discharge
  - Colicky pain relieved by discharge
  - Adnexal mass
- Hydrops tubae profluens
  - Intermittent discharge of clear or blood-tinged fluid spontaneously or on pressure followed by shrinkage of adnexal mass
  - Pathognomonic feature

FALLOPIAN TUBE CARCINOMA

- Occurs in 5% of patients
- Clinical symptoms of PFTC and EOC are otherwise similar and nonspecific
  - Vaginal bleeding or spotting (50-60%)
  - Abdominal or pelvic mass (60%)
  - Ascites (15%)

Cancer Natural History & Prognosis

- Often diagnosed at earlier stage than EOC
  - Because of colicky abdominal pain resulting from tubal distension
  - Frequency of different stages at diagnosis
    - Stage I (20-35%)
    - Stage II (20-24%)
    - Stage III (45-50%)
    - Stage IV (3-10%)
- Better survival compared to EOC
- 5-year relative survival by stage
  - Stage 0 (70%)
  - Stage IA (85%)
  - Stage IB: Not enough information to derive survival rate
  - Stage IC (89%)
  - Stage IIA (71%)
  - Stage IIB (62%)
  - Stage IIC (61%)
  - Stage IIIA (52%)
  - Stage IIIB (43%)
  - Stage IIIC (38%)
  - Stage IV (22%)

Treatment Options

- Treatment options by stage
  - Stage I
    - Total abdominal hysterectomy and bilateral salpingo-oophorectomy with omentectomy
    - Systematic pelvic and paraaortic nodal dissection is preferred to sampling (because of tendency for early lymphatic spread)
    - Undersurface of diaphragm should be visualized and biopsied; pelvic and abdominal peritoneal biopsies and peritoneal washings should be obtained routinely
    - In patients who desire childbearing and have grade I tumors, unilateral salpingo-oophorectomy may be associated with a low risk of recurrence
    - No further treatment if low-grade cancer, possible chemotherapy if high grade
  - Stage II
    - Total abdominal hysterectomy and bilateral salpingo-oophorectomy + tumor debulking + pelvic and paraaortic nodal dissection
    - Following surgery, combination chemotherapy ± radiation therapy
  - Stage III
    - Same as stage II; possible follow-up surgery to remove any remaining tumor
  - Stage VI
    - Debulking surgery to remove as much of tumor as possible, followed by combination chemotherapy

REPORTING CHECKLIST

T Staging

- Characteristic imaging feature of PFTC is change in appearance on serial imaging
  - Due to accumulation of fluid within tube and subsequent decompression into uterus or around fimbrial end
- Evaluate tumor extension to adjacent pelvic structures
  - Ovaries, uterus, bladder, and rectum
- Close attention to peritoneal implants
  - Both pelvic and abdominal implants

N Staging

- Paraaortic, pelvic, and inguinal nodes

M Staging

- Attention to pleura, liver, vagina, and lungs

SELECTED REFERENCES

1. American Joint Committee on Cancer: AJCC Cancer Staging Manual. 7th ed. New York: Springer, 2010
2. Rabban JT et al: Ovarian pathology in risk-reducing salpingo-oophorectomies from women with BRCA mutations, emphasizing the differential diagnosis of occult primary and metastatic carcinoma. Am J Surg Pathol. 33(8):1125-36, 2009
3. Wethington SL et al: Improved survival for fallopian tube cancer: a comparison of clinical characteristics and outcome for primary fallopian tube and ovarian cancer. Cancer. 113(12):3298-306, 2008
4. Pectasides D et al: Fallopian tube carcinoma: a review. Oncologist. 11(8):902-12, 2006
5. Kosary C et al: Treatment and survival for women with Fallopian tube carcinoma: a population-based study. Gynecol Oncol. 86(2):190-1, 2002
6. Makhija S et al: Positron emission tomography/computed tomography imaging for the detection of recurrent ovarian and fallopian tube carcinoma: a retrospective review. Gynecol Oncol. 85(1):53-8, 2002
7. Patel PV et al: PET-CT localizes previously undetectable metastatic lesions in recurrent fallopian tube carcinoma. Gynecol Oncol. 87(3):323-6, 2002
8. van Leeuwen BL et al: Liver metastasis as a first sign of fallopian tube carcinoma and the role of positron emission tomography in preoperative diagnosis. Scand J Gastroenterol. 37(12):1473-4, 2002
9. Gadducci A et al: Analysis of treatment failures and survival of patients with fallopian tube carcinoma: a cooperation task force (CTF) study. Gynecol Oncol. 81(2):150-9, 2001
10. Baekelandt M et al: Carcinoma of the fallopian tube. Cancer. 89(10):2076-84, 2000
11. Slanetz PJ et al: Imaging of fallopian tube tumors. AJR Am J Roentgenol. 169(5):1321-4, 1997

FALLOPIAN TUBE CARCINOMA

Stage IA (T1a N0 M0)

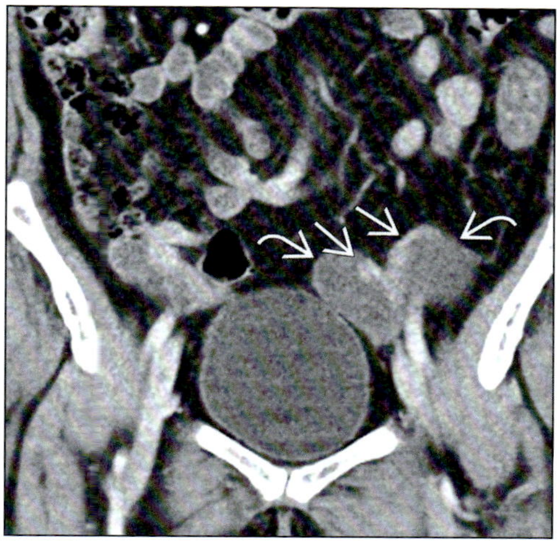

Stage IA (T1a N0 M0)

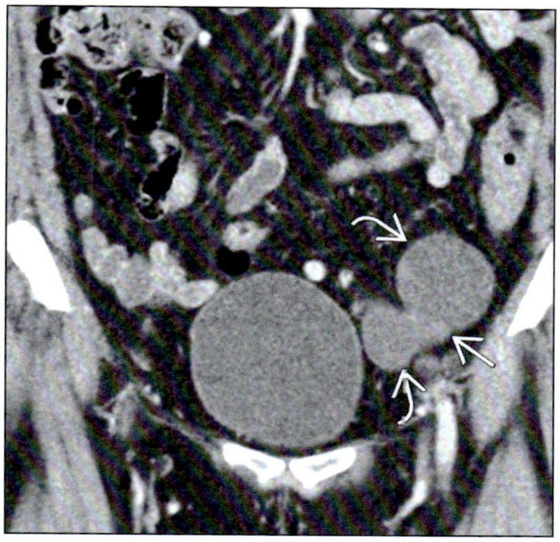

(Left) *Coronal CECT shows a left side hydrosalpinx with nodular enhancing mural lesions in a 70-year-old woman who presented with bloody vaginal bleeding and crampy abdominal pain.* ***(Right)*** *Coronal CECT in the same patient at a more anterior level shows hydrosalpinx and enhancing mural nodule. This was interpreted as a multilocular adnexal mass suspicious for cystic epithelial ovarian neoplasm. The patient refused surgery.*

Stage IA (T1a N0 M0)

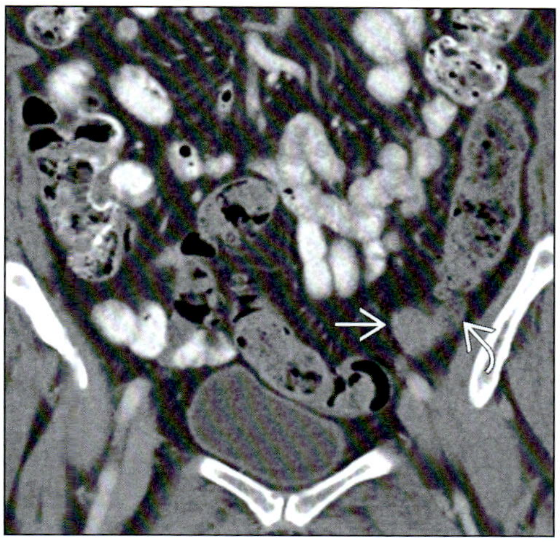

Stage IA (T1a N0 M0)

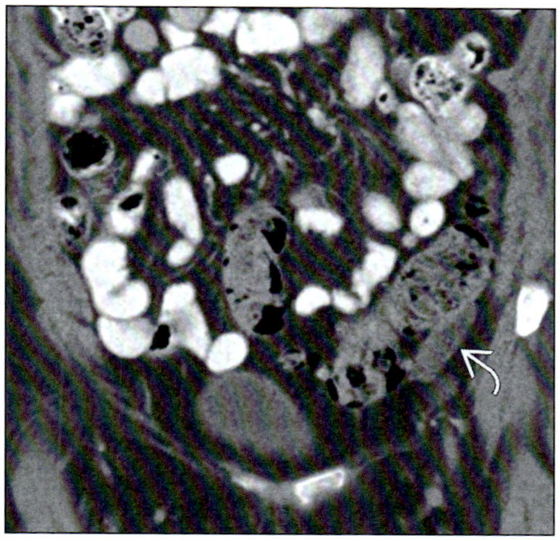

(Left) *Coronal CECT in the same patient, 6 months later, shows interval decrease in the size of the left hydrosalpinx and increase in the size of the enhancing soft tissue component.* ***(Right)*** *Coronal CECT in the same patient shows interval decrease in the size of left side hydrosalpinx. The decrease in size of hydrosalpinx is the radiological equivalent of "hydrops tubae profluens," in which the tube decompresses into the uterus resulting in less tubal dilatation.*

Stage IA (T1a N0 M0)

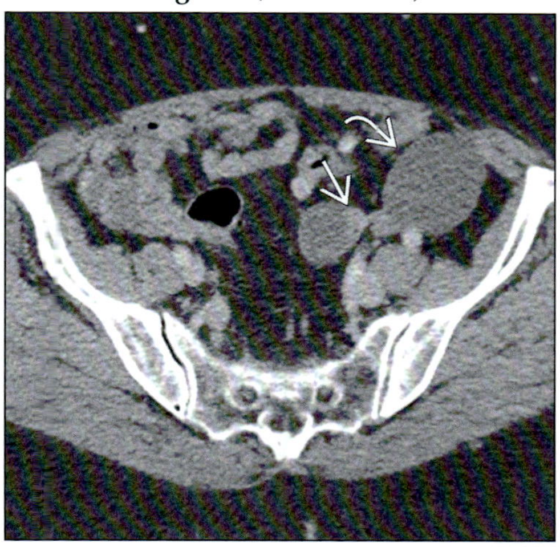

Stage IA (T1a N0 M0)

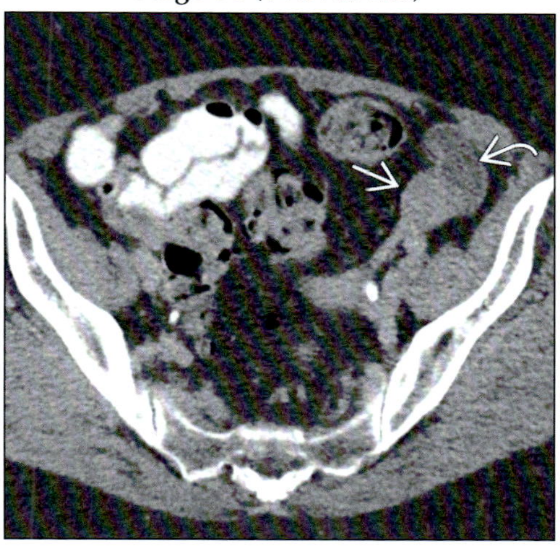

(Left) *Axial CECT in the same patient on her initial presentation shows marked hydrosalpinx with small mural enhancing nodule.* ***(Right)*** *Axial CECT in the same patient, 6 months later, shows decrease in the size of hydrosalpinx and increased size of enhancing solid component. The patient finally agreed to undergo surgery and was found to have stage I (T1 N0 M0) serous fallopian tube carcinoma.*

FALLOPIAN TUBE CARCINOMA

*(**Left**) Longitudinal transvaginal ultrasound shows severe tubal dilatation (hydrosalpinx) with an echogenic mural nodule. (**Right**) Transverse color Doppler ultrasound in the same patient shows hydrosalpinx with an echogenic mural nodule, which demonstrates low resistance arterial flow. The low resistance arterial flow is not specific for fallopian tube carcinoma and is also seen in both benign and malignant ovarian lesions.*

Stage IA (T1a N0 M0)

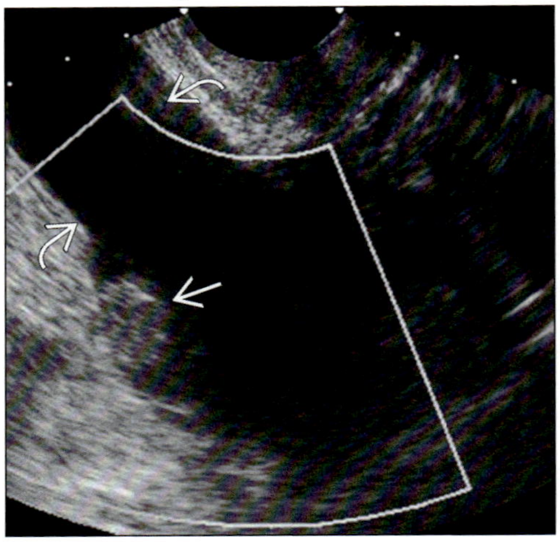

Stage IA (T1a N0 M0)

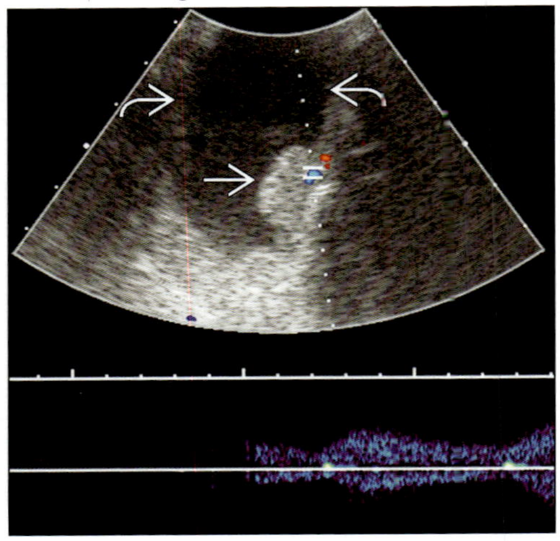

*(**Left**) Axial NECT of the pelvis obtained as part of PET/CT for the staging of breast cancer shows normal-appearing left adnexa without identifiable mass. (**Right**) Axial PET/CT in the same patient shows an area of increased metabolic activity in the left adnexa that appears elongated. It is difficult on this image to identify whether the location of increased activity is the left ovary or fallopian tube.*

Stage IA (T1a N0 M0)

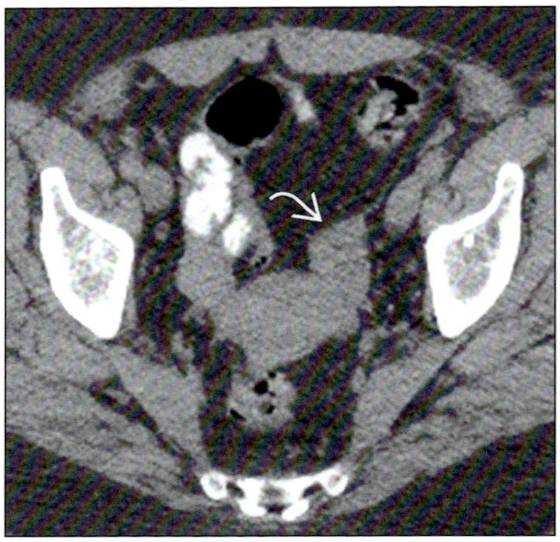

Stage IA (T1a N0 M0)

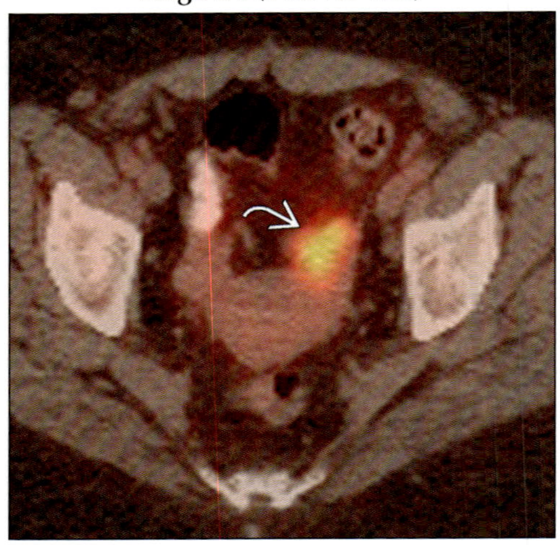

*(**Left**) Coronal fused PET/CT in the same patient shows that the area of increased metabolic activity has a tubular configuration, suggesting tubal origin. (**Right**) Coronal PET in the same patient shows tubular, comma-shaped configuration of the area of increased metabolic activity within the left adnexa. No other areas of abnormal metabolic activity were detected. Fallopian tube adenocarcinoma confined to the tube was confirmed during surgery.*

Stage IA (T1a N0 M0)

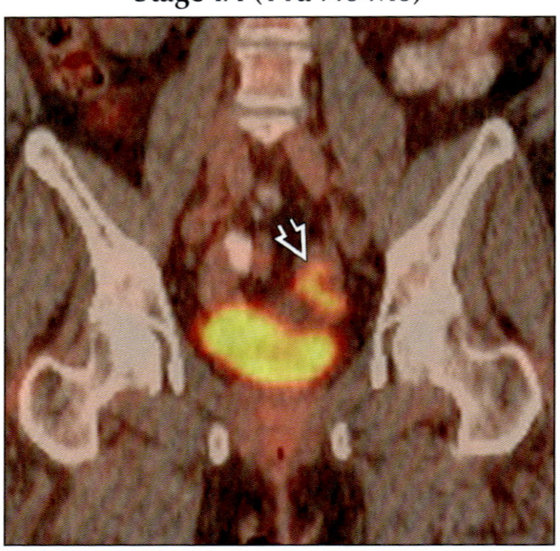

Stage IA (T1a N0 M0)

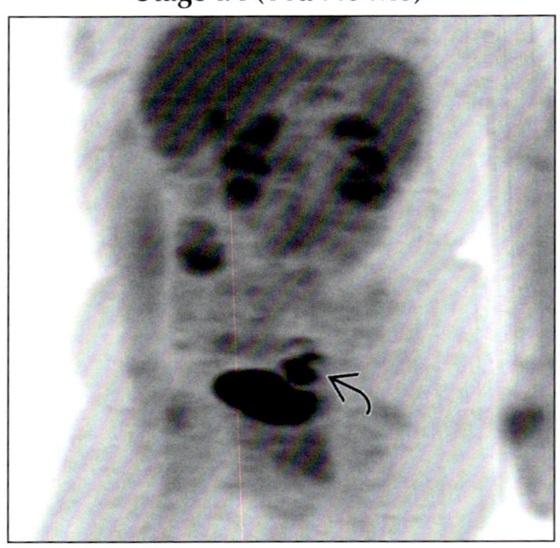

FALLOPIAN TUBE CARCINOMA

Stage IA (T1a N0 M0)

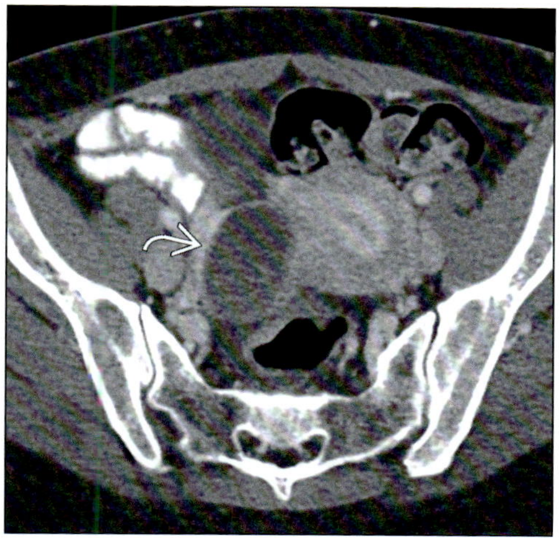

Stage IA (T1a N0 M0)

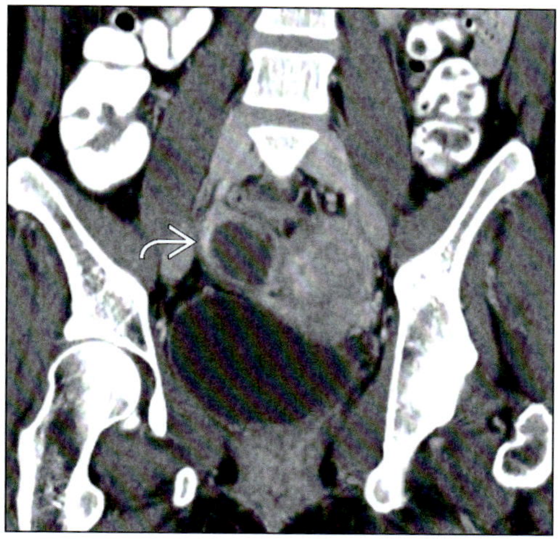

*(**Left**) Axial CECT in a 45-year-old woman who presented with lower abdominal pain shows a right adnexal cystic structure → without obvious mural nodules. The density of the lesion was 30 HU. (**Right**) Coronal CECT in the same patient shows the right adnexal cystic structure →. The radiological interpretation was a cystic adnexal mass, likely hydrosalpinx or ovarian cyst. Follow-up ultrasound in 6 weeks was recommended.*

Stage IA (T1a N0 M0)

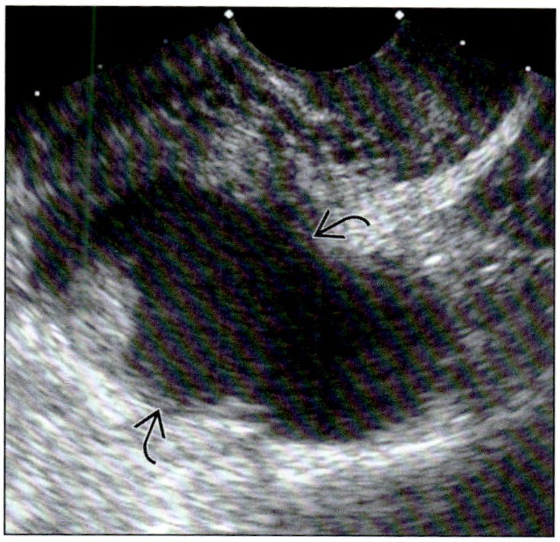

Stage IA (T1a N0 M0)

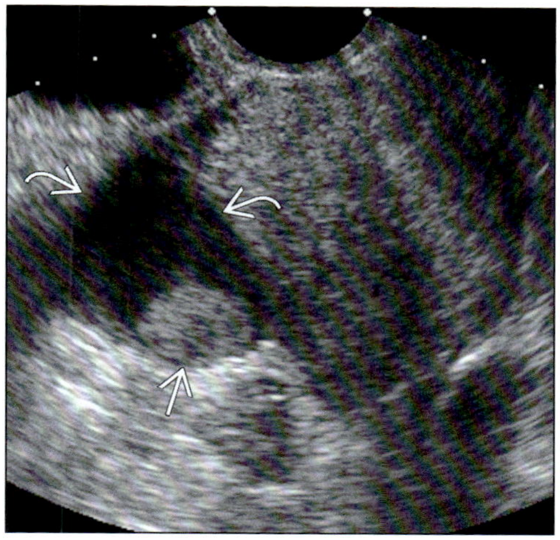

*(**Left**) Longitudinal transvaginal ultrasound in the same patient 6 weeks after the CECT shows the dilated adnexal structure to be a dilated tube → with echogenic mural nodule. (**Right**) Transverse transvaginal ultrasound in the same patient shows hydrosalpinx → with a mural nodule →. This was found at surgery to be serous adenocarcinoma limited to the fallopian tube.*

Stage IIA (T2a N0 M0)

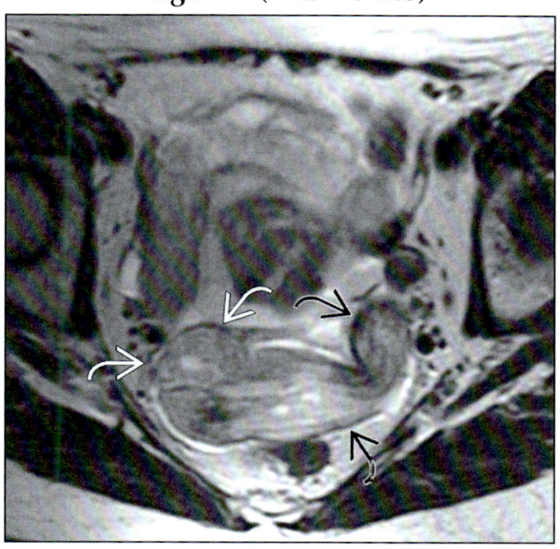

Stage IIA (T2a N0 M0)

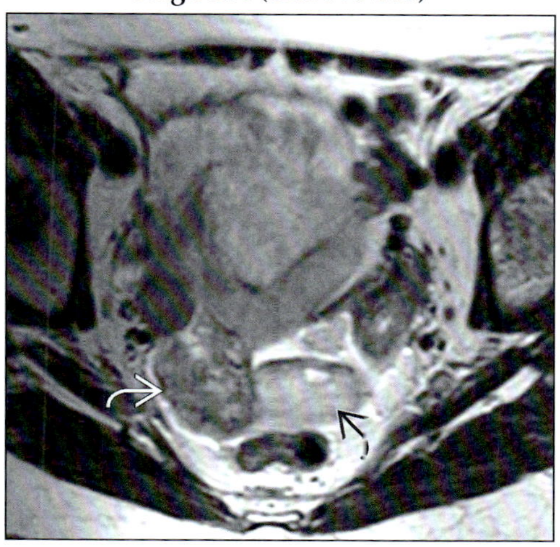

*(**Left**) Axial T2WI MR shows dilated left fallopian tube → containing mixed signal intensity material. The left ovary → is enlarged, pushed toward the right side, and cannot be separated from the fimbrial end of the tube. (**Right**) Axial T2WI MR in the same patient at a slightly lower level shows the dilated heterogeneous tube → and the enlarged heterogeneous ovary →.*

FALLOPIAN TUBE CARCINOMA

(Left) *Axial T1WI MR in the same patient shows left side hydrosalpinx ⇨ and filling of the tube with material that has low signal intensity similar to that of fluid. The subsequent gadolinium-enhanced images help separate enhancing tumor from fluid/mucous filling the tube.* **(Right)** *Sagittal T1WI C+ FS MR in the same patient shows hydrosalpinx ➡ with irregular thickening and enhancement of the wall of the fallopian tube.*

Stage IIA (T2a N0 M0)

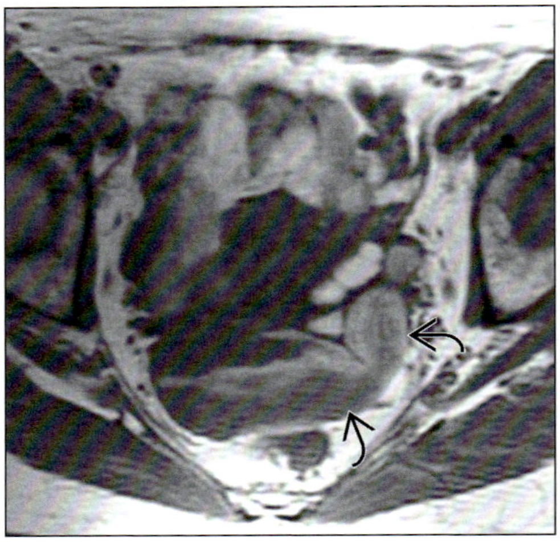

Stage IIA (T2a N0 M0)

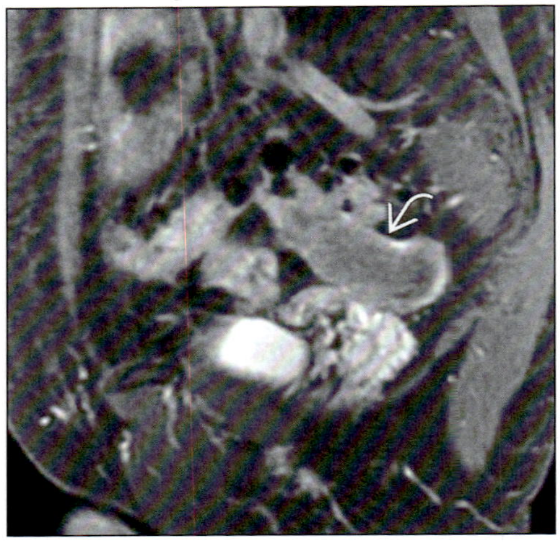

(Left) *Axial T1WI C+ FS MR in the same patient shows enhancement and nodular thickening of the fallopian tube wall ➡ as well as heterogeneous enhancement of the enlarged ovary ➡.* **(Right)** *Axial T1WI C+ FS MR shows enhancement and nodular thickening of the fallopian tube wall ➡ as well as heterogeneous enhancement of the enlarged ovary ➡. The dilated tube is filled with tumor and bloody fluid ➡.*

Stage IIA (T2a N0 M0)

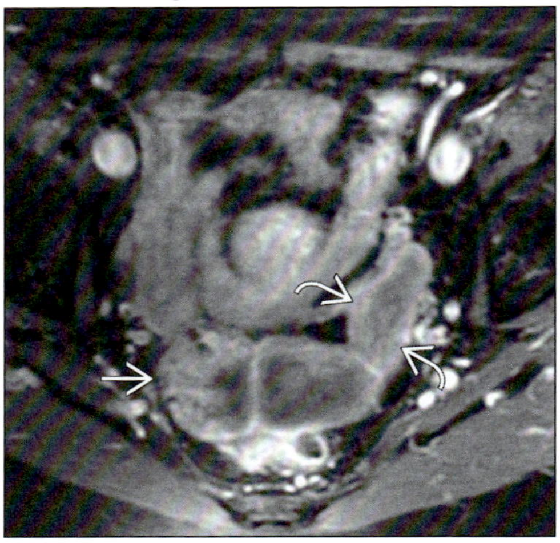

Stage IIA (T2a N0 M0)

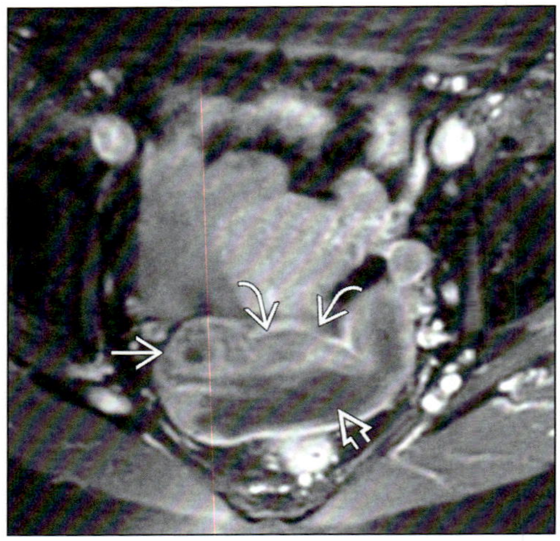

(Left) *Transverse transabdominal ultrasound in a 56-year-old woman presenting with increasing abdominal girth shows a left adnexal sausage-shaped solid mass ⇨ with blood flow ➡ within the mass.* **(Right)** *Transverse transabdominal ultrasound in the same patient shows ascites ⇨ with low-level internal echoes. Abnormal anterior soft tissue ➡ underneath the anterior abdominal wall represents omental metastases (caking).*

Stage IIC (T2c N0 M0)

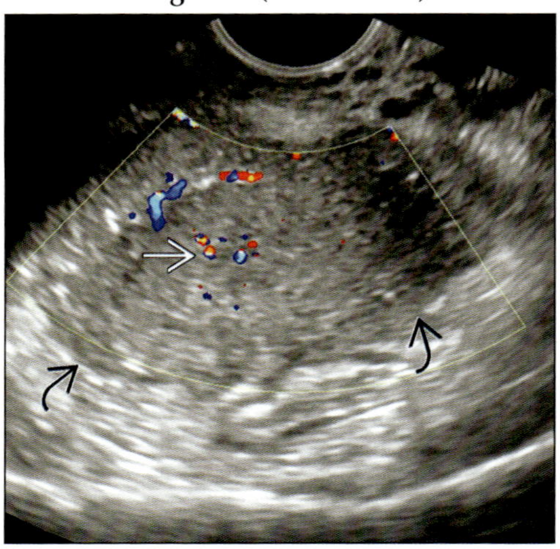

Stage IIC (T2c N0 M0)

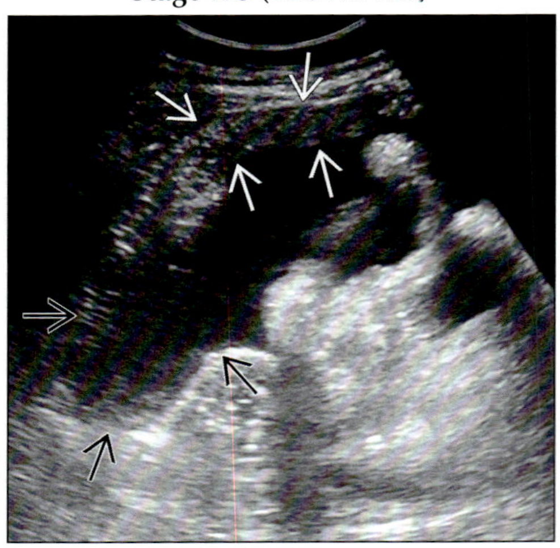

FALLOPIAN TUBE CARCINOMA

Stage IIC (T2c N0 M0)

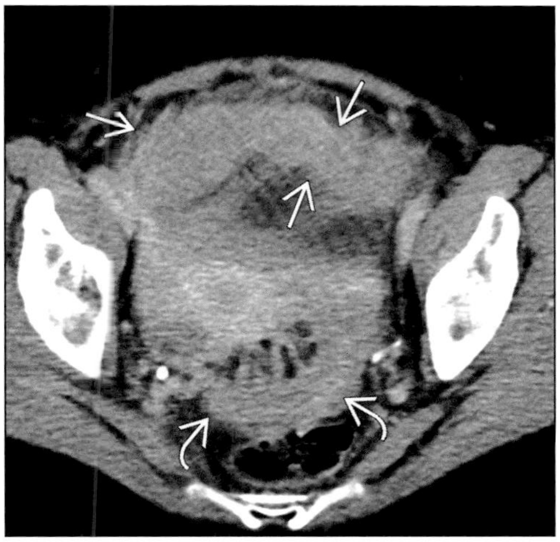

Stage IIC (T2c N0 M0)

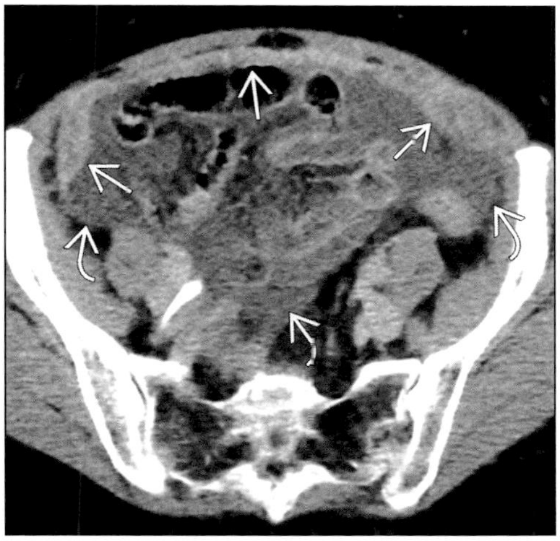

(Left) *Axial CECT in the same patient shows a solid left adnexal mass between the uterus and rectum. Extensive omental metastatic disease is seen anteriorly.* **(Right)** *Axial CECT in the same patient shows ascites and enhancing omental metastatic disease (omental caking) forming a sheet of abnormal tissue anterior to the bowel.*

Stage IIIC (T2a N1 M0)

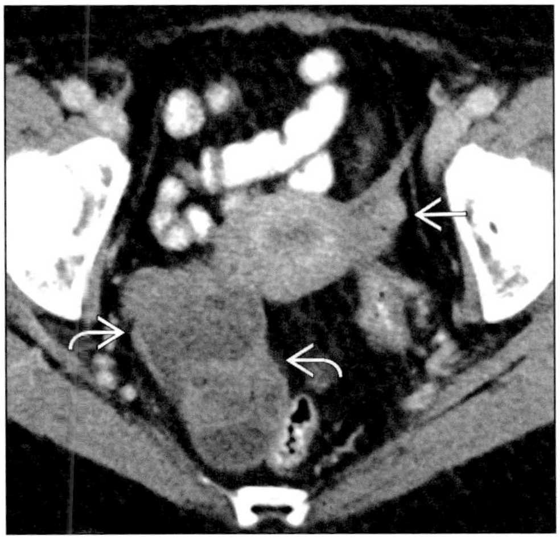

Stage IIIC (T2a N1 M0)

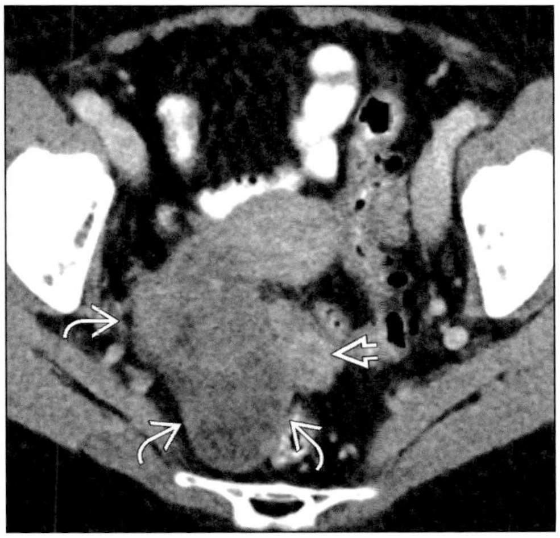

(Left) *Axial CECT in a middle-aged woman shows a sausage-shaped, mixed solid/cystic right adnexal mass. An enhancing left ovarian nodule was found at surgery to be a metastatic tumor.* **(Right)** *Axial CECT in the same patient shows the sausage-shaped right adnexal mass separate from the enhancing right ovary. During surgery the right ovary was involved (T2a), but the main bulk of the mass was within the fallopian tube and arising from the endosalpinx.*

Stage IIIC (T2a N1 M0)

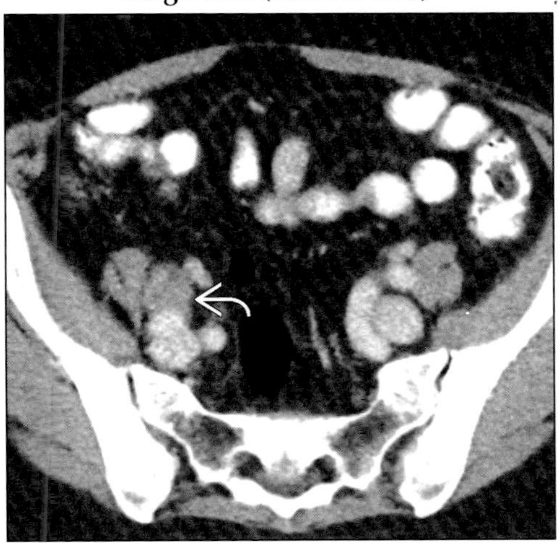

Stage IIIC (T2a N1 M0)

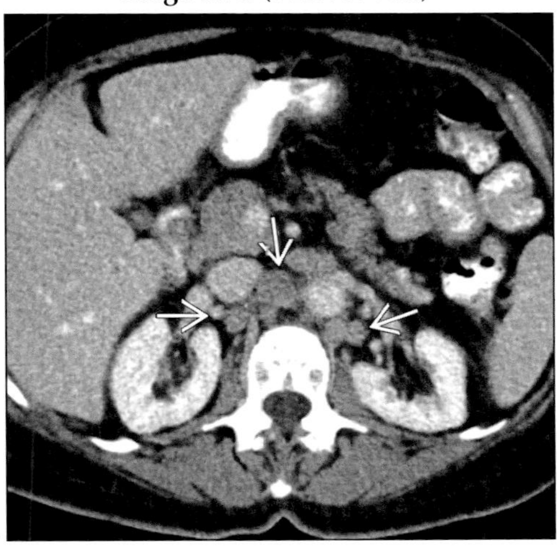

(Left) *Axial CECT in the same patient shows right iliac lymphadenopathy.* **(Right)** *Axial CECT in the same patient at the level of the kidneys shows retroperitoneal lymphadenopathy. The lymphatic drainage of the fallopian tubes is similar to the lymphatic drainage of the ovaries, and tumor spreads along the ovarian veins to the retroperitoneal lymph nodes.*

FALLOPIAN TUBE CARCINOMA

(Left) Axial CECT in a 54-year-old woman who presented with vague pelvic pain shows a fluid-filled sausage-shaped tubular structure (hydrosalpinx) anterior to the vagina and superior to the urinary bladder. *(Right)* Axial CECT in the same patient shows the proximal part of hydrosalpinx with enhancing mural nodule. The medial end of the hydrosalpinx shows ill-defined enhancement that cannot be separated from the uterus.

Stage IIIC (T2a N1 M0)

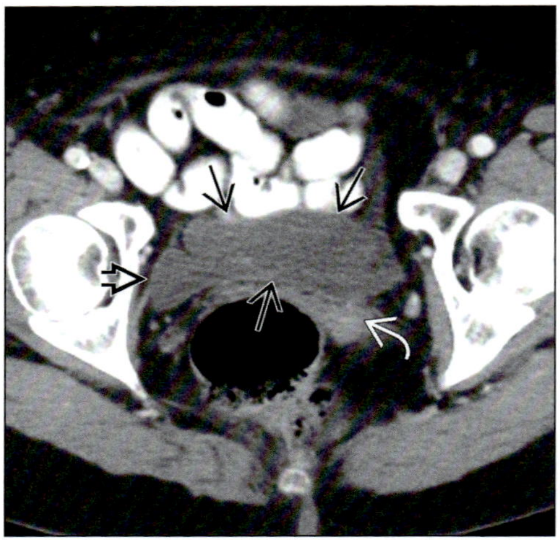

Stage IIIC (T2a N1 M0)

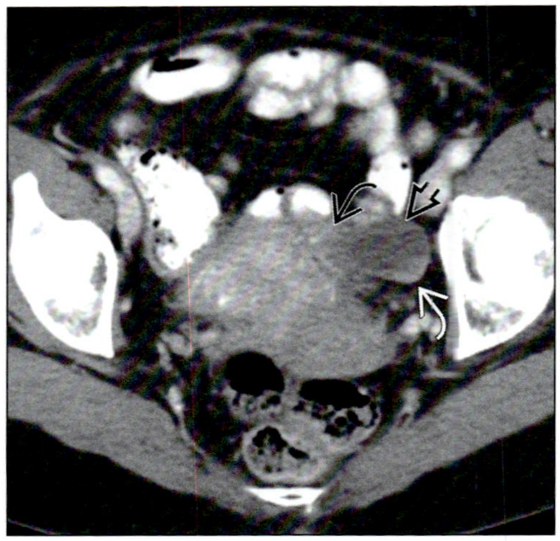

(Left) Axial CECT in the same patient shows extensive left paraaortic and aortocaval lymphadenopathy. *(Right)* Coronal CECT in the same patient shows the sausage-shaped hydrosalpinx with enhancing soft tissue tumor at its uterine end. The location of the hydrosalpinx inferior to the uterus is unusual and is likely due to the increased weight of the mucus-filled fallopian tube.

Stage IIIC (T2a N1 M0)

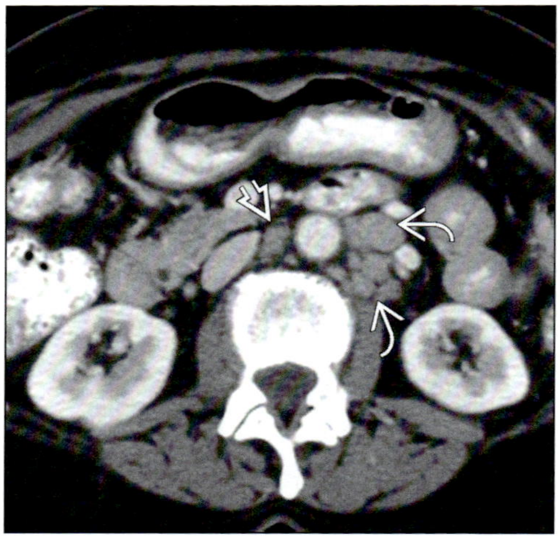

Stage IIIC (T2a N1 M0)

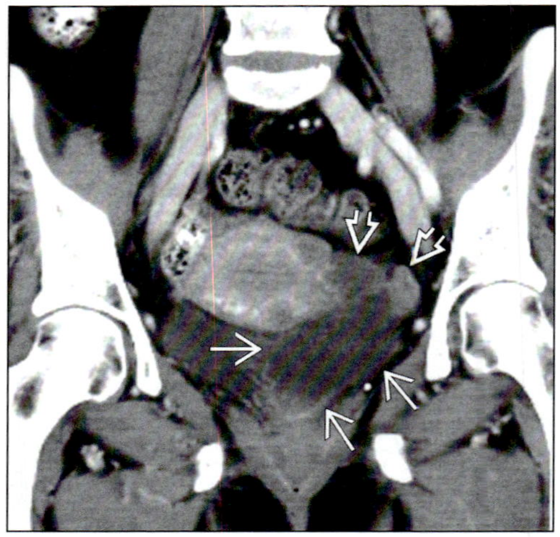

(Left) Coronal CECT in the same patient shows almost the entire length of the fluid-filled fallopian tube located between the uterus and the partially filled urinary bladder. *(Right)* Coronal CECT in the same patient shows left paraaortic and aortocaval lymphadenopathy. Left tubal adenocarcinoma involving the uterus with retroperitoneal metastatic disease was confirmed during surgery.

Stage IIIC (T2a N1 M0)

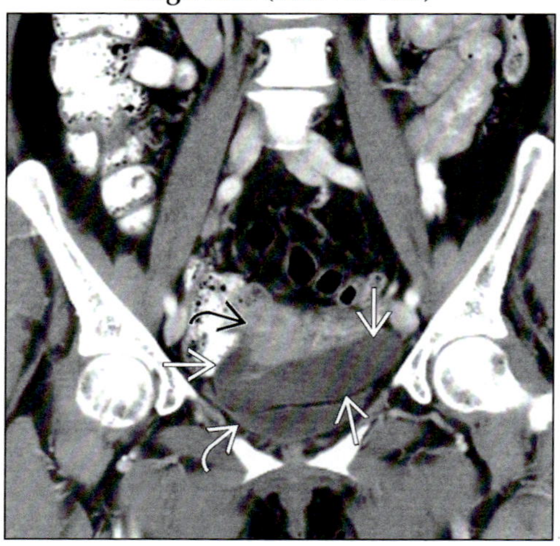

Stage IIIC (T2a N1 M0)

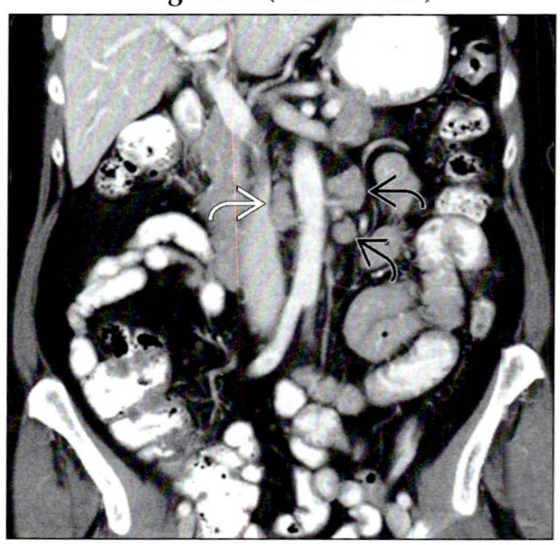

FALLOPIAN TUBE CARCINOMA

Stage IIIC (T2b N1 M0)

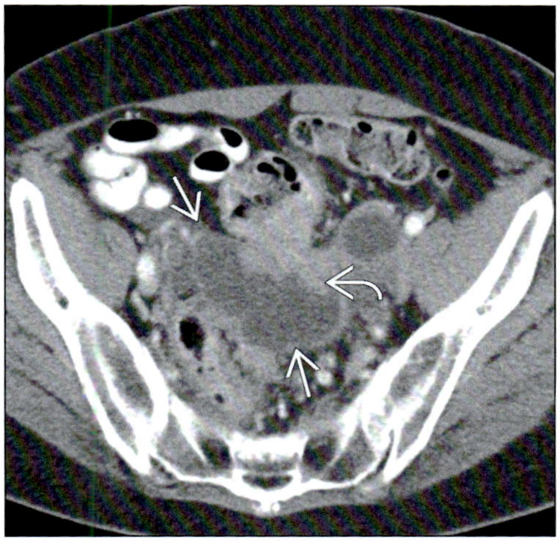

Stage IIIC (T2b N1 M0)

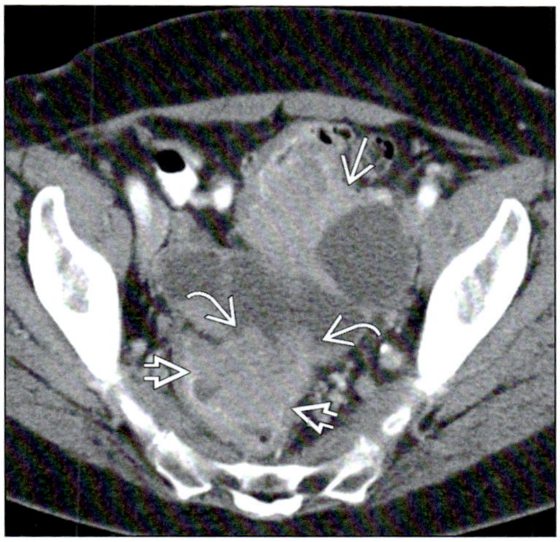

(Left) *Axial CECT in a 73-year-old woman who presented with abdominal pain shows a sausage-shaped, predominantly cystic mass with mural papillary projections.* ***(Right)*** *Axial CECT in the same patient shows the cystic mass arising from the left cornu of the uterus. The solid component of the mass extends through the wall and invades the rectum.*

Stage IIIC (T2b N1 M0)

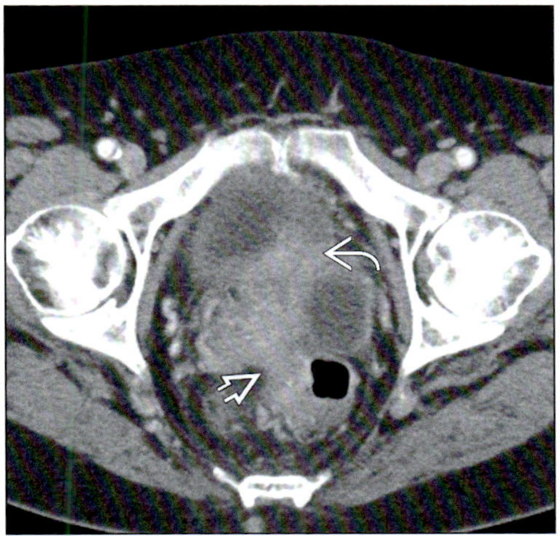

Stage IIIC (T2b N1 M0)

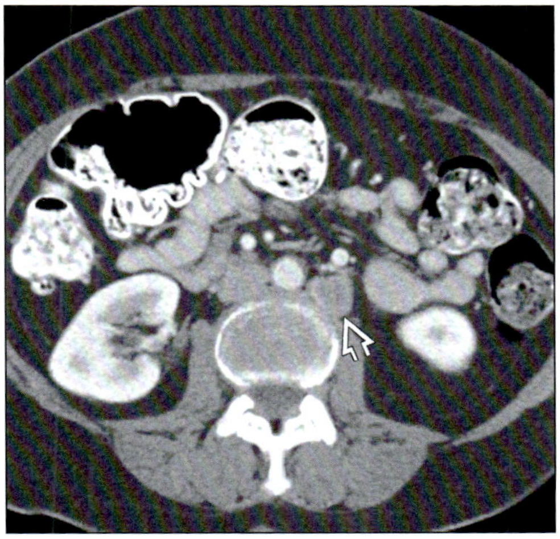

(Left) *Axial CECT in the same patient at a lower level shows tumor invading the posterior wall of the urinary bladder as well as the rectum.* ***(Right)*** *Axial CECT in the same patient shows an enlarged necrotic left paraaortic lymph node.*

Stage IIIC (T2b N1 M0)

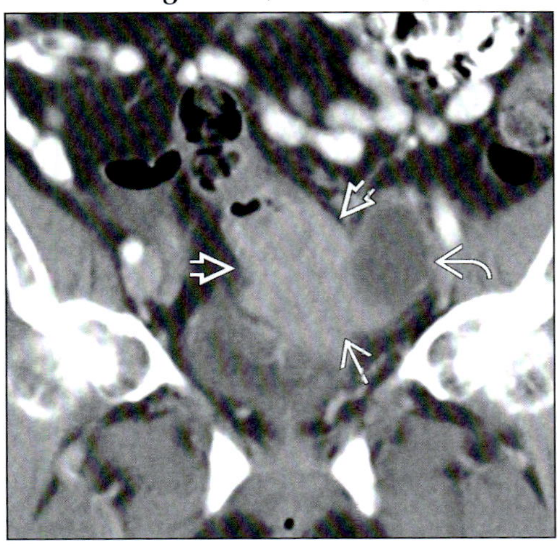

Stage IIIC (T2b N1 M0)

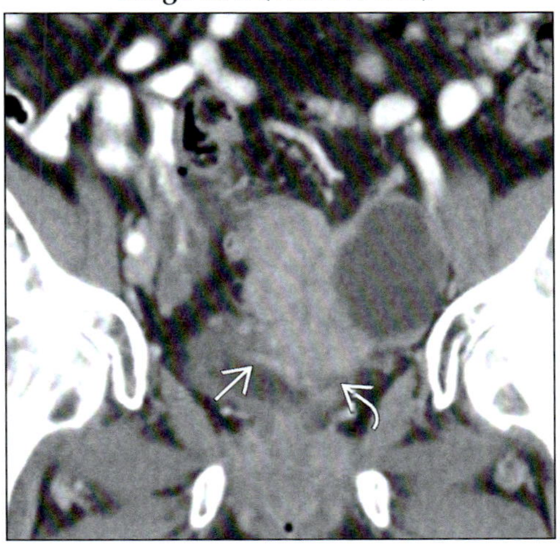

(Left) *Coronal CECT in the same patient shows the cystic component of the mass as well as the solid component invading the wall of the rectum.* ***(Right)*** *Coronal CECT in the same patient shows tumor invading the wall of the urinary bladder with enhancement of the bladder mucosa. Tumor extension to pelvic organs other than the uterus and ovaries constitutes T2b disease.*

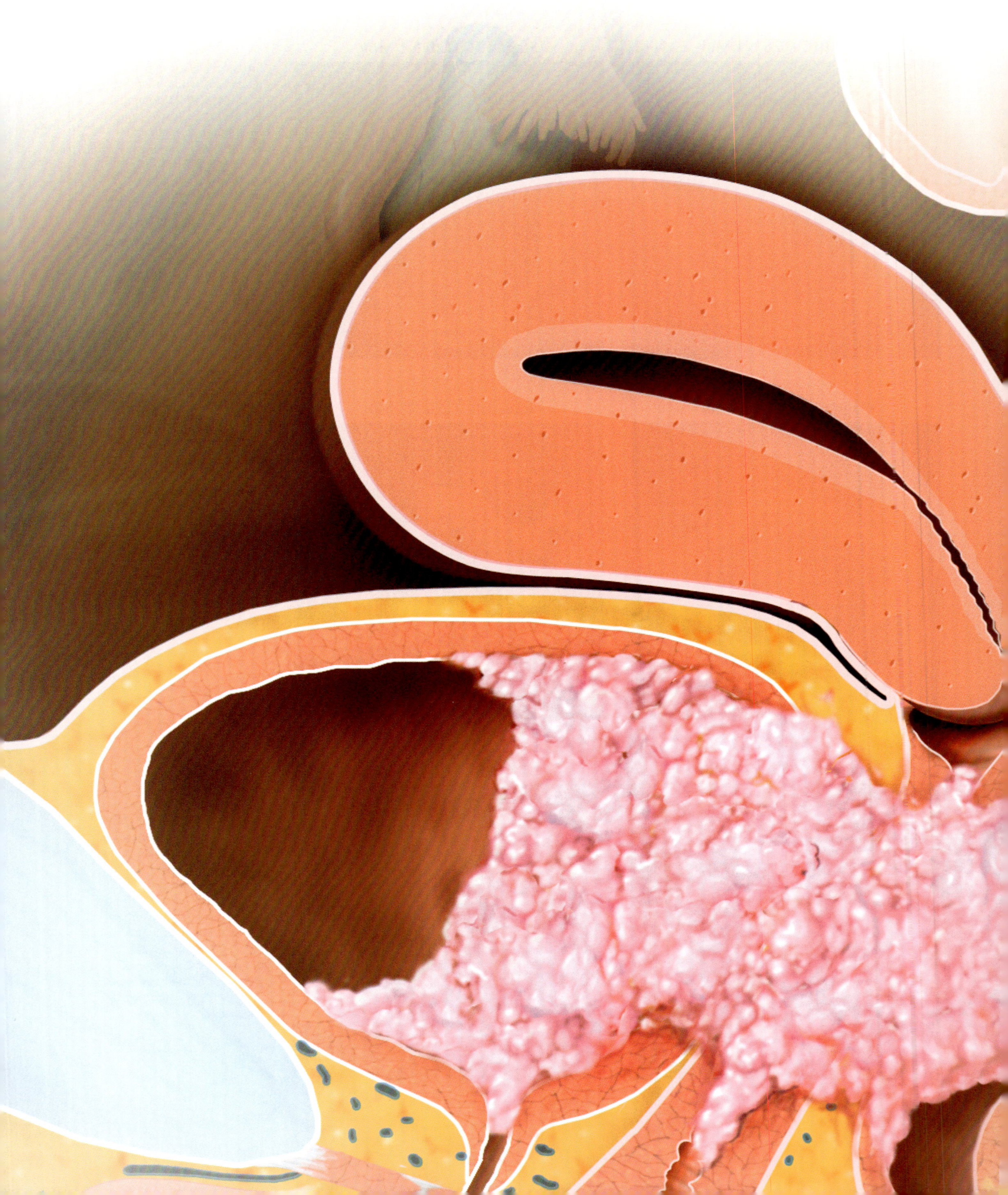

Vaginal Carcinoma

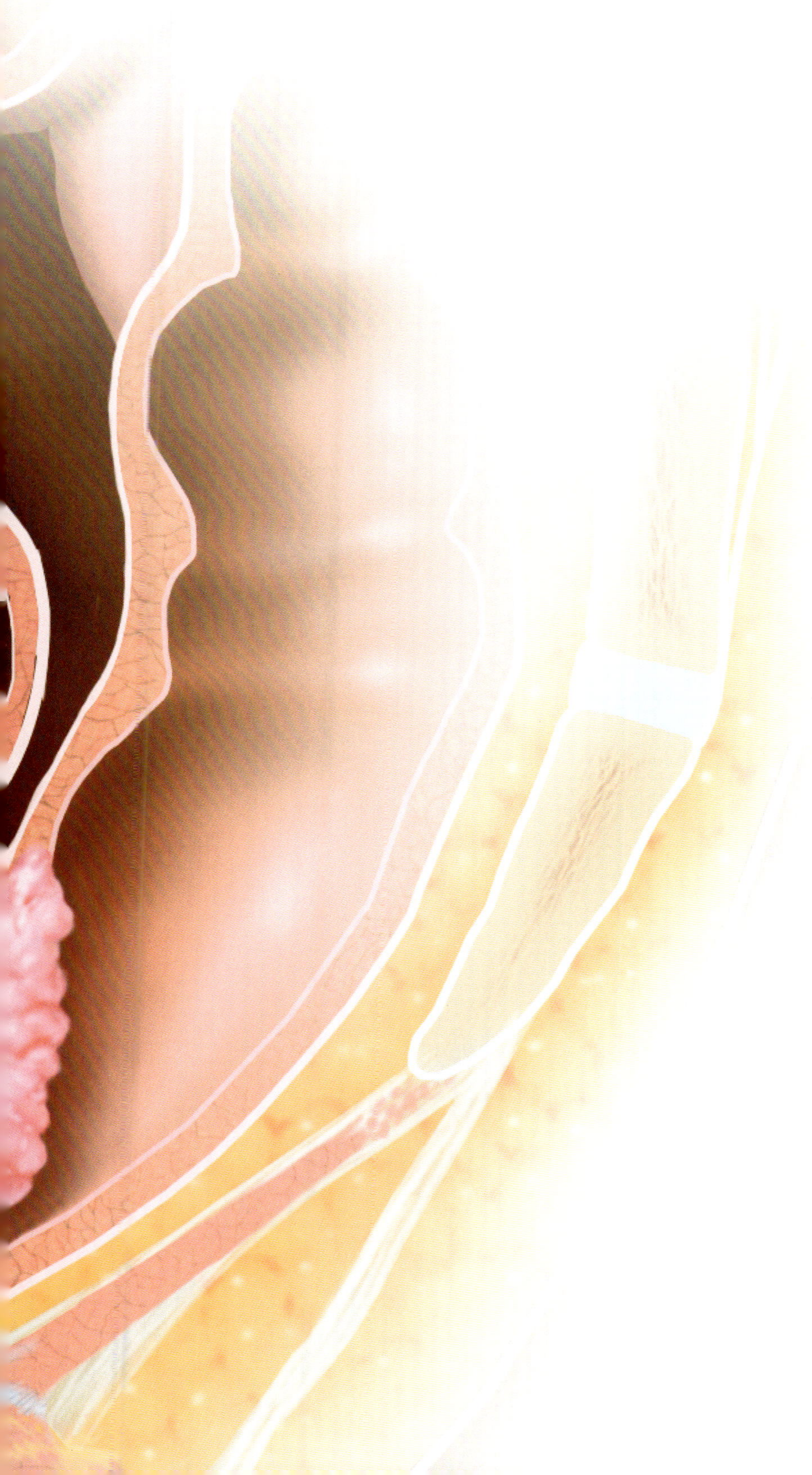

VAGINAL CARCINOMA

(T) Primary Tumor

Adapted from 7th edition AJCC Staging Forms.

TNM	*FIGO*	*Definitions*
TX		Primary tumor cannot be assessed
T0		No evidence of primary tumor
Tis[1]		Carcinoma in situ (preinvasive carcinoma)
T1	I	Tumor confined to vagina
T2	II	Tumor invades paravaginal tissues but not to pelvic wall
T3	III	Tumor extends to pelvic wall[2]
T4	IVA	Tumor invades mucosa of the bladder or rectum &/or extends beyond true pelvis (bullous edema is not sufficient evidence to classify a tumor as T4)

(N) Regional Lymph Nodes

NX		Regional lymph nodes cannot be assessed
N0		No regional lymph node metastasis
N1	III	Pelvic or inguinal lymph node metastasis

(M) Distant Metastasis

M0		No distant metastasis
M1	IVB	Distant metastasis

[1]FIGO no longer includes stage 0 (Tis). [2]Pelvic wall is defined as muscle, fascia, neurovascular structures, or skeletal portions of the bony pelvis. On rectal examination, there is no cancer-free space between the tumor and pelvic wall.

AJCC Stages/Prognostic Groups

Adapted from 7th edition AJCC Staging Forms.

Stage	*T*	*N*	*M*
0	Tis	N0	M0
I	T1	N0	M0
II	T2	N0	M0
III	T1-T3	N1	M0
	T3	N0	M0
IVA	T4	Any N	M0
IVB	Any T	Any N	M1

VAGINAL CARCINOMA

Tis

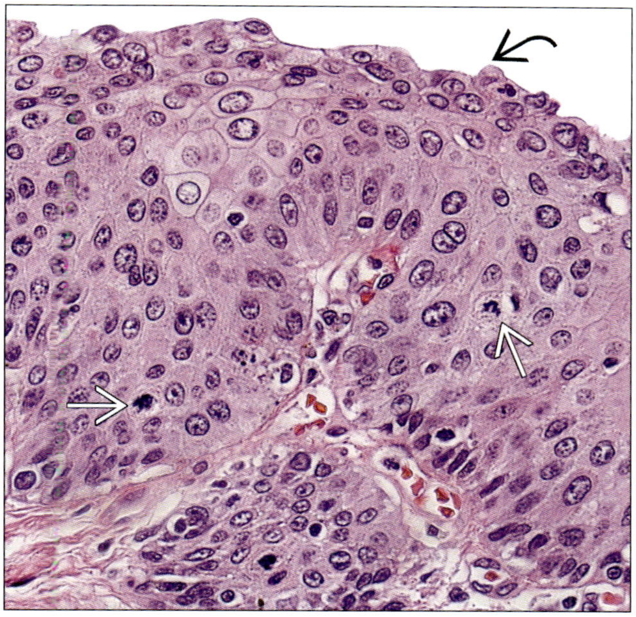

H&E stain shows dysplastic cells with enlarged and pleomorphic nuclei and high nuclear-to-cytoplasmic ratio involving the full thickness of the mucosa. Numerous dysplastic cells extend all the way to the surface →. Mitotic figures are evident ➔. (Original magnification 400x.)

Invasive Sqamous Cell Carcinoma (T1)

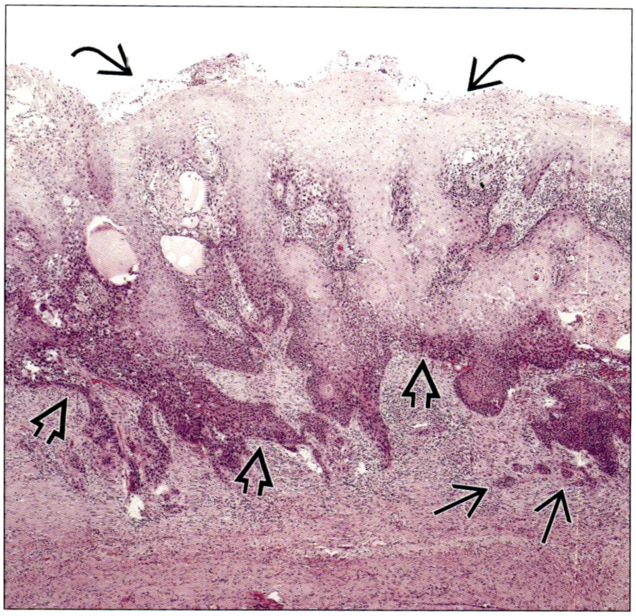

Low-power magnification of H&E stain shows nonstratified squamous epithelium of vaginal mucosa with invasive squamous cell carcinoma. Both the mucosal surface → and irregular basement membrane ⇨ are highlighted. Few nests are noted deeper in the submucosa →. (Original magnification 20x.)

Invasive Sqamous Cell Carcinoma (T1)

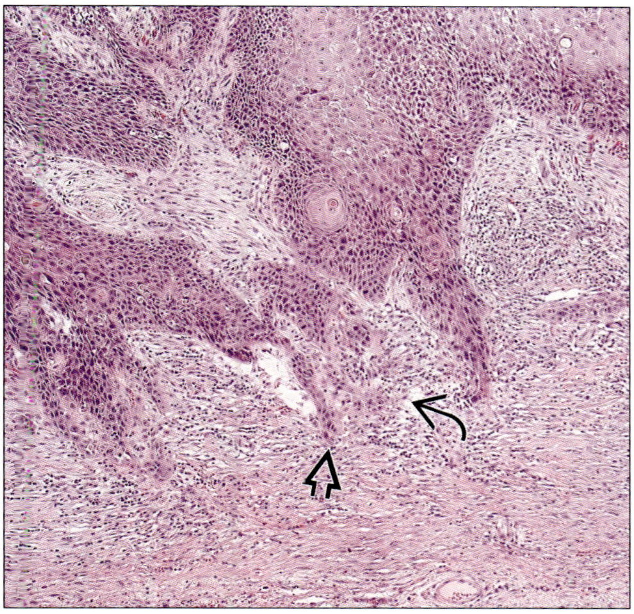

Higher magnification of the lower aspect of the mucosa shows irregular basement membrane with projections of cords ⇨ and nests → of cells indicating an invasive component to the submucosa. (Original magnification 100x.)

T3

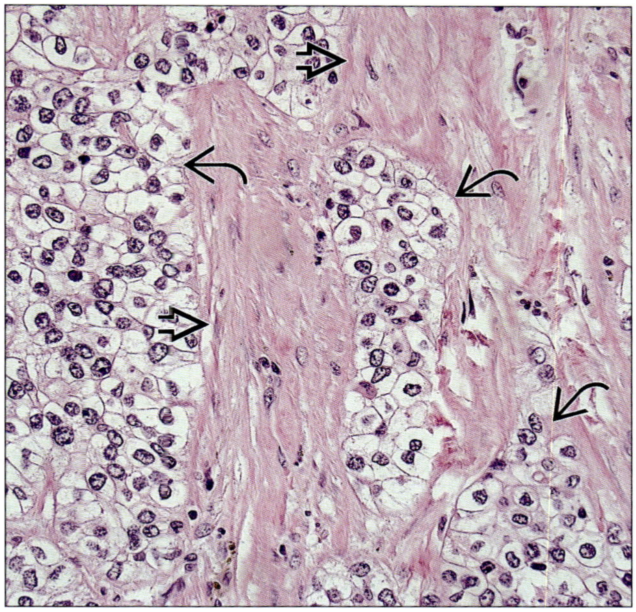

Tumor extends to the pelvic wall (T3). H&E stain from pelvic wall nodule shows vaginal squamous carcinoma. Note the nests and sheets of neoplastic squamous cells → invading into the fibroconnective tissue and fascia ⇨ of the pelvic wall. (Original magnification 400x.)

VAGINAL CARCINOMA

T1

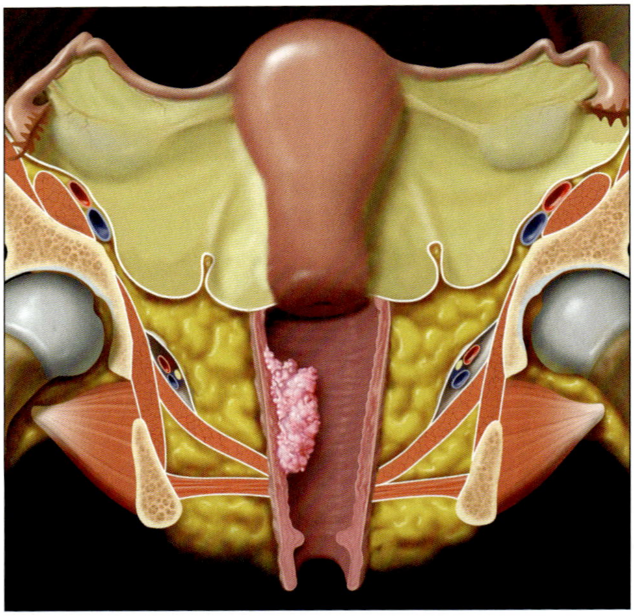

Graphic illustrates T1 tumor. Tumor is confined to the vagina without invasion of the paravaginal tissues.

T2

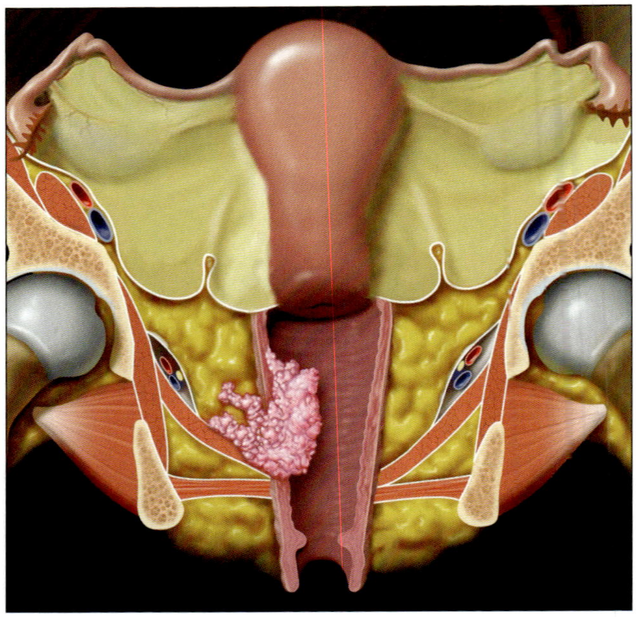

Graphic illustrates T2 tumor. Tumor invades paravaginal tissues but does not reach to the pelvic wall.

T3

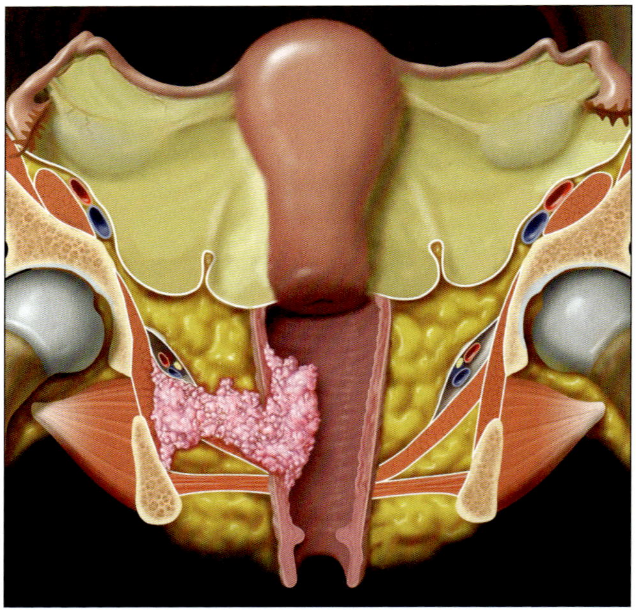

Graphic illustrates T3 tumor. Tumor invades paravaginal tissues and extends to the pelvic wall. Pelvic wall is defined as muscle, fascia, neurovascular structures, or bony pelvis.

T4

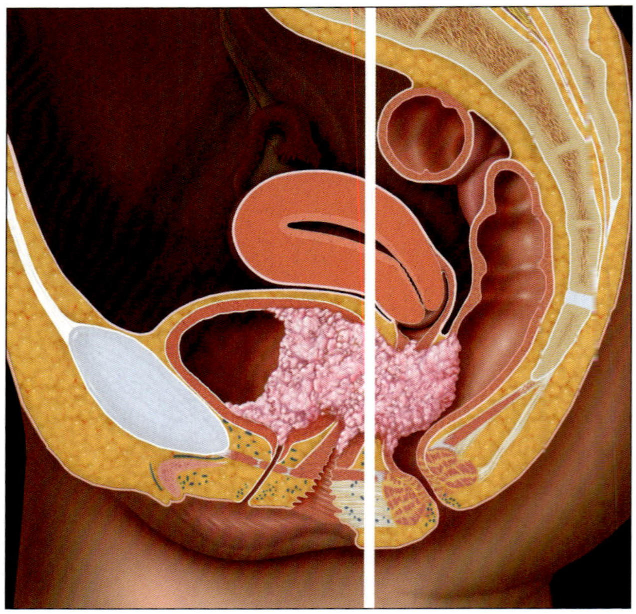

Graphic illustrates T4 tumor. Tumor invades mucosa of bladder (to the left of the divider) or rectum (to the right of the divider) &/or extends beyond the true pelvis.

Nodal Drainage of the Vagina

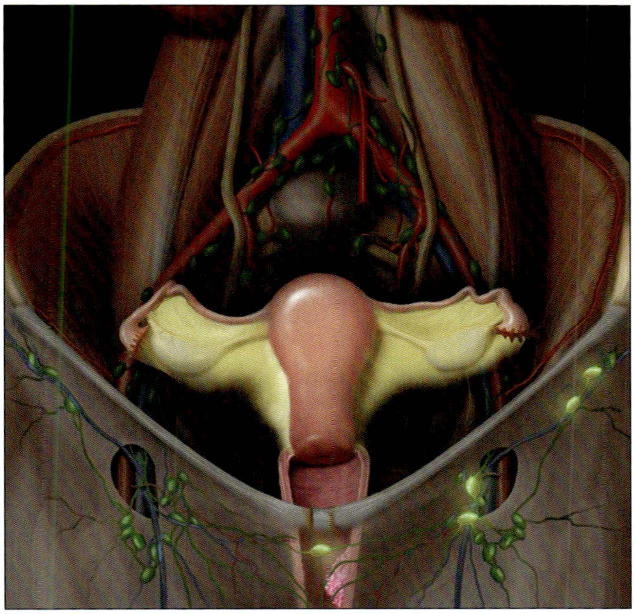

Graphic illustrates nodal drainage of tumors arising in the lower 1/3 of the vagina. Those tumors spread to inguinal and femoral lymph nodes.

Nodal Drainage of the Vagina

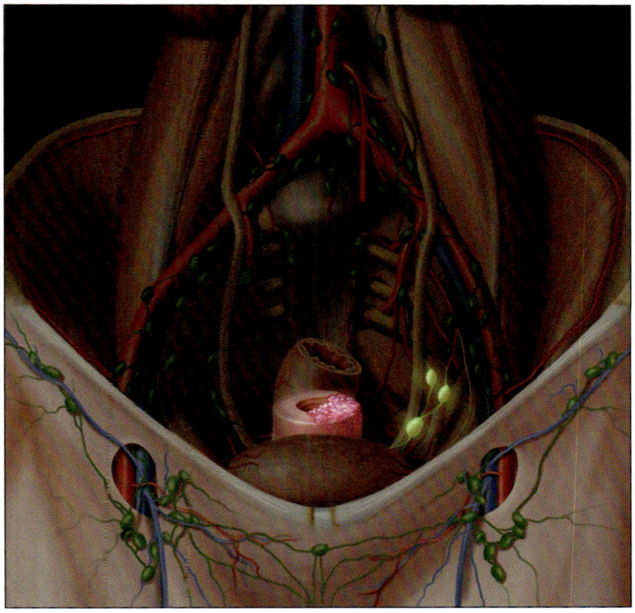

Graphic illustrates nodal drainage of tumors arising in the upper 2/3 of the vagina. Those tumors spread to pelvic lymph nodes, including obturator and internal and external iliac nodes.

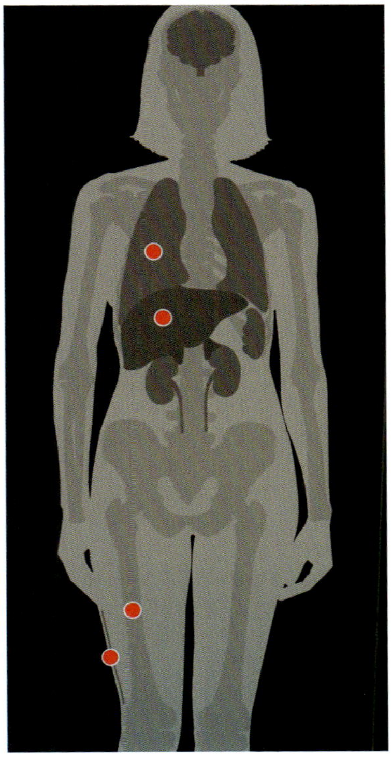

METASTASES, ORGAN FREQUENCY

Lungs

Liver

Bones

Skin

Because vaginal carcinoma is a rare tumor, there are no data present in the literature describing the incidence of distant metastases. Metastatic sites described in the literature include lungs, liver, bones, and skin.

VAGINAL CARCINOMA

OVERVIEW

General Comments

- Vaginal involvement with malignant disease occurs more commonly from metastatic spread
  - Most commonly due to direct local invasion from female urogenital tract
- Vaginal carcinoma should be diagnosed only if other gynecologic malignancies have been excluded
  - Tumor involving cervix, including external os, should always be assigned to carcinoma of cervix
  - Tumor involving vulva and extending to vagina should always be assigned to carcinoma of vulva
  - Different clinical approaches in treatment of cervical and vulvar carcinoma

Classification

- Tumors involving vagina can be
  - Squamous cell carcinoma
    - Approximately 85-90% of cases
  - Adenocarcinoma
    - Approximately 10% of cases
  - Adenosquamous carcinoma
    - Approximately 1-2% of cases
  - Melanoma
  - Sarcoma

PATHOLOGY

Routes of Spread

- Local spread
  - Tumor spreads locally into paravaginal soft tissues and eventually to pelvic side wall, mucosa of bladder, or rectum
- Lymphatic spread
  - Early spread to regional lymph nodes
    - 1/3 of patients have pelvic or groin lymph node involvement at diagnosis
  - Nodal spread usually depends on site of primary tumor
    - Expected nodal disease
      - Upper and middle 1/3 → pelvic obturator nodes, internal and external iliac nodes, and paraaortic nodes
      - Lower 1/3 → inguinal and femoral nodes
      - Disease progression or tumor involving whole length of vagina may → inguinal and iliac nodes
  - Lymphatic drainage does not always follow expected lymphatic channels predicted anatomically based on tumor location
- Hematogenous spread
  - Most common sites of distant metastases are lung, liver, and bone

General Features

- Etiology
  - Squamous cell carcinoma
    - Squamous carcinoma of vagina is associated with human papilloma virus (HPV)
      - HPV viral particles can be identified in approximately 60% of invasive squamous cancers of vagina
      - Up to 30% of patients have history of intraepithelial or invasive carcinoma of cervix or vulva
  - Adenocarcinoma
    - Thought to arise from
      - Areas of vaginal adenosis
      - Foci of endometriosis
      - Wolffian rest remnants
      - Periurethral glands
    - Develop in up to 2% of women exposed in utero to diethylstilbestrol (DES)
      - 2/3 have history of in utero exposure to DES
      - Associated with congenital T-shaped uterus
- Epidemiology & cancer incidence
  - Uncommon tumor comprising 1-2% of gynecologic malignancies
    - 5th in frequency behind carcinoma of ovary, uterus, cervix, and vulva
  - 2,160 estimated new cases in USA in 2009
    - Highest incidence among African-American women (1.24 per 100,000 person-years)
  - 770 estimated deaths in USA in 2009
  - Age of presentation depends on histological type
    - Squamous cell carcinoma
      - Predominantly in postmenopausal women
      - Mean age ± standard deviation at diagnosis was 65.7 ± 14.3 years
    - Adenocarcinoma
      - Typically occurs in younger women ages 14–21 years (peak age: 19 years)
      - Majority are clear cell histology
- Associated diseases, abnormalities
  - Vaginal carcinoma frequently found in association with vaginal intraepithelial neoplasia

Gross Pathology & Surgical Features

- Most common patterns of presentation of vaginal squamous cell carcinoma are
  - Ulcerating lesion (50%)
  - Fungating mass (30%)
  - Annular constricting mass (20%)
- Tumor location in vagina depends on tumor histologic type
  - Squamous cell carcinoma
    - Occurs mainly in upper 1/3 on posterior wall
  - Adenocarcinoma
    - Occurs mainly in upper 1/3 on anterior wall

Microscopic Pathology

- Squamous cell carcinoma
  - Tumor composed of malignant squamous cells
  - Tumors can be graded as
    - Well differentiated
    - Moderately differentiated
    - Poorly differentiated
    - Undifferentiated
  - Squamous cell carcinoma can be
    - Keratinizing
    - Nonkeratinizing
  - Subtypes of squamous cell carcinoma include
    - Verrucous
    - Warty
    - Spindle
- Adenocarcinoma
  - Clear cell adenocarcinoma

- Tumor cells have clear or eosinophilic cytoplasm
- Type of vaginal adenocarcinoma related to DES exposure
- May be seen next to areas of adenosis in older women

○ Endometrioid adenocarcinoma
- Closely resemble morphology of uterine endometrial carcinoma
- May be seen in association with adenosis or endometriosis

○ Mucinous adenocarcinoma
- Rare in vagina
- Can be of endocervical or enteric (contain goblet cells) types

○ Mesonephric adenocarcinoma

IMAGING FINDINGS

Detection

- CT
  - Detection of vaginal carcinoma is difficult with CT
    - In 1 study, CT detected vaginal carcinoma in only 43% of patients
  - Tumors are only seen if large enough to alter vaginal contour
- MR
  - Location and extent best assessed with high-resolution T2-weighted imaging
  - Improved detection of vaginal pathology by intravaginal instillation of ultrasound gel
  - Appearance on MR imaging correlates with macroscopic patterns of disease
    - Ill-defined, irregular, diffuse mass (ulcerating pattern of disease)
    - Well-defined lobulated mass (fungating pattern of disease)
    - Circumferential thickening (annular constricting pattern of disease)
  - T1WI
    - Isointense to muscle
    - May be difficult to see unless large enough to alter vaginal contour
  - T2WI
    - Mass of homogeneous intermediate signal intensity distinct from low signal intensity of vaginal wall
    - Hyperintense to muscles, lower than that of fat
    - Presence of high signal intensity foci likely due to tumoral necrosis should raise possibility of
      - Poorly differentiated squamous cell carcinoma
      - Adenosquamous carcinoma
      - Mucinous adenocarcinoma
- FDG PET
  - In 1 study, FDG PET identified abnormal vaginal uptake in 100% of patients with primary vaginal carcinoma

Staging

- **Local disease**
  - MR
    - Crucial in demonstrating
      - Tumor location
      - Parametrial extension
      - Pelvic sidewall involvement
      - Local extension to bladder or urethra and rectum
      - Regional lymph node involvement
    - T1
      - Tumor limited to vaginal mucosa
      - Appears as mass or plaque of tissue of intermediate signal intensity on T2WI, expanding and filling vagina
      - Preservation of low signal intensity of outer vaginal muscularis layer
    - T2
      - Extension into paravaginal tissue
      - Paravaginal fat is of abnormal low signal intensity on T1WI
      - Loss of low signal intensity of vaginal muscularis layer
    - T3
      - Tumor extends to pelvic sidewall (defined as muscle, fascia, neurovascular structures, or skeletal portions of bony pelvis)
      - Best seen on axial and coronal T2WI
      - Intermediate signal intensity tumor extends to and infiltrates low signal intensity muscles of pelvic sidewall and floor
    - T4
      - Invasion of bladder or rectal mucosa
      - Spreads beyond pelvis and may involve peritoneum and small or large bowel loops
      - Best evaluated on T2-weighted images
      - Invasion through low signal intensity of bladder or rectal wall
      - Loss of fat planes between vagina and bladder or rectum
      - Presence of bullous edema is not sufficient evidence to classify a tumor as T4
  - CT
    - Except in advanced disease CT is not helpful for local staging
      - Poor soft tissue characterization
- **Nodal metastases**
  - CT and MR can be equally useful in evaluating regional lymph nodes
  - PET/CT is superior to CT in identification of nodal metastases
  - Lymphoscintigraphy can be helpful in detection of nodal metastases
    - Nodal metastases do not always follows predicted patterns
    - May result in change of radiation field
- **Distant metastases**
  - CT or PET/CT are modalities of choice for evaluation of distant metastases
  - Lung metastatic nodules from squamous cell carcinoma frequently cavitate

Restaging

- CT or PET/CT is useful for detection of recurrent or metastatic tumor

CLINICAL ISSUES

Presentation

- Patients usually present with following symptoms
  - Painless vaginal bleeding (65-80%)

VAGINAL CARCINOMA

- Abnormal discharge (30%)
- Urinary symptoms (20%)
- Pelvic pain (15-30%)
- Feeling of vaginal mass (10%)
- Asymptomatic (10-27%)

Cancer Natural History & Prognosis

- 5-year survival depends on stage
  - Stage 0 (85%)
  - Stage I (61%)
  - Stage II (48%)
  - Stage III (34%)
  - Stage IVA (22%)
  - Stage IVB (11%)
- Exophytic tumors are associated with significantly better prognosis than infiltrative ones
  - Possibly because exophytic tumors tend to grow more superficially, while ulcerative lesions are more likely to invade adjacent pelvic structures

Treatment Options

- Treatment options by stage
  - Squamous cell carcinoma in situ
    - Wide local excision ± skin grafting
    - Partial or total vaginectomy with skin grafting for multifocal or extensive disease
    - Intravaginal chemotherapy with 5% fluorouracil cream
    - Laser therapy
    - Intracavitary radiation therapy delivering 60-70 Gy to mucosa
      - Entire vaginal mucosa should be treated
  - Stage I squamous cell carcinoma
    - Superficial lesions < 0.5 cm thick
      - Intracavitary radiation therapy
      - External beam radiation therapy (EBRT) for bulky lesions
      - For lesions of lower 1/3 of vagina, elective radiation therapy to pelvic ± inguinal lymph nodes
      - Wide local excision or total vaginectomy with vaginal reconstruction, especially in lesions of upper vagina
      - In cases with close or positive surgical margins, adjuvant radiation therapy should be considered
    - Lesions > 0.5 cm thick
      - Upper 1/3: Radical vaginectomy + pelvic lymphadenectomy ± construction of neovagina
      - Lower 1/3: Radical vaginectomy + inguinal lymphadenectomy
      - Adjuvant radiation therapy in cases with close or positive surgical margins
      - Combination of interstitial (single-plane implant) and intracavitary therapy
      - EBRT for poorly differentiated or infiltrating tumors
      - Elective radiation therapy to pelvic ± inguinal lymph nodes
  - Stage I adenocarcinoma
    - Total radical vaginectomy + hysterectomy with lymph node dissection
      - Upper vagina: Deep pelvic nodes dissection
      - Lower vagina: Inguinal nodes dissection
    - Adjuvant radiation therapy in cases with close or positive surgical margins
    - Combination of interstitial (single-plane implant) and intracavitary therapy
    - For lesions of lower 1/3 of vagina, elective radiation therapy to pelvic ± inguinal lymph nodes
    - Combined local therapy in selected cases, which may include wide local excision, lymph node sampling, and interstitial therapy
  - Stage II squamous cell carcinoma or adenocarcinoma
    - Combination of brachytherapy and EBRT
    - For lesions of lower 1/3 of vagina, elective radiation therapy to pelvic &/or inguinal lymph nodes
    - Radical vaginectomy or pelvic exenteration ± radiation therapy
  - Stage III, IVA squamous cell carcinoma or adenocarcinoma
    - Combination of interstitial, intracavitary, and EBRT
    - Rarely, surgery may be combined with above
  - Stage IVB squamous cell carcinoma or adenocarcinoma
    - Radiation (for palliation of symptoms) ± chemotherapy

REPORTING CHECKLIST

T Staging

- MR is imaging modality of choice for assessment of local tumor
  - Tumor limited to vaginal mucosa is T1
  - Extension into paravaginal tissue is T2
  - Extension to pelvic sidewall is T3
  - Invasion of bladder or rectal mucosa or spread beyond pelvis or involvement of peritoneum and small or large bowel loops

N Staging

- CT, MR, PET/CT, or lymphoscintigraphy for detection of nodal disease
- May involve inguinal, femoral, pelvic, or paraaortic nodes

M Staging

- CT or PET/CT for detection of distal metastases
- Lung is most common site for distal metastases

SELECTED REFERENCES

1. American Joint Committee on Cancer: AJCC Cancer Staging Manual. 7th ed. New York: Springer, 2010
2. Shah CA et al: Factors affecting risk of mortality in women with vaginal cancer. Obstet Gynecol. 113(5):1038-45, 2009
3. Griffin N et al: Magnetic resonance imaging of vaginal and vulval pathology. Eur Radiol. 18(6):1269-80, 2008
4. Parikh JH et al: MR imaging features of vaginal malignancies. Radiographics. 28(1):49-63; quiz 322, 2008
5. Taylor MB et al: Magnetic resonance imaging of primary vaginal carcinoma. Clin Radiol. 62(6):549-55, 2007
6. Lamoreaux WT et al: FDG-PET evaluation of vaginal carcinoma. Int J Radiat Oncol Biol Phys. 62(3):733-7, 2005

VAGINAL CARCINOMA

Stage I (T1 N0 M0)

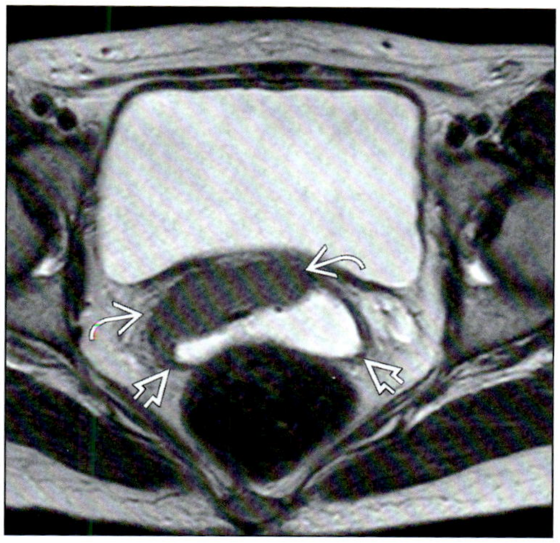

Stage I (T1 N0 M0)

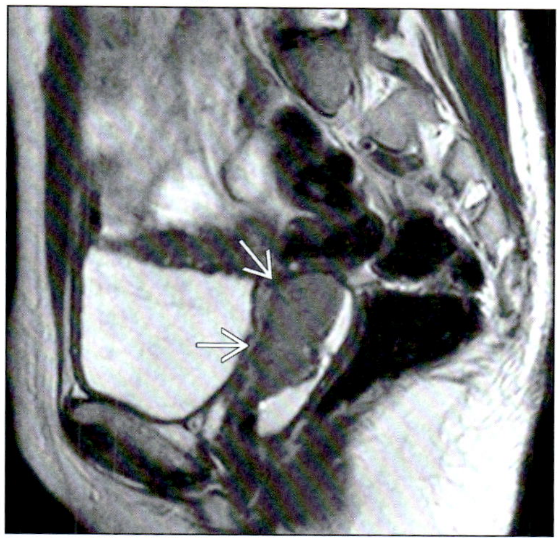

(Left) *Axial T2WI MR in a 52-year-old woman who had a hysterectomy at the age of 40 due to uterine leiomyomas shows an intermediate signal tumor ➔ involving the right anterior aspect of the gel-filled vagina ➔. Tumor is limited by the vaginal wall with no invasion of the paravaginal tissues.* ***(Right)*** *Sagittal T2WI MR in the same patient shows the tumor ➔ involving the upper and middle 1/3 of the vagina.*

Stage I (T1 N0 M0)

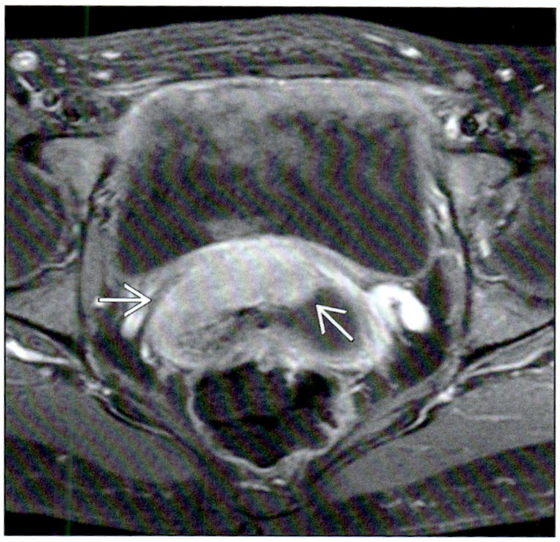

Stage I (T1 N0 M0)

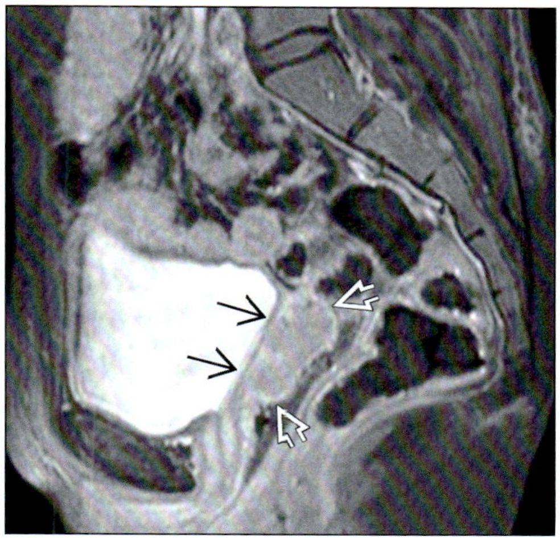

(Left) *Axial T1WI C+ FS MR in the same patient shows enhancement of the vaginal tumor ➔ with no enhancing nodules extending into the paravaginal fat.* ***(Right)*** *Sagittal T1WI C+ FS MR in the same patient shows enhancing tumor ➔ with clear plane ➔ between the vaginal tumor and the contrast-filled urinary bladder.*

Stage I (T1 N0 M0)

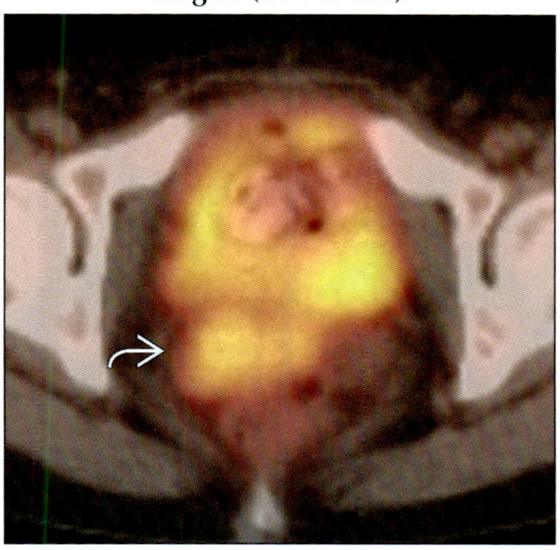

Stage I (T1 N0 M0)

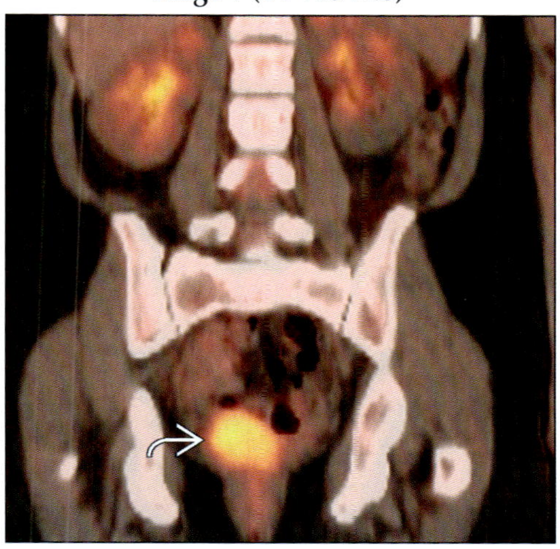

(Left) *Axial PET/CT in the same patient shows increased metabolic activity within the vaginal mass ➔.* ***(Right)*** *Coronal PET/CT in the same patient shows increased metabolic activity within the vaginal mass ➔. No other metastatic lesions were detected. Tumor limited to the vagina without paravaginal involvement constitutes T1 disease.*

VAGINAL CARCINOMA

(**Left**) *Sagittal T2WI MR shows a lobulated mass → of intermediate signal intensity filling the left posterior vaginal fornix. There is no extension outside the vagina.* (**Right**) *Axial T2WI MR in the same patient shows a polypoidal vaginal carcinoma → filling the left side of the posterior vaginal fornix. The low signal intensity cervical stroma → is intact without evidence of invasion.*

Stage I (T1 N0 M0)

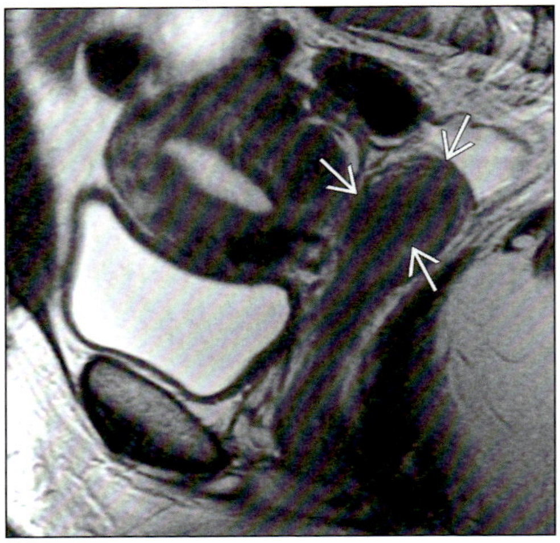

Stage I (T1 N0 M0)

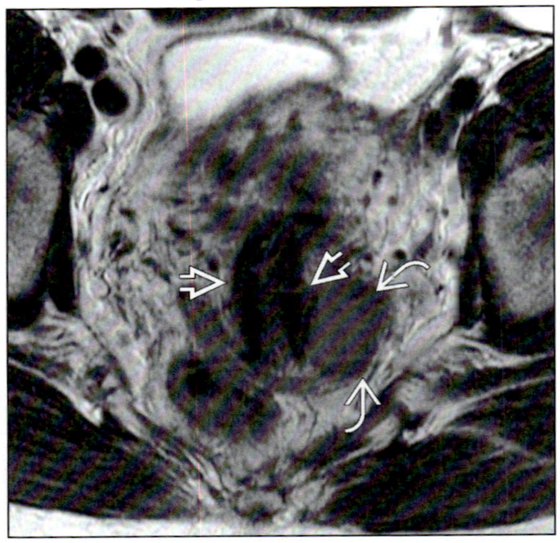

(**Left**) *Sagittal T2WI MR shows a large polypoid mass → expanding the vaginal lumen. The cervix → is not involved.* (**Right**) *Coronal T2WI MR in the same patient shows a vaginal mass → with irregular nodular interface → with the paravaginal tissues due to paravaginal fat invasion. Paravaginal fat invasion without extension to pelvic wall represents T2 disease.*

Stage II (T2 N0 M0)

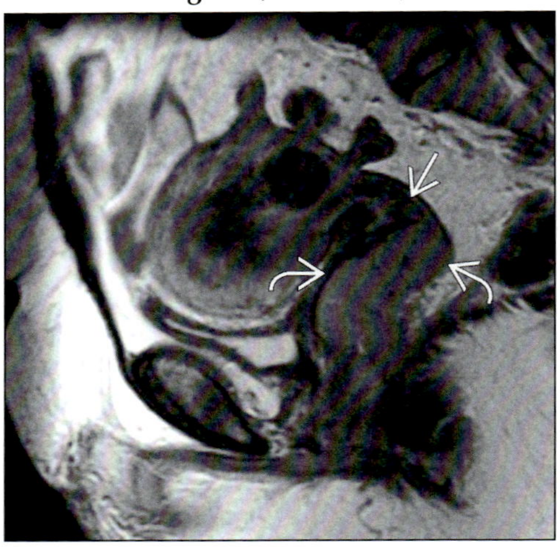

Stage II (T2 N0 M0)

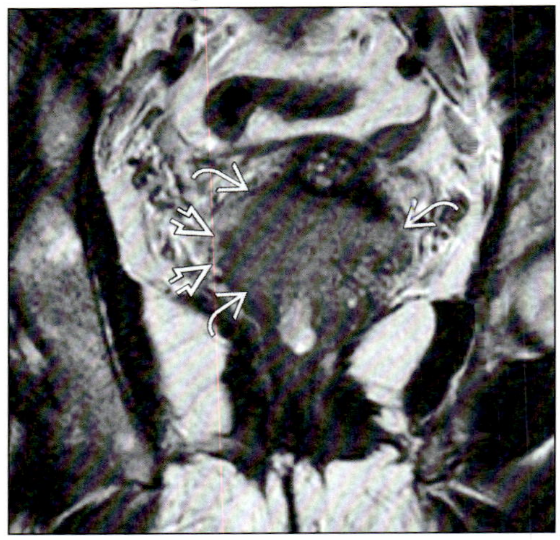

(**Left**) *Axial T2WI MR in the same patient shows a tumor → filling the vagina, with paravaginal invasion → disrupting the low signal intensity vaginal wall.* (**Right**) *Axial T1WI C+ MR shows an enhancing vaginal mass → with bilateral extension into the paravaginal fat →. Note the clear interface → anteriorly between the vagina and the posterior wall of the urinary bladder.*

Stage II (T2 N0 M0)

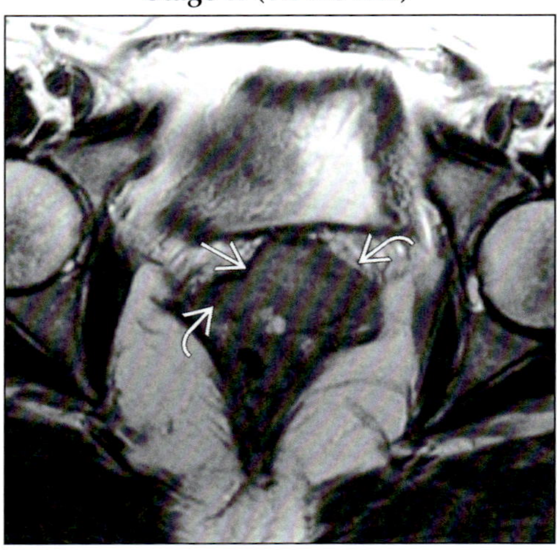

Stage II (T2 N0 M0)

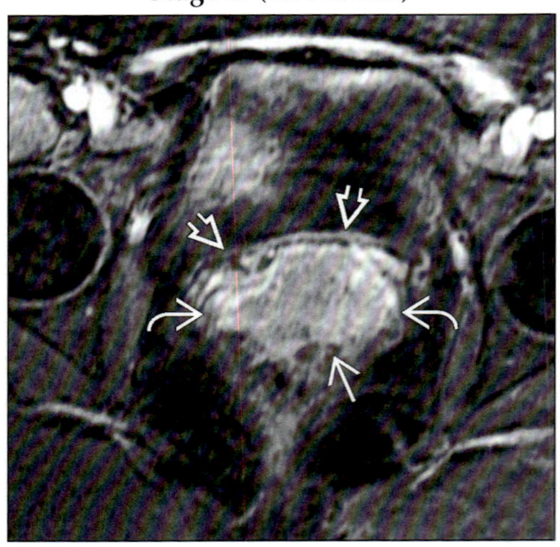

VAGINAL CARCINOMA

Stage IVA (T4 N1 M0)

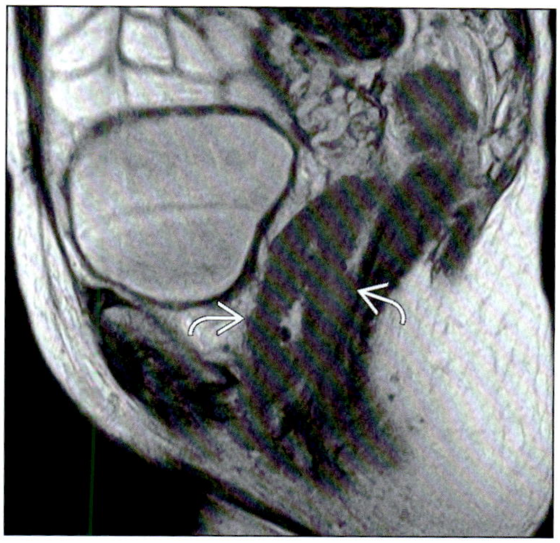

Stage IVA (T4 N1 M0)

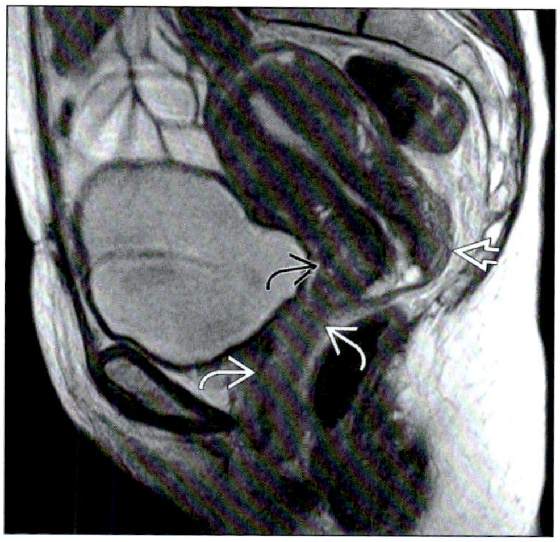

(Left) *Sagittal T2WI MR to the right of the midline in a 45-year-old woman, who presented with vaginal bleeding and discharge, shows circumferential thickening of the vaginal wall involving almost the entire length of the vagina.* ***(Right)*** *Sagittal T2WI MR in the same patient close to the midline shows thickening of the vaginal wall. The cervix is normal. Tumor extends into the anterior vaginal fornix.*

Stage IVA (T4 N1 M0)

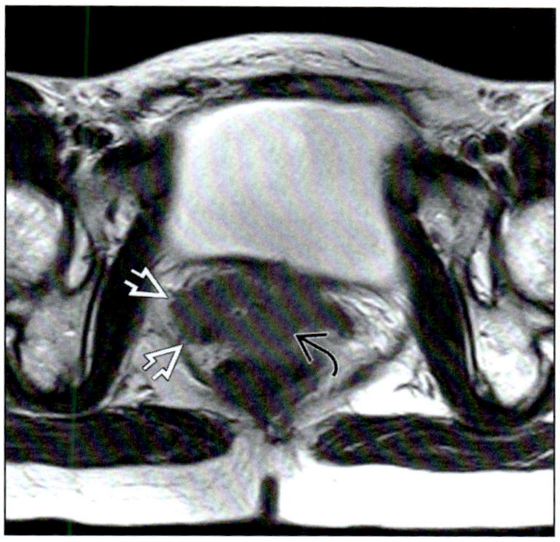

Stage IVA (T4 N1 M0)

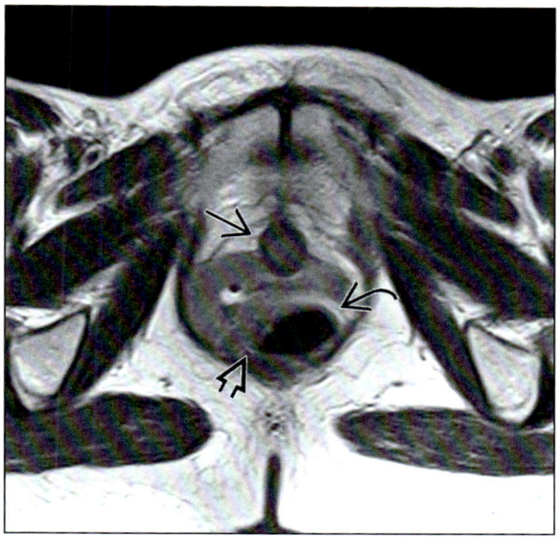

(Left) *Axial T2WI MR in the same patient shows thickening of the vaginal wall with extension into the right paravaginal fat.* ***(Right)*** *Axial T2WI MR in the same patient shows tumor extension to involve the right side of the rectum. Compare this to the clear fat plane between the vagina and anterior aspect of the rectum. The low signal intensity around the urethra is preserved with no evidence of tumor invasion.*

Stage IVA (T4 N1 M0)

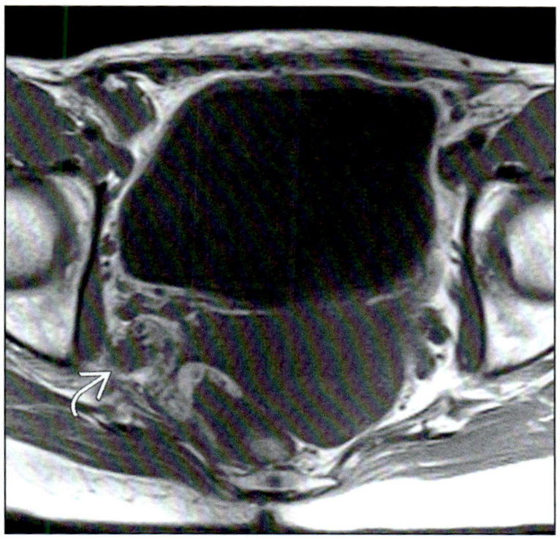

Stage IVA (T4 N1 M0)

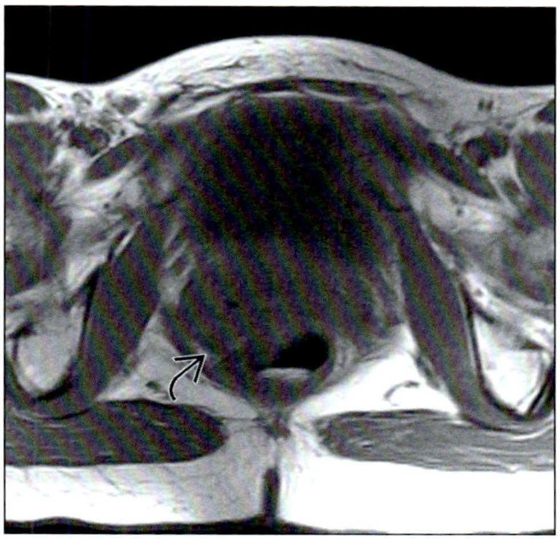

(Left) *Axial T1WI MR in the same patient shows a rounded and irregular right pelvic lymph node.* ***(Right)*** *Axial T1WI MR in the same patient shows tumor extending into the paravaginal fat. MR imaging should include imaging without fat suppression to allow visualization of intermediate signal linear or nodular tumor extension into paravaginal fat.*

VAGINAL CARCINOMA

Stage IVA (T4 N1 M0)

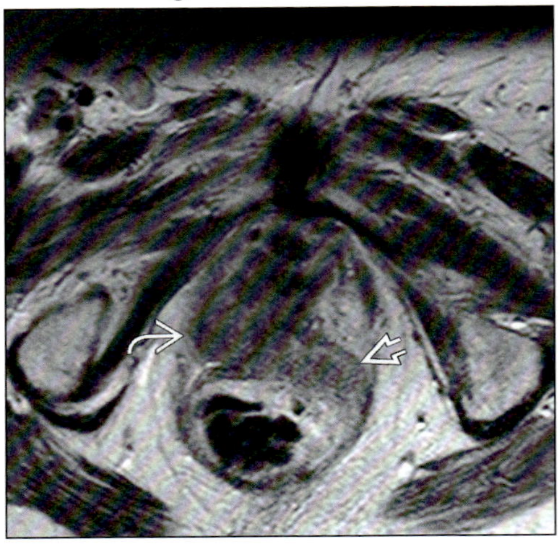

Stage IVA (T4 N1 M0)

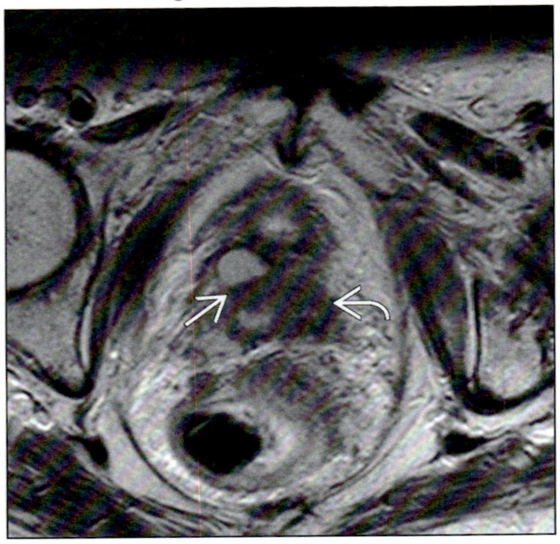

(Left) *Axial T2WI MR in an 85-year-old woman with ureteric duplication who presented with vaginal bleeding shows a slightly hyperintense heterogeneous vaginal mass with extension into the rectum .* ***(Right)*** *Axial T2WI MR in the same patient shows the vaginal mass with extension to involve a right side low inserting ectopic ureter.*

Stage IVA (T4 N1 M0)

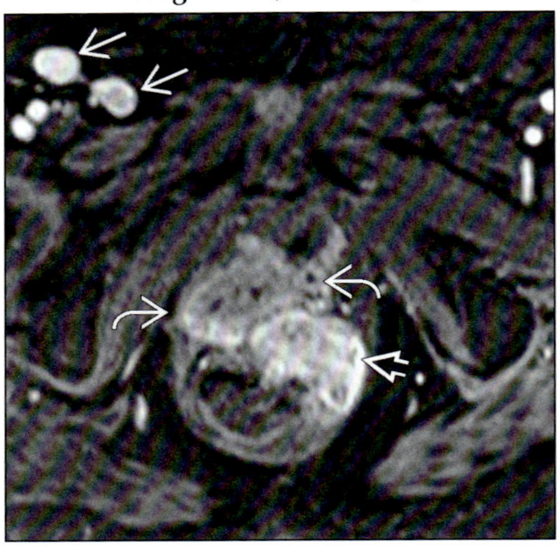

Stage IVA (T4 N1 M0)

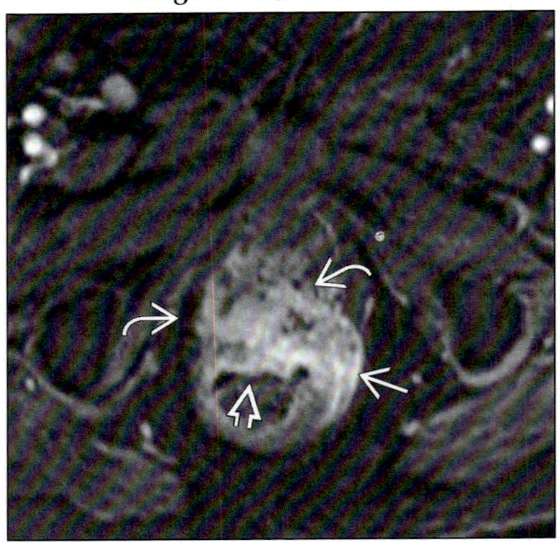

(Left) *Axial T1WI C+ FS MR in the same patient shows an enhancing vaginal mass with extension into the rectum . Note also the rounded right inguinal enhancing lymph nodes .* ***(Right)*** *Axial T1WI C+ FS MR in the same patient shows the vaginal enhancing mass extending into the rectal wall with enhancement of the rectal mucosa .*

Stage IVA (T4 N0 M0)

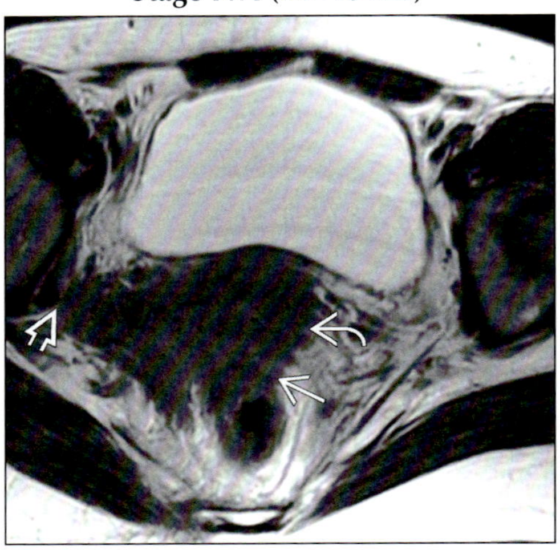

Stage IVA (T4 N0 M0)

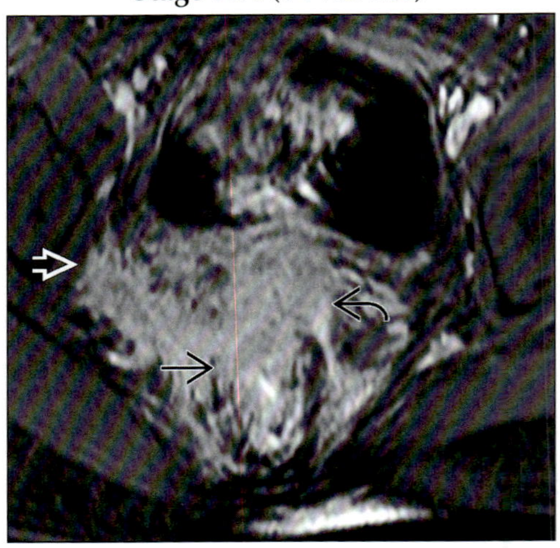

(Left) *Axial T2WI MR in a 65-year-old woman who presented with vaginal bleeding shows a vaginal mass of intermediate signal intensity that extends through the paravaginal fat to involve the pelvic side wall and rectum .* ***(Right)*** *Axial T1WI C+ FS MR in the same patient shows intense enhancement of the vaginal mass with enhancing soft tissue extending to involve the pelvic side wall and rectum .*

VAGINAL CARCINOMA

Stage IVA (T4 N0 M0)

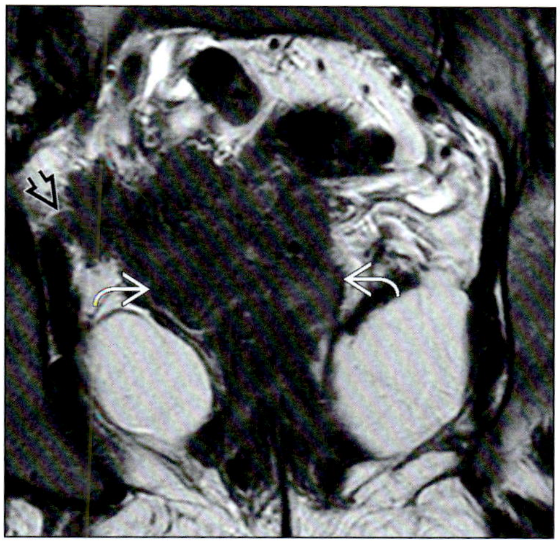

Stage IVA (T4 N0 M0)

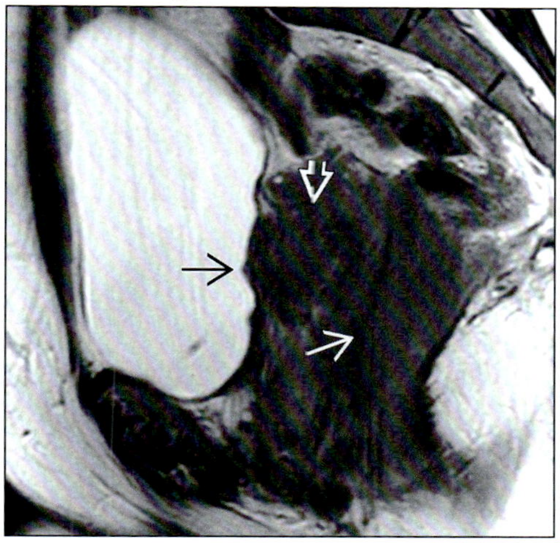

(Left) *Coronal T2WI MR in the same patient shows the vaginal mass with lateral extension to the pelvic side wall.* ***(Right)*** *Sagittal T2WI MR in the same patient shows a vaginal mass with anterior extension to involve the posterior wall of the urinary bladder and posterior extension to involve the rectum.*

Metastatic Vaginal Carcinoma

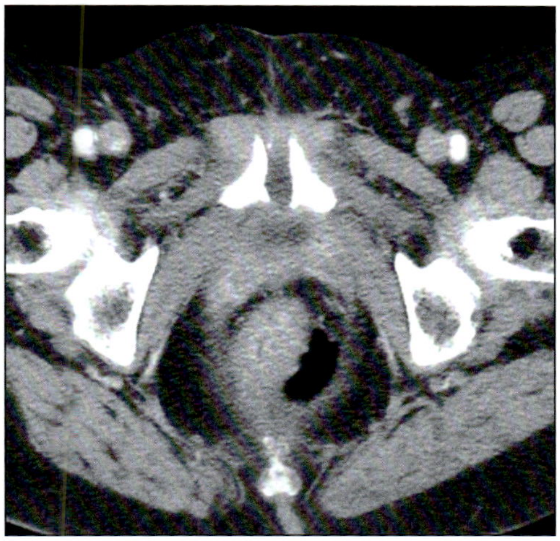

Metastatic Vaginal Carcinoma

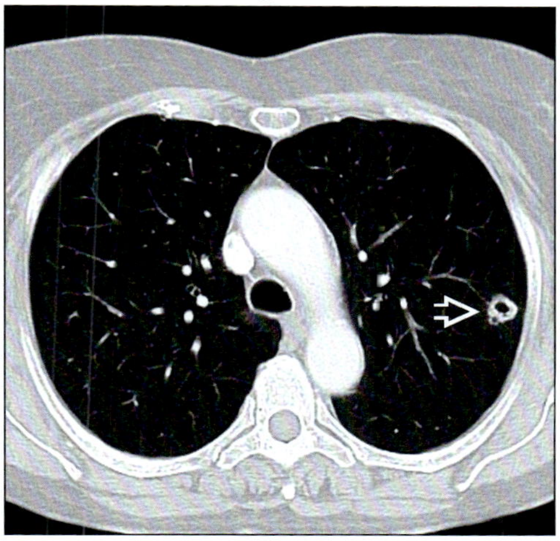

(Left) *Axial CECT in a 79-year-old woman who underwent radical vaginectomy for stage II vaginal squamous carcinoma shows no evidence of local recurrence.* ***(Right)*** *Axial CECT lung window in the same patient shows a cavitary lung lesion. Metastases from squamous carcinoma frequently cavitate. CT is useful for follow-up in patients with vaginal carcinoma for detection of local recurrence or metastatic disease.*

Local Recurrent Vaginal Carcinoma

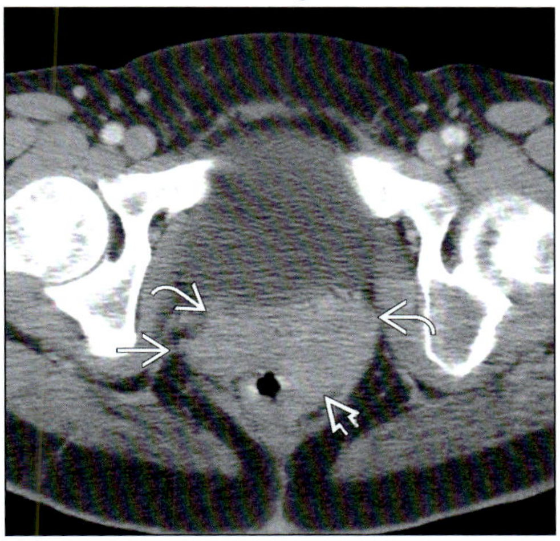

Local Recurrent Vaginal Carcinoma

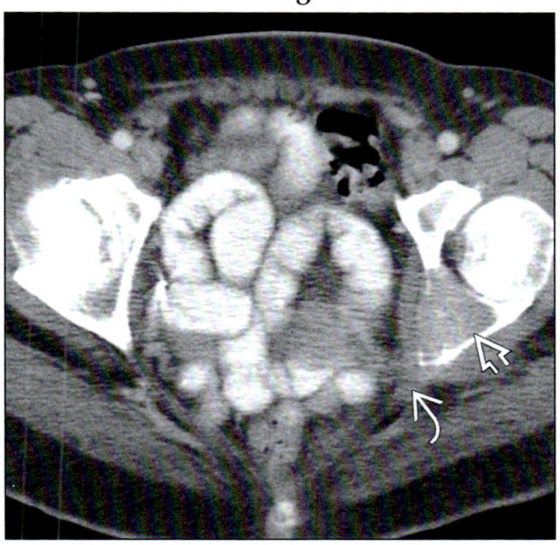

(Left) *Axial CECT in a 75-year-old woman who presented with stage III vaginal carcinoma and underwent radiation treatment shows a vaginal mass with extension to the paravaginal tissue and to the rectum.* ***(Right)*** *Axial CECT in the same patient also shows extension to the pelvic muscles and left ischium.*

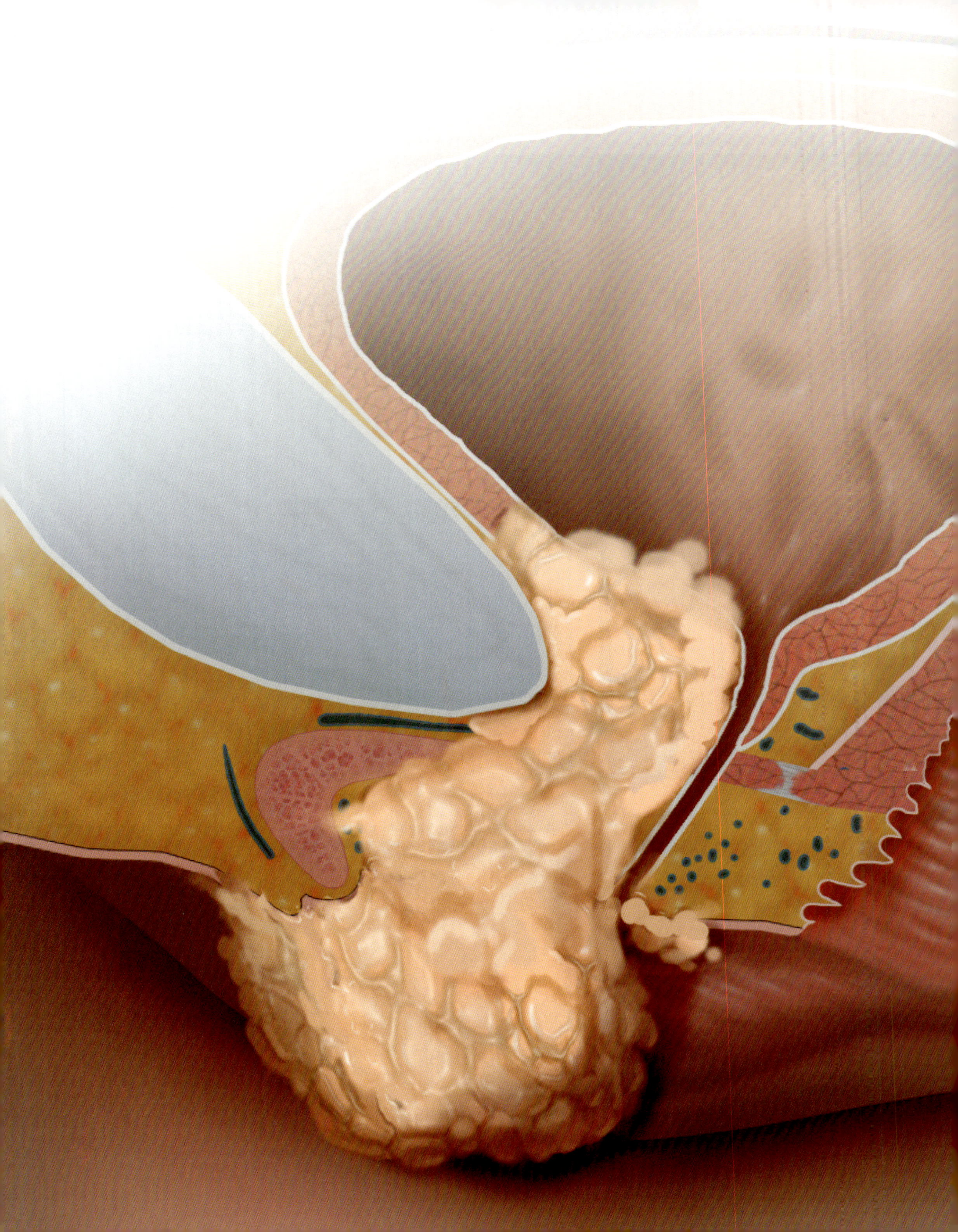

Vulvar Carcinoma

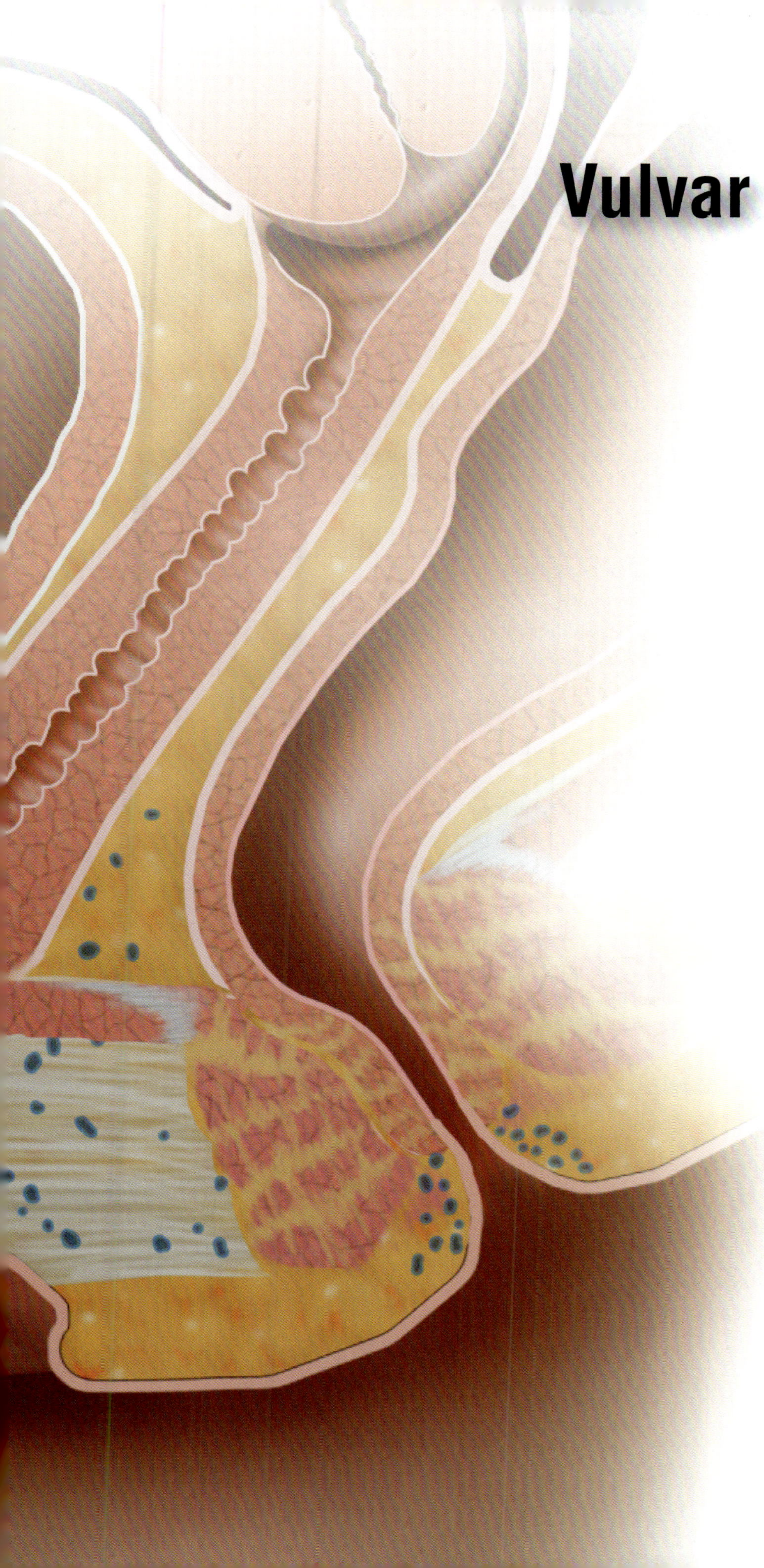

VULVAR CARCINOMA

(T) Primary Tumor

Adapted from 7th edition AJCC Staging Forms.

TNM	*FIGO*	*Definitions*
TX		Primary tumor cannot be assessed
T0		No evidence of primary tumor
Tis[1]		Carcinoma in situ (preinvasive carcinoma)
T1a	IA	Lesions ≤ 2 cm in size, confined to the vulva or perineum and with stromal invasion ≤ 1.0 mm[2]
T1b	IB	Lesions > 2 cm in size **or** any size with stromal invasion > 1.0 mm, confined to the vulva or perineum
T2[3]	II/III	Tumor of any size with extension to adjacent perineal structures (lower/distal 1/3 urethra, lower/distal 1/3 vagina, anal involvement)
T3[4]	IVA	Tumor of any size with extension to any of the following: Upper/proximal 2/3 of urethra, upper/proximal 2/3 vagina, bladder mucosa, rectal mucosa, or fixed to pelvic bone

(N) Regional Lymph Nodes

NX		Regional lymph nodes cannot be assessed
N0		No regional lymph node metastasis
N1		1 or 2 regional lymph nodes with the following features
N1a	IIIA	1 or 2 lymph node metastases each < 5 mm
N1b	IIIA	1 lymph node metastasis ≥ 5 mm
N2	IIIB	Regional lymph node metastasis with the following features
N2a	IIIB	≥ 3 lymph node metastases each < 5 mm
N2b	IIIB	≥ 2 lymph node metastases ≥ 5 mm
N2c	IIIC	Lymph node metastasis with extracapsular spread
N3	IVA	Fixed or ulcerated regional lymph node metastasis

(M) Distant Metastasis

M0		No distant metastasis
M1	IVB	Distant metastasis (including pelvic lymph node metastasis)

[1]FIGO no longer includes stage 0 (Tis). [2]The depth of invasion is defined as the measurement of the tumor from the epithelial-stromal junction of the adjacent most superficial dermal papilla to the deepest point of invasion. [3]FIGO uses the classification T2/T3. This is defined as T2 in TNM. [4]FIGO uses the classification T4. This is defined as T3 in TNM.

AJCC Stages/Prognostic Groups

Adapted from 7th edition AJCC Staging Forms.

Stage	*T*	*N*	*M*
0	Tis	N0	M0
I	T1	N0	M0
IA	T1a	N0	M0
IB	T1b	N0	M0
II	T2	N0	M0
IIIA	T1, T2	N1a, N1b	M0
IIIB	T1, T2	N2a, N2b	M0
IIIC	T1, T2	N2c	M0
IVA	T1, T2	N3	M0
	T3	Any N	M0
IVB	Any T	Any N	M1

VULVAR CARCINOMA

Tis

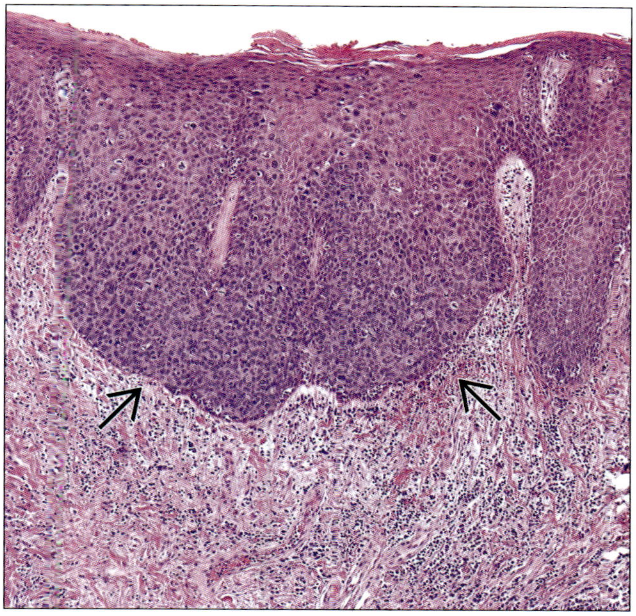

Low-power magnification of H&E section from vulvar biopsy specimen shows the surface of the stratified squamous epithelium. Deep to the surface is the intraepithelial lesion characterized by cellular disarray with lack of maturation that involves almost the full thickness of the epithelium →. (Original magnification 100x.)

Tis

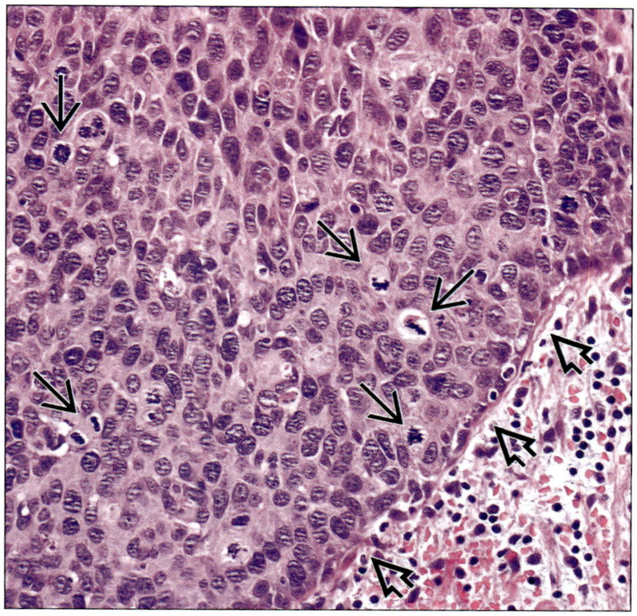

Higher magnification shows the crowded, pleomorphic, and dysplastic cells that lack maturation. The nuclei are hyperchromatic with many mitotic figures →. Note that the basement membrane ⇨ is intact with no invasive component. (Original magnification 400x.)

T1a

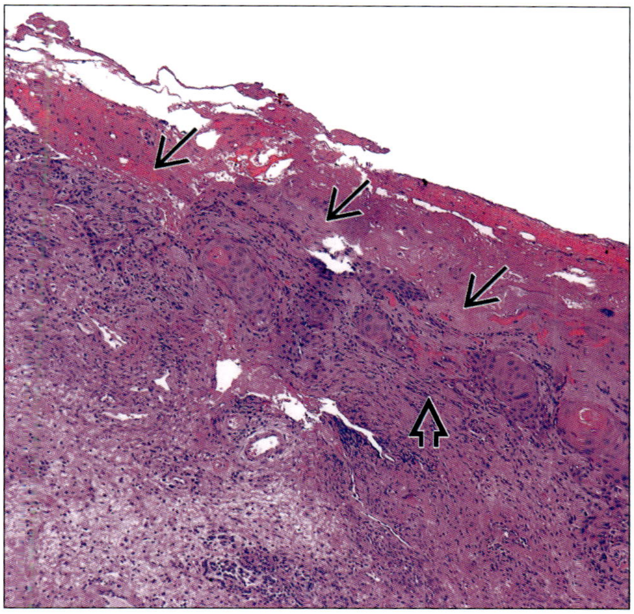

H&E stain of a biopsy specimen from an ulcerated skin lesion → shows invasive squamous cell carcinoma with superficial stromal invasion of < 1 mm depth (⇨ = 0.7 mm depth of invasion). (Original magnification 40x.)

T1a

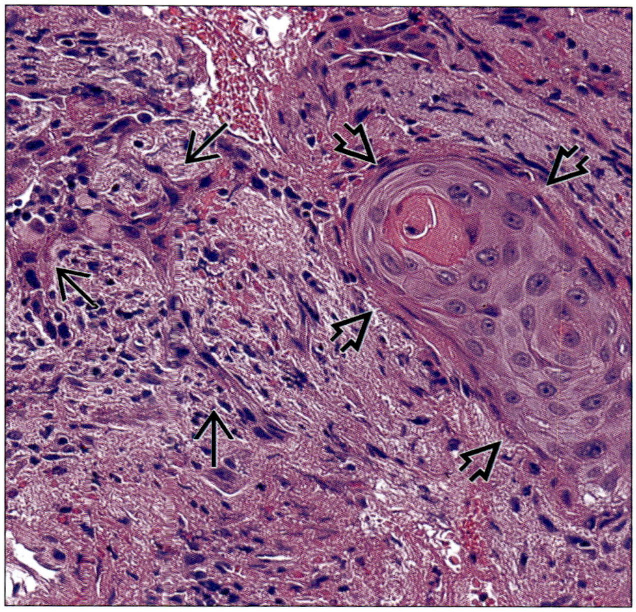

Higher magnification shows invasion of squamous cords and nests → into the superficial dermis. Note the keratinized nest on the right side ⇨. (Original magnification 400x.)

VULVAR CARCINOMA

T1b

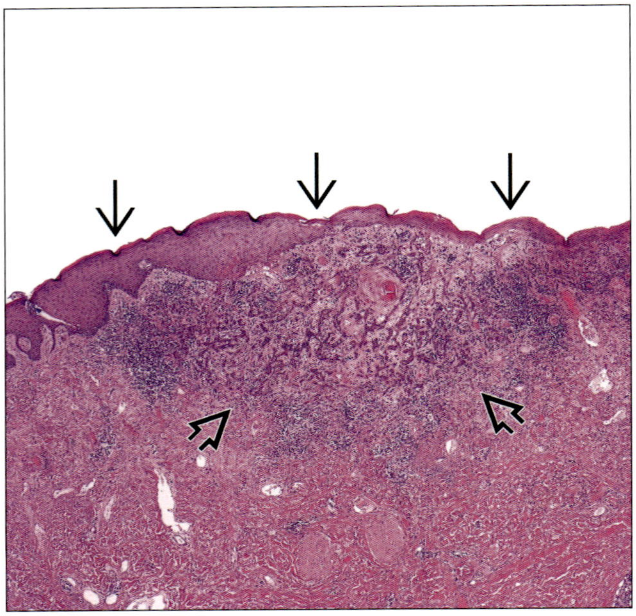

Low magnification of H&E stain from vulvar biopsy specimen shows overlying stratified squamous epithelium → with an invasive squamous cell carcinoma ⇨ infiltrating to a depth of 3 mm. (Original magnification 40x.)

T1b

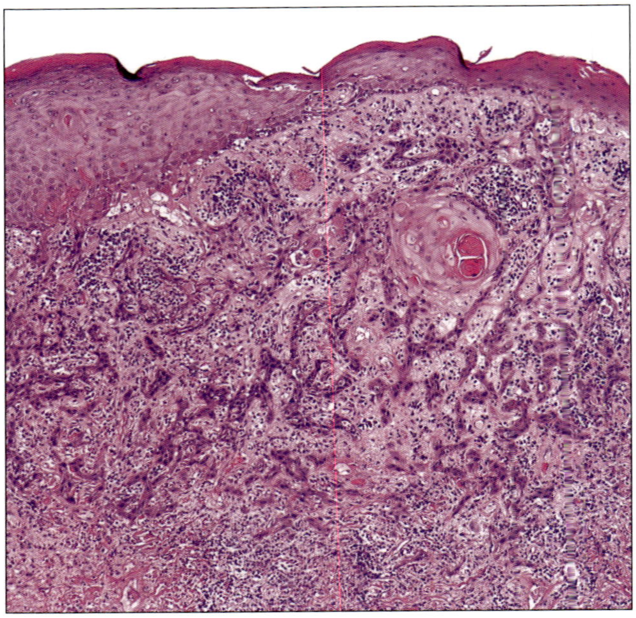

Higher magnification of the invasive component shows nonkeratinized cords and nests of malignant cells in a desmoplastic stroma. (Original magnification 100x.)

T3

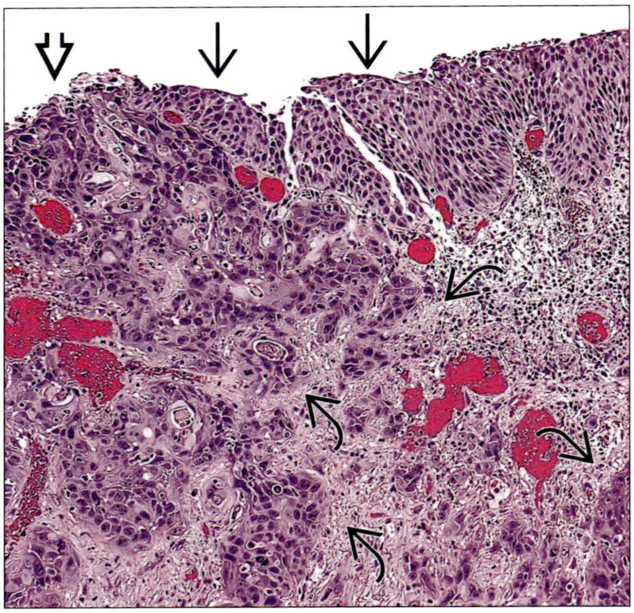

H&E stain of a biopsy specimen from the urinary bladder shows bladder mucosa with transitional epithelium →. Invasive vulvar carcinoma involves the wall of the bladder ↷ and extends to involve the bladder mucosa in the left upper corner ⇨. (Original magnification 100x.)

T3

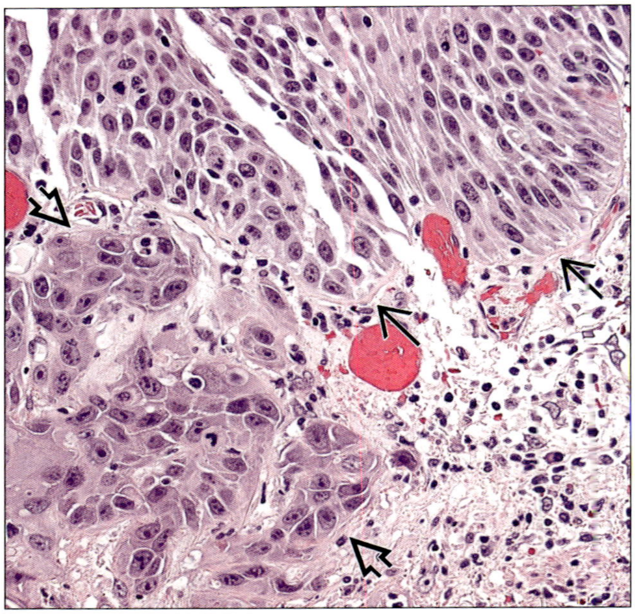

Higher magnification image depicts transitional epithelium → with squamous cell carcinoma of vulvar primary ⇨ in close approximation. (Original magnification 400x.)

VULVAR CARCINOMA

T1a

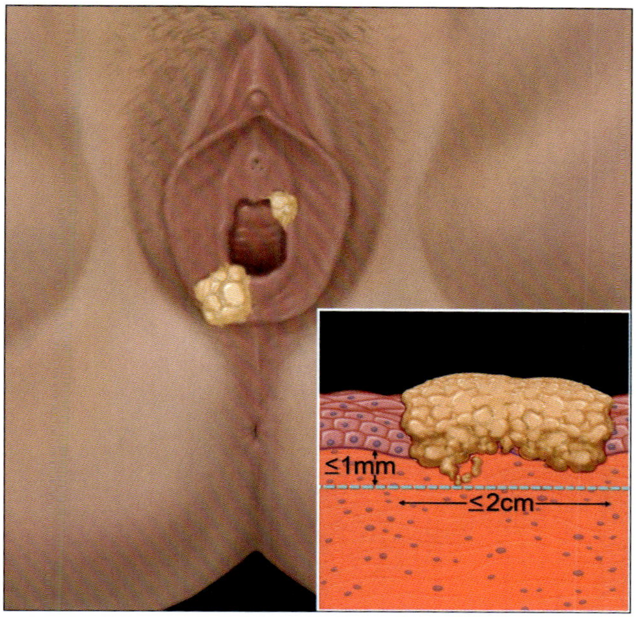

External view of the female genitalia depicts tumor confined to the vulva or vulva and perineum measuring ≤ 2 cm in greatest dimension. In addition, depth of tumor invasion must be ≤ 1 mm for tumor stage T1a.

T1b

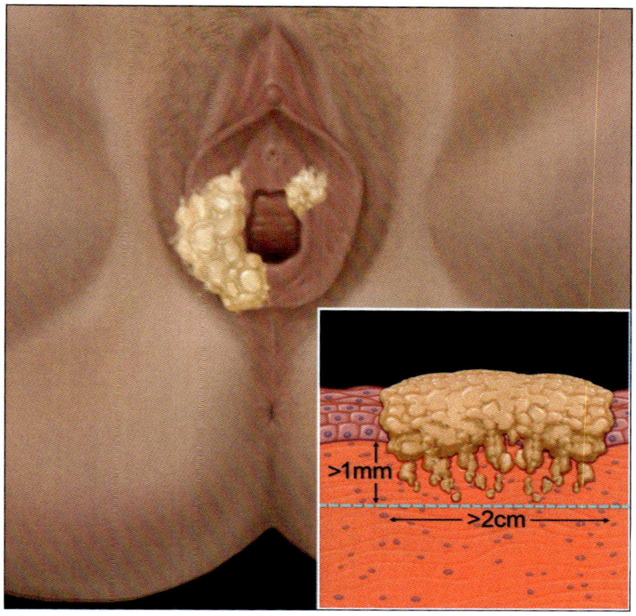

External view of the female genitalia depicts tumor confined to the vulva or vulva and perineum measuring > 2 cm in greatest dimension. In addition, tumor of any size with depth of invasion > 1 mm is stage T1b.

T2

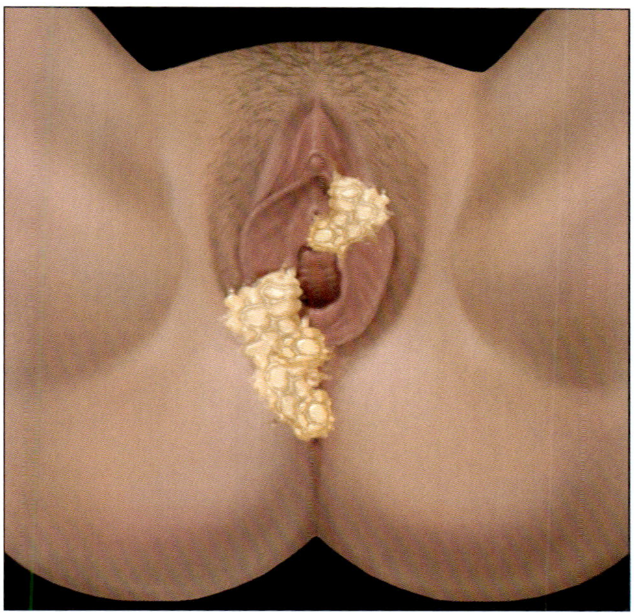

External view of the female genitalia depicts tumor extending to adjacent perineal structures. T2 tumors can be any size while invading the lower urethra, lower vagina, and anus.

T2

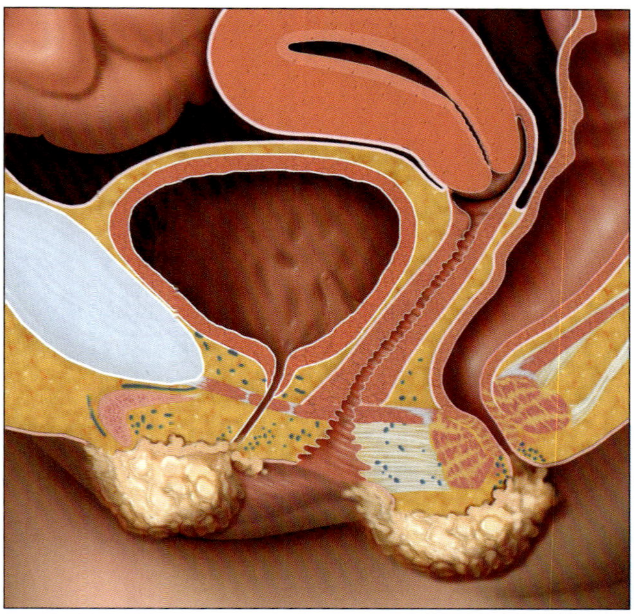

Sagittal view of the pelvis depicts vulvar tumor invading the lower urethra, lower vagina, and anus. Invasion of the distal 1/3 of adjacent perineal structures characterizes tumor stage T2.

VULVAR CARCINOMA

T3

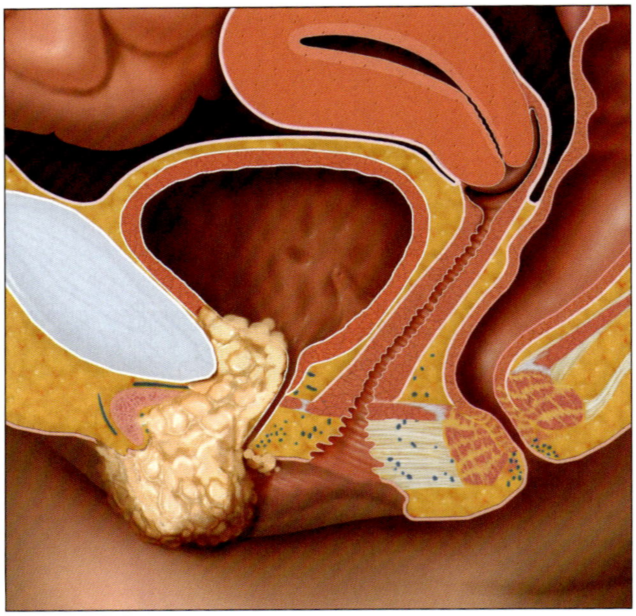

Sagittal view of the pelvis depicts vulvar tumor extending to the upper urethra, urinary bladder, and pubic bone. Invasion of the proximal urethra and bladder mucosa constitutes tumor stage T3, as does tumor fixed to the pelvic bone.

T3

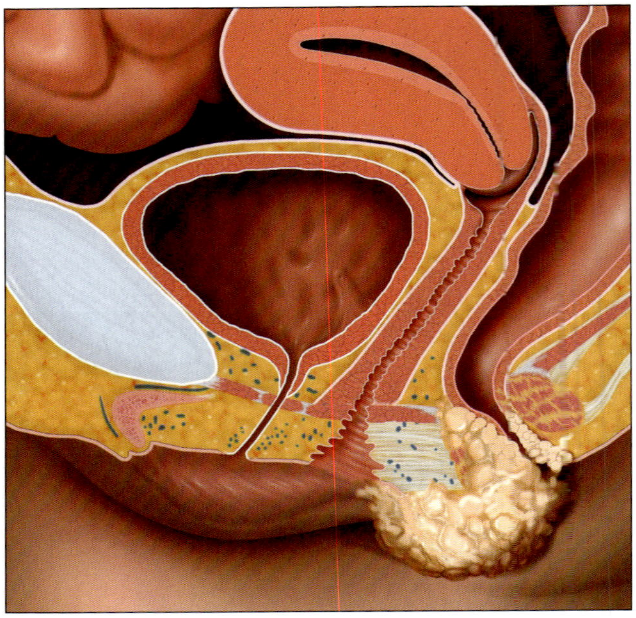

Sagittal view of the pelvis depicts vulvar tumor invading the rectum. Extension to the rectal mucosa constitutes tumor stage T3.

N1a and N1b

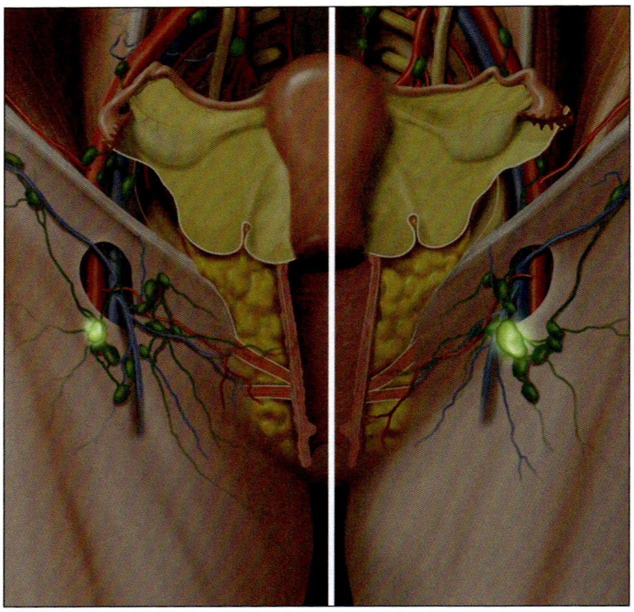

This graphic shows the inguinofemoral lymph node basin. Image on the left depicts 1 lymph node metastasis ≤ 5 mm. Only 1 or 2 regional lymph nodes with metastases ≤ 5 mm can be involved for nodal stage N1a. Image on the right depicts 1 lymph node metastasis ≥ 5 mm, which constitutes stage N1b.

N2a and N2b

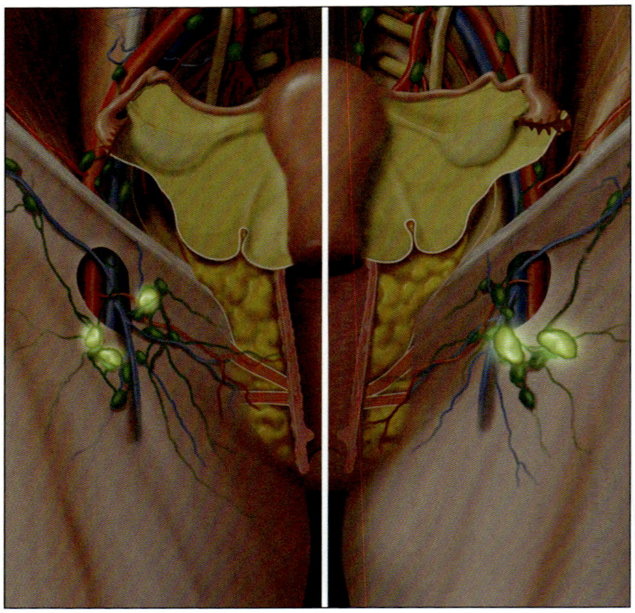

Image on the left depicts 3 lymph node metastases, each < 5 mm. For nodal stage N2a, 3 or more regional lymph nodes with metastases < 5 mm can be involved. Image on the right depicts 2 lymph node metastases ≥ 5 mm. For nodal stage N2b, 2 or more lymph nodes with metastases ≥ 5 mm can be involved.

N2c

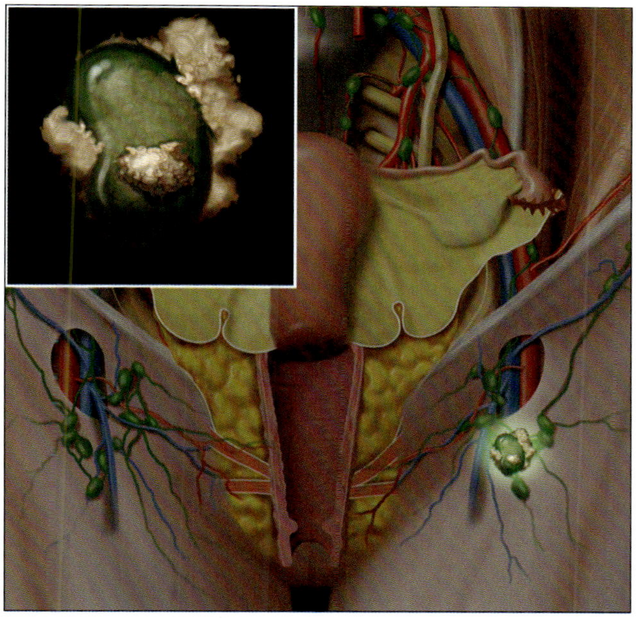

This graphic shows the inguinofemoral lymph node basin with a magnified lymph node inset. Regional lymph node metastases with extracapsular spread of tumor constitute nodal stage N2c.

N3

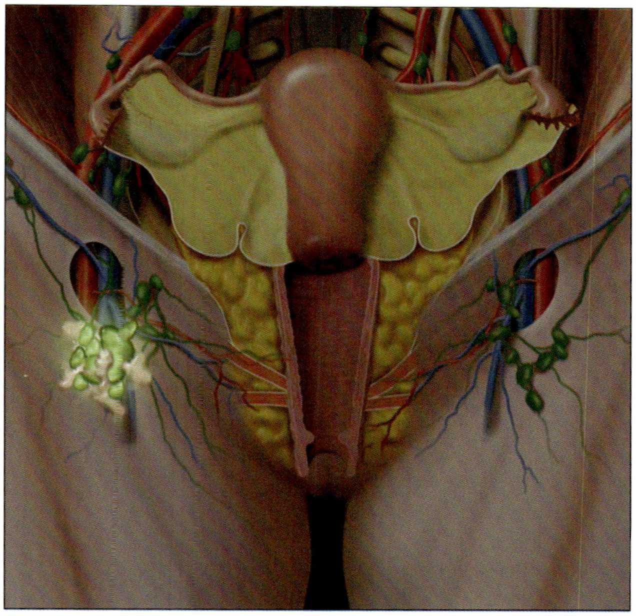

Graphic of the inguinofemoral lymph node basin depicts regional lymph node metastases with the nodal mass fixed to surrounding tissues. Fixation or ulceration of adjacent tissues constitutes nodal stage N3.

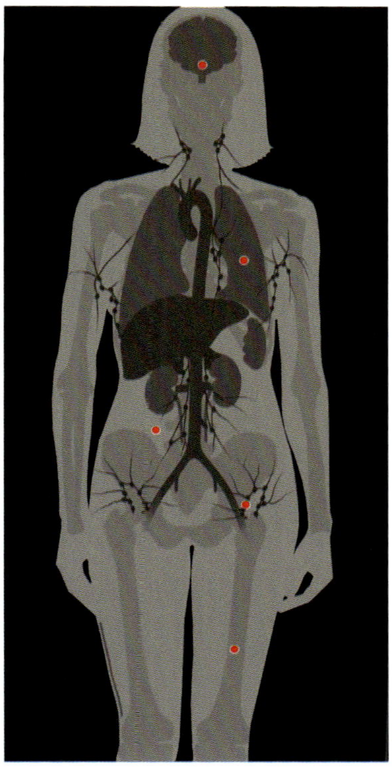

METASTASES, ORGAN FREQUENCY

Pelvic lymph nodes

Intraabdominal sites

Lung

Bone

Central nervous system

Distant metastatic disease beyond the pelvic lymph nodes is rare. The number is not sufficiently significant to determine organ frequency.

VULVAR CARCINOMA

OVERVIEW

General Comments

- 4th most common gynecologic malignancy
- 4% of female genital tract malignancies
- 90% are squamous cell carcinoma

Classification

- Histopathologic types
  - Squamous cell carcinoma
  - Verrucous carcinoma
  - Paget disease of vulva
  - Adenocarcinoma, NOS
  - Basal cell carcinoma, NOS
  - Bartholin gland carcinoma
- Mucosal malignant melanoma is not included in this classification and staging

PATHOLOGY

Routes of Spread

- **Contiguous spread**
  - Influenced by histology
    - Well differentiated: Superficial spread with minimal invasion
    - Anaplastic: More likely to be deeply invasive
  - Posteriorly to anus and rectum
  - Anteriorly to urethra, rarely to urinary bladder and pubic bone
  - Cranially to vagina
  - Usually slowly infiltrates local tissues, followed by lymph node spread
- **Lymphatic spread**
  - Typical lymphatic drainage
    - Superficial inguinal → deep femoral → external iliac lymph nodes
    - Superficial inguinal lymph nodes
      - Subcutaneous along medial inguinal ligament
      - Along saphenous vein, near saphenofemoral junction
    - Deep femoral lymph nodes
      - Along femoral artery and vein, within femoral sheath
      - Can be involved without superficial inguinal adenopathy
    - External iliac lymph nodes
      - Cloquet node: Most caudal lymph node in this chain, at entrance of femoral canal
      - Cloquet node signals likelihood of pelvic node metastases
  - Drainage based on tumor location
    - Lateral lesions spread to ipsilateral lymph nodes
    - Central lesions may spread to ipsilateral, contralateral, or both lymph nodes
      - Lesions within 1 cm of vulvar midline
      - Anterior lesions (area immediately posterior to clitoris)
  - Likelihood of lymphatic spread increases with each millimeter of depth of invasion
    - ≤ 1 mm → 0%
    - 1.1-2 mm → 5.4%
    - > 5 mm → 32%
  - Other patterns of lymphatic spread
    - Bilateral groin metastasis
      - Drainage from midline structures: Perineum and clitoris
    - Contralateral groin metastasis
      - Bartholin cancer
    - Direct spread to pelvic nodes
      - Rarely occurs with central cancers
      - Direct drainage via internal pudendal chain to internal iliac nodes
    - Subcutaneous and dermal lymphatics
      - Obstruction of typical lymphatic drainage
      - Involves vulva, upper thighs, lower abdomen
    - Obturator or internal iliac nodes
      - Involved if invasion of vagina or bladder
  - Risk factors for lymph node metastases
    - Clinical node status
    - Age
    - Degree of differentiation
    - Tumor stage
    - Tumor thickness
    - Depth of stromal invasion
    - Presence of lymphovascular invasion
- **Hematogenous spread**
  - Distant metastases are rare and usually fatal
  - Occur late and rarely without nodal metastases
  - 1 series showed significantly lower risk of hematogenous metastases with < 3 positive lymph nodes at time of diagnosis

General Features

- Comments
  - 3-5% of gynecologic malignancies
  - 4th most common gynecologic malignancy
- Genetics
  - S-phase fraction (proliferation index)
    - ↑ in tumors from patients with lymphatic spread
  - HPV-encoded oncoproteins E6 and E7
    - Can bind tumor suppressor gene products (p53 protein and retinoblastoma)
    - Loss of growth suppression
  - Epidermal growth factor receptor
    - ↑ expression in vulvar tumor is associated with nodal metastases and ↓ patient survival
  - HER-2/neu
    - Positivity associated with ↑ risk of nodal metastases
- Etiology
  - Risk factors
    - Cigarette smoking
    - Vulvar dystrophy
    - Vulvar intraepithelial neoplasia (VIN)
    - Cervical intraepithelial neoplasia (CIN)
    - Human papilloma virus infection
    - Immunodeficiency syndromes
    - History of cervical cancer
    - Northern European ancestry
- Epidemiology & cancer incidence
  - 3,580 new cases each year in USA
  - 900 deaths each year in USA
  - Rate of invasive cancer has been stable for 2 decades
  - Incidence of vulvar intraepithelial neoplasia (in situ) has doubled
- Associated diseases, abnormalities
  - Synchronous 2nd malignancy in up to 22%
    - Most commonly cervical neoplasia

VULVAR CARCINOMA

- Human papilloma virus (HPV)
  - Responsible for 60% of vulvar cancers
  - HPV 16, 18, and 33 are most common
  - HPV-related cancer found in younger women
    - Increasing incidence of HPV-related VIN in young women
    - Tend to present with earlier stage disease
  - Risk factors associated with HPV infection
    - Early age at 1st intercourse
    - Multiple sexual partners
    - HIV infection
    - Cigarette smoking
- Vulvar dystrophies
  - Includes lichen sclerosus and squamous cell hyperplasia
  - Cancer occurs in older women
  - Not associated with HPV

Gross Pathology & Surgical Features

- Location
  - 50% in labia majora
  - 15-20% in labia minora
  - 10-15% in clitoris
  - Infrequently in other sites (Bartholin glands)
  - 10% of lesions are too extensive to determine site of origin
- 5% of cases are multifocal
- Verrucous cancer is typically exophytic
  - May be large, infiltrates locally

Microscopic Pathology

- H&E
  - Squamous cell carcinoma is most common
  - Usually well differentiated
  - If high grade, may have areas of glandular differentiation
  - Clitoral tumors may be more anaplastic
  - VIN and keratosis may occur at margins
    - Better prognosis
  - Fibromyxoid stromal response
    - Older age
    - Worse survival rates
    - More extensive nodal metastases

IMAGING FINDINGS

Detection

- **Ultrasound**
  - No role in primary tumor detection
- **CT**
  - Small superficial tumors
    - Often not seen
    - May appear as irregularity of vulvar surface
  - Large exophytic tumors
    - Exophytic enhancing solid mass
    - Surface irregularity may indicate ulceration
- **MR**
  - Tumor characteristics
    - Hypointense on T1WI
    - Intermediate to high signal on T2WI
  - IV contrast not helpful for tumor detection
  - Limited visualization of small tumors & plaque-like lesions

Staging

- Surgically staged malignancy
- Stage cannot be changed on basis of disease progression, response, or recurrence
- **Primary tumor**
  - Vulva is area immediately external to vagina
    - Includes labia and perineum
  - T1a: Tumor confined to vulva & perineum, ≤ 2 cm in greatest dimension, ≤ 1 mm stromal invasion
  - T1b: Tumor confined to vulva & perineum, > 2 cm in greatest dimension, or any size with > 1 mm stromal invasion
  - T2: Tumor extension to lower perineal structures
  - T3: Tumor extension to upper perineal structures or pelvic bone
  - Imaging of limited utility in early stage (small superficial) tumors
  - Tumor stage T2 & T3
    - CT
      - May demonstrate gross invasion of adjacent structures
      - Limited for depth of invasion
      - Limited for tumor size
    - MR
      - May be helpful for deeply invading tumor
      - May be useful to evaluate invasion of adjacent structures
      - T2WI are most useful for extent of tumor
      - IV contrast not helpful for tumor staging
- **Lymphatic metastasis**
  - Regional lymph nodes → femoral & inguinal
  - Likelihood of lymphatic spread is very low if ≤ 1 mm stromal invasion
    - Lymph node dissection (LND) is optional for stage IA disease
  - Unilateral lesions with ≥ 3 mm stromal invasion have ≥ 2.8% rate of bilateral groin metastases
  - Traditionally nodal staging has been surgical
    - Inguinal-femoral lymphadenectomy
    - Up to 70% of patients have node-negative disease
    - Incur undue morbidity of surgical dissection
      - Lower extremity lymphedema (most common, in up to 69%)
      - Wound breakdown or infection
      - Lymphocysts
      - Psychosexual consequences
  - Unilateral dissection performed if < 1% risk of contralateral metastasis
    - Unifocal tumor < 2 cm
    - Lateral lesion (> 1 cm from vulvar midline)
    - No palpable adenopathy in either groin
    - No lymph node metastases at time of unilateral LND
  - Bilateral dissection performed if
    - Tumor > 2 cm
    - Small but central lesion (< 1 cm from vulvar midline)
    - Metastases found at unilateral LND
  - Clinical palpation is unreliable
    - Sensitivity is 57%, specificity is 62%
    - Allows evaluation of only superficial lymph nodes
    - May be limited by body habitus, small lymph node size, scar tissue

VULVAR CARCINOMA

- Ultrasound
  - Helpful for evaluation of groin adenopathy
    - Sensitivity is 86%, specificity is 96%
  - Characteristics of malignant lymph nodes
    - Round shape, irregular contour
    - Short axis diameter > 8 mm
    - Long axis/short axis ratio < 2
    - Loss of echogenic fatty hilum
    - ↑ thickness & ↓ echogenicity of cortex
    - Peripheral vascularity, high resistance flow
  - Advantages
    - Can evaluate superficial and deep lymph nodes
    - Can guide surgery or cytology
  - Limitations
    - Operator dependent
    - May be difficult to reproduce findings
    - False-positives due to reactive lymph nodes
    - Morphologically normal lymph nodes may harbor micrometastases
- Ultrasound-guided fine needle aspiration cytology
  - Most reliable: Combines morphology & cytology
    - Sensitivity is 93%, specificity is 100%
  - More sensitive than cytology alone
    - Sensitivity of 75% due to sampling error
  - Limitations
    - Operator dependent
    - Micrometastases
- CT
  - Inferior to US and guided FNA in detecting malignant adenopathy
- MR
  - Sensitivity is inconsistent among studies
    - 40-50% in 1 study, but 86% and 89% in others
    - Significant overlap in size of benign and malignant lymph nodes
  - High specificity, 97-100%
  - Malignant lymph node characteristics
    - Short axis diameter > 8 mm
    - Irregular or round shape
    - ↑ SI on STIR or heterogeneous SI on T2WI
  - Advantages
    - Not operator dependent, reproducible
    - Multiplanar imaging allows assessment of size, shape, and signal intensity
  - Future directions: MR lymphography
    - Ultra-small iron particles accumulate in normal lymph nodes
    - ↓ SI in normal lymph nodes on T2WI post contrast
    - Metastatic lymph nodes are replaced by tumor cells → do not accumulate iron oxide → no change in SI post contrast
    - May improve sensitivity of MR
    - May be able to detect micrometastases
- PET
  - Poor sensitivity for metastatic lymph nodes
    - Sensitivity is 67%, specificity is 95%
  - Limitations
    - False-positives (acute or chronic inflammation, post-radiotherapy reactions)
    - Micrometastases
- Lymphoscintigraphy & sentinel node biopsy (SNB)
  - Injection of radiotracer within or around lesion
  - Highly accurate in predicting nodal metastases
  - Learning curve for successful application
  - Absence of tracer uptake may indicate lymph node completely replaced by tumor
- Future directions
  - Imaging in lieu of surgical dissection
  - US surveillance every 3 months
  - US-guided FNA of morphologically abnormal lymph nodes

- **Distant metastasis**
  - Any site beyond regional lymph nodes, including pelvic nodes
    - Lung, extragenital skin, bone, intraabdominal sites, heart, central nervous system
  - Rare in most common types of vulvar cancer
  - Can be seen with melanoma and rare sarcomas

Restaging

- Recurrence
  - Poor prognosis, usually fatal
  - Predictors of recurrence
    - Size of lesion
    - Close margins at resection
      - Need > 10 mm tumor-free margin
    - Metastases in ≥ 2 groin nodes
  - 80% of recurrence occurs within 2 years of primary treatment
  - Location
    - Vulva
    - Groin
    - Skin bridge
      - Between vulvar & groin incisions
    - Pelvic lymph nodes
    - Distant sites
      - Rare except with melanoma or sarcoma

CLINICAL ISSUES

Presentation

- Elderly women, mean age of 65 at diagnosis
  - Data suggest age at diagnosis is trending down
    - May be related to ↑ in VIN in young women
- Signs and symptoms
  - Asymptomatic
  - Vulvar plaque, ulcer, or mass
  - Pruritus
  - Bleeding or discharge
  - Dysuria
  - Enlarged groin lymph node

Cancer Natural History & Prognosis

- Lymph nodes are most important prognostic indicator
  - 90% survival if negative groin nodes
  - 50-60% survival if positive groin nodes
  - Poor prognostic indicators
    - Bilateral malignant nodes
    - Unilateral malignant adenopathy involving multiple nodes
    - Tumor penetration of lymph node capsule
    - Increasing size of metastatic focus in node
- Tumor characteristics are important in prognosis
  - Tumor size
    - Recently thought to be less important in predicting survival (independent of other factors)
  - Depth of tumor invasion

- Measured from epithelial-stromal junction of adjacent most superficial dermal papilla to deepest point of invasion
- Lymphovascular space invasion
  - Documented at histologic evaluation
  - Correlates with incidence of nodal metastases

Treatment Options

- Major treatment alternatives
  - Surgery
    - Radical vulvectomy
      - Removal of vulva to level of deep thigh fascia
      - Removal of periosteum of pubis
      - Removal of inferior fascia of urogenital diaphragm
    - Radical local excision
    - Inguinofemoral lymphadenectomy
      - En bloc resection with vulvectomy
      - Morbidity reduced with separate groin incisions
  - Radiation therapy
    - Primary radiation therapy
      - Unable to tolerate surgery
    - Adjuvant radiation therapy
      - Surgical margin < 8 mm, lymphovascular invasion, > 5 mm thickness
      - Radiation therapy to groin if node positive
- Treatment options by stage
  - Early stage disease
    - Microinvasive disease (< 1 mm invasion)
      - Wide excision (5-10 mm)
    - Lateralized tumor confined to vulva < 2 cm, invasion < 5 mm, clinically node negative
      - Radical local excision
      - Unilateral lymphadenectomy
    - Tumor confined to vulva & perineum > 2 cm
      - Modified radical vulvectomy
      - Bilateral inguinofemoral LND
      - Adjuvant local radiation therapy if surgical margin < 8 mm, lymphovascular invasion, > 5 mm thickness, positive lymph nodes
    - If patient is unable to tolerate surgery → radiation
  - Advanced stage disease
    - Radical vulvectomy + en bloc inguinofemoral LND
      - Depending on tumor extent, may require removal of involved structures or pelvic exenteration
      - Radiation therapy to vulva if large tumor, margins narrow, lymphovascular invasion, or thickness > 5 mm
      - Radiation therapy to groin if positive lymph nodes → improves survival
    - If patient is unable to tolerate surgery → radiation therapy ± chemotherapy
  - Survival predominantly determined by lymph node metastases
    - Unilateral lymphadenopathy, 70% 5-year survival
    - ≥ 3 unilateral lymph nodes involved, 30% 5-year survival
  - Recurrent disease
    - Local recurrence without regional LND
      - Radical excision: 5-year survival is 56%
    - Local recurrence > 2 years after treatment
      - Excision & radiation: 5-year survival > 50%

REPORTING CHECKLIST

T Staging

- Size
- Depth of invasion
- Invasion of adjacent structures
  - Urethra: Lower or upper
  - Urinary bladder
  - Vagina: Lower or upper
  - Anus
  - Rectal mucosa
  - Pubic bone

N Staging

- Location
  - Superficial inguinal
  - Deep femoral
- Morphology
  - Size & shape
  - Fatty hilum & cortex
  - Vascularity
- Extracapsular spread
- Fixed or ulcerated
- Unilateral or bilateral

M Staging

- Pelvic lymph nodes
- Distant metastasis

SELECTED REFERENCES

1. American Joint Committee on Cancer: AJCC Cancer Staging Manual. 7th ed. New York: Springer, 2010
2. McMahon CJ et al: Lymphatic metastases from pelvic tumors: anatomic classification, characterization, and staging. Radiology. 254(1):31-46, 2010
3. Oonk MH et al: The role of sentinel node biopsy in gynecological cancer: a review. Curr Opin Oncol. 21(5):425-32, 2009
4. Bipat S et al: Is there a role for magnetic resonance imaging in the evaluation of inguinal lymph node metastases in patients with vulva carcinoma? Gynecol Oncol. 103(3):1001-6, 2006
5. Land R et al: Routine computerized tomography scanning, groin ultrasound with or without fine needle aspiration cytology in the surgical management of primary squamous cell carcinoma of the vulva. Int J Gynecol Cancer. 16(1):312-7, 2006
6. Oonk MH et al: Prediction of lymph node metastases in vulvar cancer: a review. Int J Gynecol Cancer. 16(3):963-71, 2006
7. Singh K et al: Accuracy of magnetic resonance imaging of inguinofemoral lymph nodes in vulval cancer. Int J Gynecol Cancer. 16(3):1179-83, 2006
8. Hall TB et al: The role of ultrasound-guided cytology of groin lymph nodes in the management of squamous cell carcinoma of the vulva: 5-year experience in 44 patients. Clin Radiol. 58(5):367-71, 2003
9. Sohaib SA et al: Imaging in vulval cancer. Best Pract Res Clin Obstet Gynaecol. 17(4):543-56, 2003
10. Hawnaur JM et al: Identification of inguinal lymph node metastases from vulval carcinoma by magnetic resonance imaging: an initial report. Clin Radiol. 57(11):995-1000, 2002
11. Sohaib SA et al: MR imaging of carcinoma of the vulva. AJR Am J Roentgenol. 178(2):373-7, 2002

VULVAR CARCINOMA

(Left) Coronal PET/CT shows minimal soft tissue and increased FDG uptake in the left vulva. No enlarged or FDG-avid lymph nodes were seen. On physical examination this tumor was estimated to be 1 x 1 cm; however, on pathologic examination the largest diameter was 2.1 cm, making it a T1b tumor. ***(Right)*** Coronal T2WI MR shows an intermediate signal mass ⇨ arising from the labia majora and extending up to invade the lower urethra.

Stage IB (T1b N0 M0)

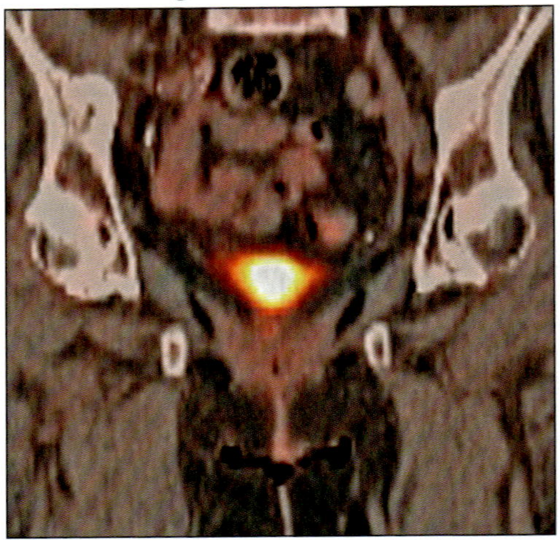

Stage II (T2 N0 M0)

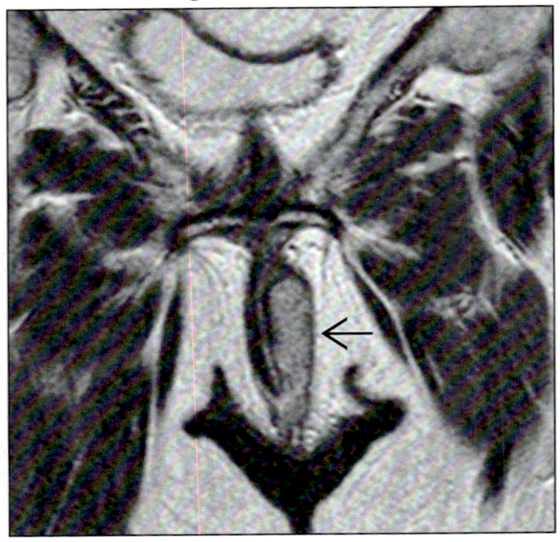

(Left) Axial T1WI C+ FS MR in the same patient shows avid enhancement of the vulvar mass. No regional or pelvic adenopathy was seen on this exam. ***(Right)*** Axial and coronal CECT images show a right inguinal lymph node ➡ with central hypodensity. The fatty hilum is obliterated, and the node is replaced by soft tissue centrally. The metastatic focus is > 5 mm; however, there is no extracapsular spread of tumor.

Stage II (T2 N0 M0)

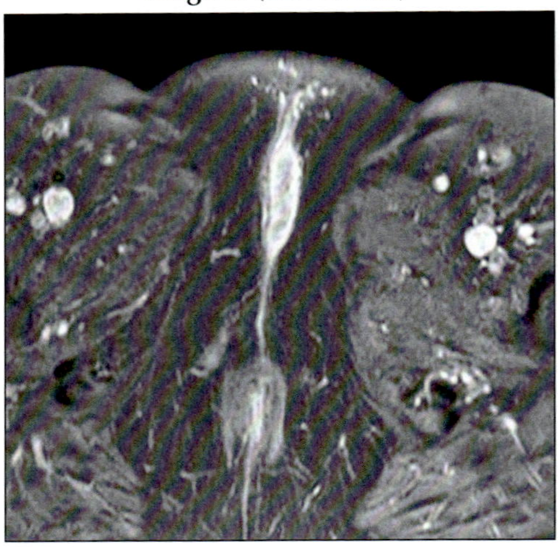

Stage IIIA (T1b N1b M0)

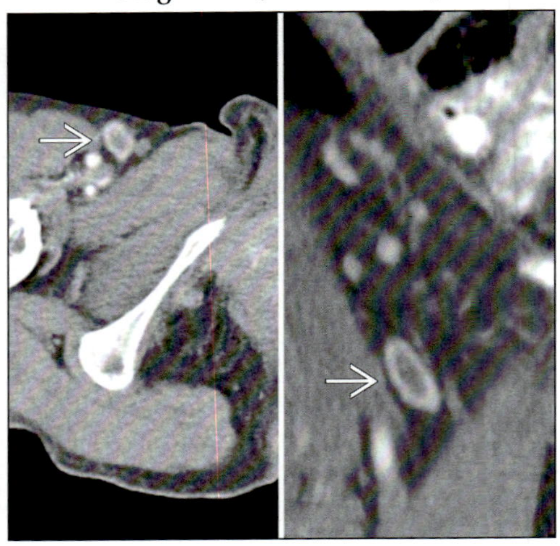

(Left) Axial T1WI C+ FS MR shows an enhancing vulvar mass ➡. ***(Right)*** Axial T1WI C+ FS MR in the same patient shows cephalad extension of the vulvar mass ➡ to invade the distal urethra. In addition, there are 2 enlarged, round, enhancing right inguinal lymph nodes ➡ with loss of the fatty hila, corresponding to nodal stage N2b.

Stage IIIB (T2 N2b M0)

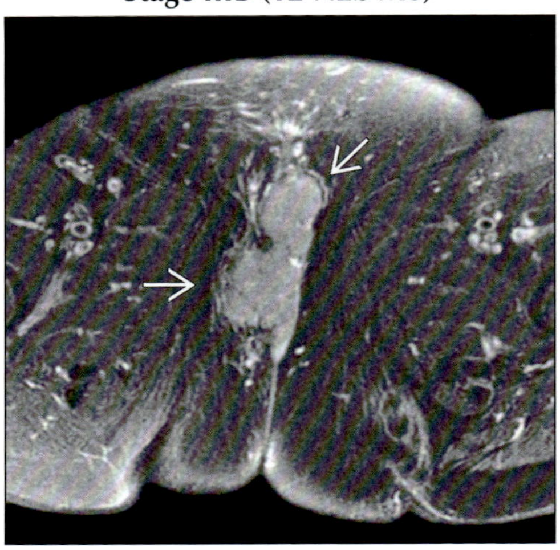

Stage IIIB (T2 N2b M0)

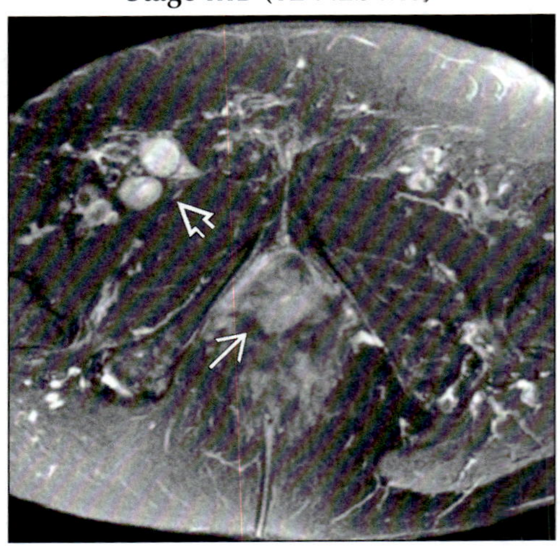

Stage IIIC (T2 N2c M0)

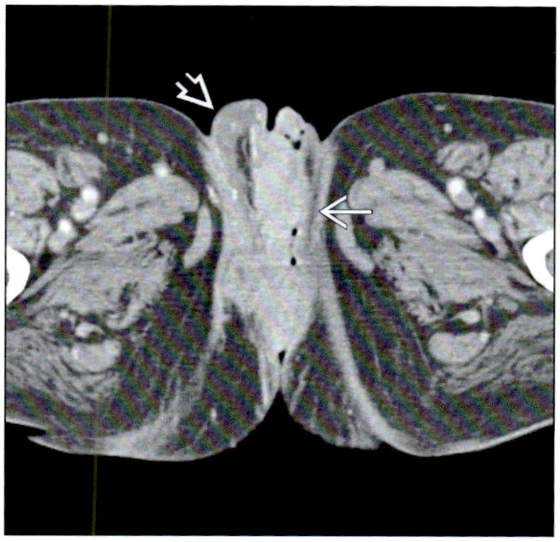

Stage IIIC (T2 N2c M0)

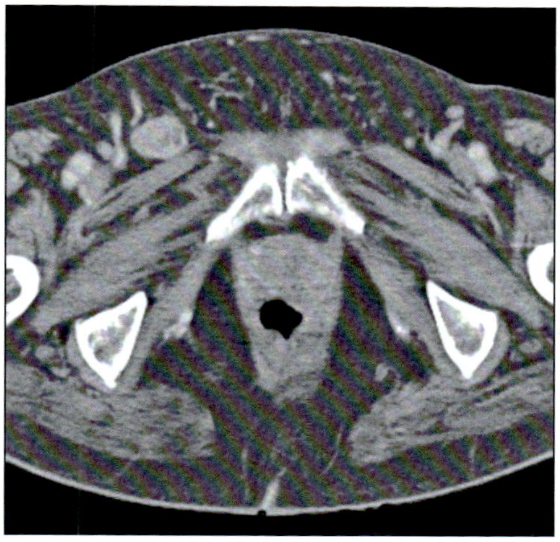

(Left) *Axial CECT shows an enhancing vulvar mass → with a large exophytic component. The right labia majora ⇨ is partially visualized with skin thickening and enhancement, concerning for dermal invasion.* ***(Right)*** *Axial CECT in the same patient shows a large right inguinal lymph node with foci of central necrosis. The lymph node margins are irregular and ill defined, suggestive of extracapsular spread.*

Stage IIIC (T2 N2c M0)

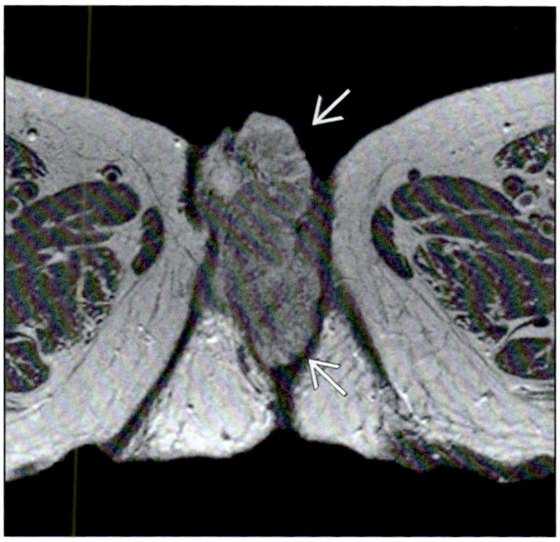

Stage IIIC (T2 N2c M0)

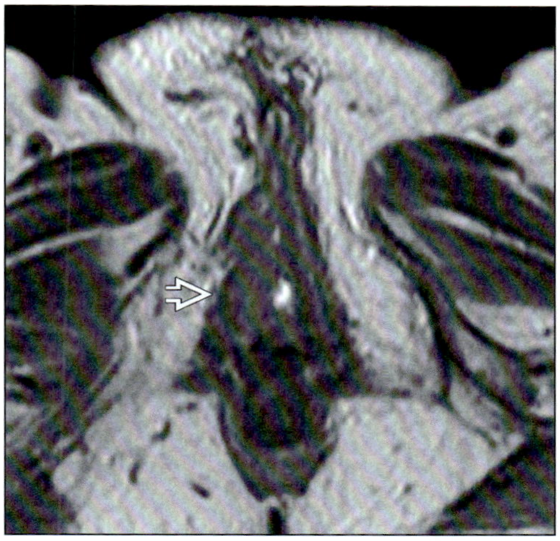

(Left) *Axial T2WI FSE MR in the same patient shows a large, exophytic, intermediate signal vulvar mass →.* ***(Right)*** *Axial T2WI FSE MR obtained more cephalad to the previous image shows the intermediate signal mass invading the right lower vaginal wall ⇨ and the right crus of the clitoris, as well as obliterating the lower urethra.*

Stage IIIC (T2 N2c M0)

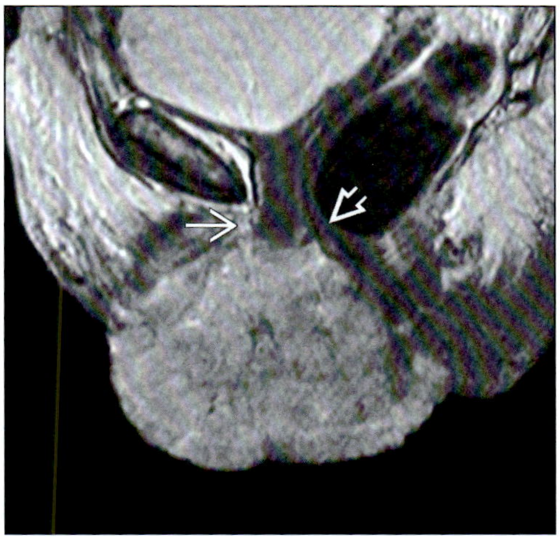

Stage IIIC (T2 N2c M0)

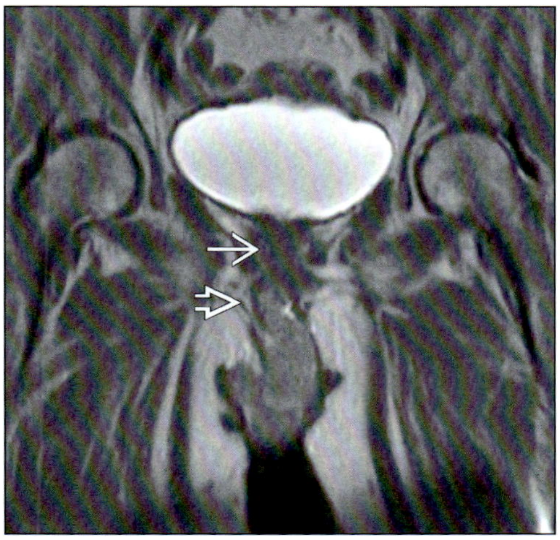

(Left) *Sagittal T2WI FSE MR in the same patient shows the large exophytic vulvar mass. Note extension to the lower urethra → and vagina ⇨.* ***(Right)*** *Coronal T2WI MR shows the vulvar mass invading the lower urethra ⇨. Note the normal, low signal upper urethra →.*

VULVAR CARCINOMA

Stage IIIC (T2 N2c M0)

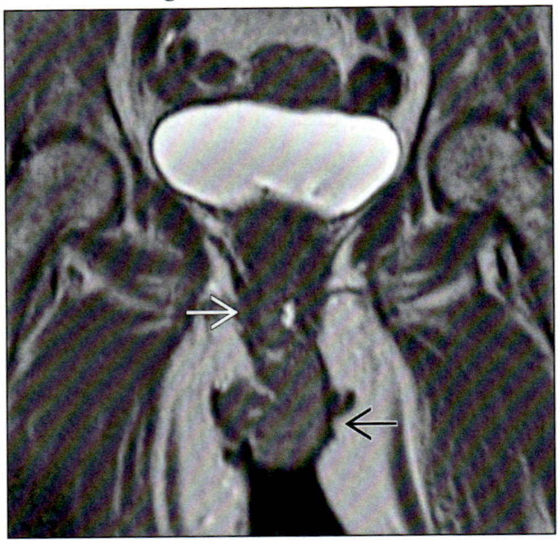

Stage IIIC (T2 N2c M0)

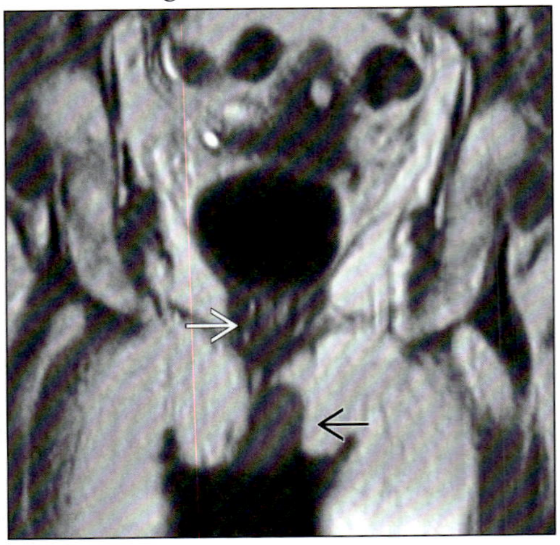

(Left) *Coronal T2WI MR in the same patient at the level of the vagina shows partially exophytic vulvar tumor → extending cephalad to invade the lower 1/3 of the vagina →.* ***(Right)*** *Coronal T2WI MR in the same patient at the level of the anus → and rectum shows no involvement by the vulvar mass →. The fat plane between the mass and anus is preserved.*

Stage IIIC (T2 N2c M0)

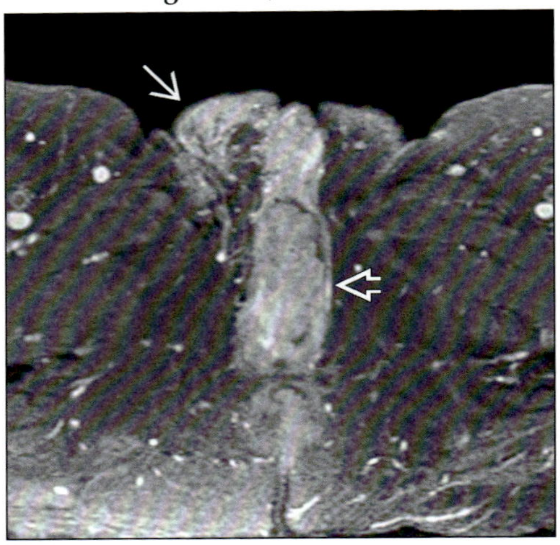

Stage IIIC (T2 N2c M0)

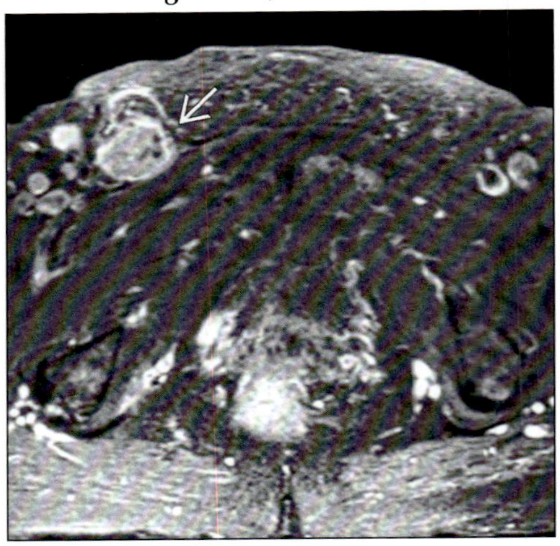

(Left) *Axial T1WI C+ FS MR through the vulvar mass → also shows dermal thickening and enhancement of the right labia majora →, consistent with dermal invasion.* ***(Right)*** *Axial T1WI C+ FS MR in the same patient shows multiple, hyperenhancing right inguinal lymph nodes. The largest → has irregular ill-defined margins, suggestive of extracapsular spread.*

Stage IIIC (T2 N2c M0)

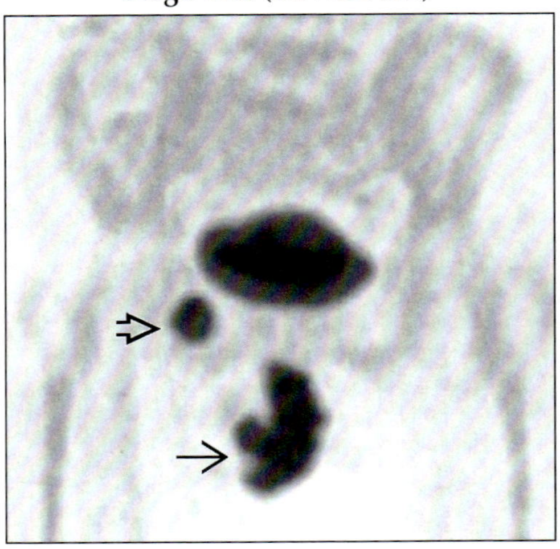

Stage IIIC (T2 N2c M0)

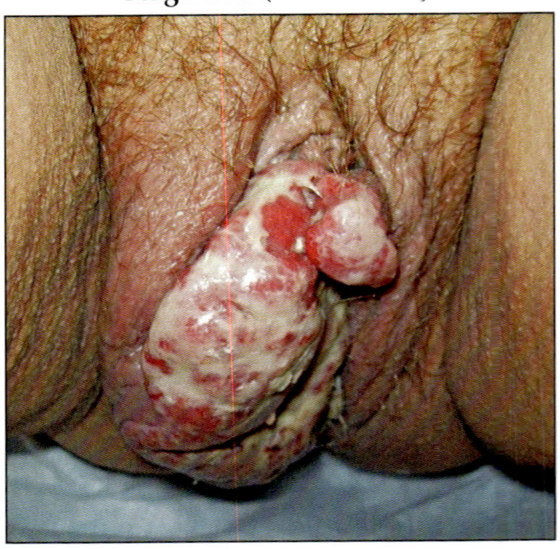

(Left) *Image of the pelvis from whole body PET shows the large hypermetabolic vulvar mass → and right inguinal lymph node →. There was no distant metastatic disease including no pelvic lymphadenopathy.* ***(Right)*** *Picture of the perineum of the same patient shows a large mass centered in the right labia majora with extensive surface ulceration and necrosis.*

VULVAR CARCINOMA

Stage IVA (T2 N3 M0)

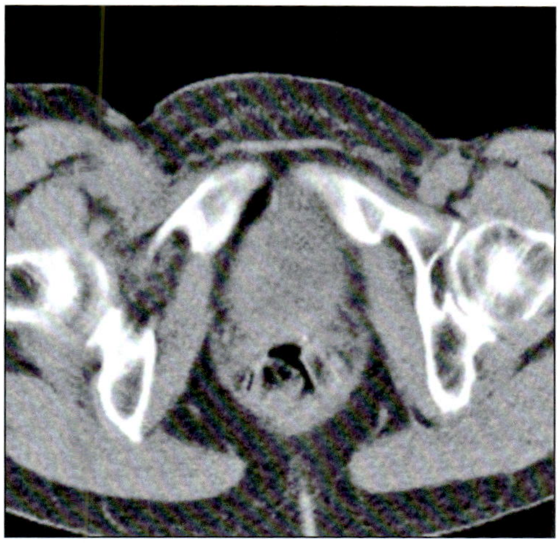

Stage IVA (T2 N3 M0)

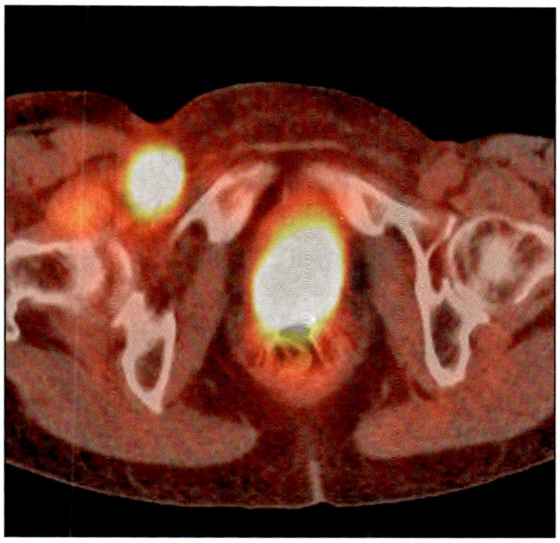

(Left) *Axial NECT shows a right femoral lymph node mass. Ill-defined infiltrative margins and encasement of the right femoral vessels are characteristic of nodal stage N3 adenopathy.* ***(Right)*** *Axial PET/CT in the same patient shows avid FDG uptake in the right femoral lymphadenopathy.*

Stage IVA (T3 N0 M0)

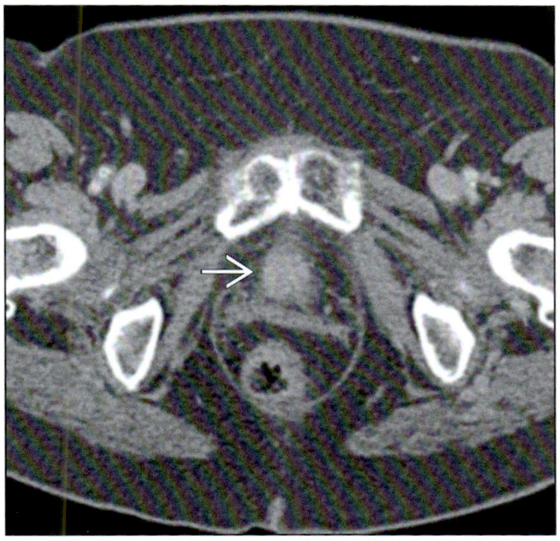

Stage IVA (T3 N0 M0)

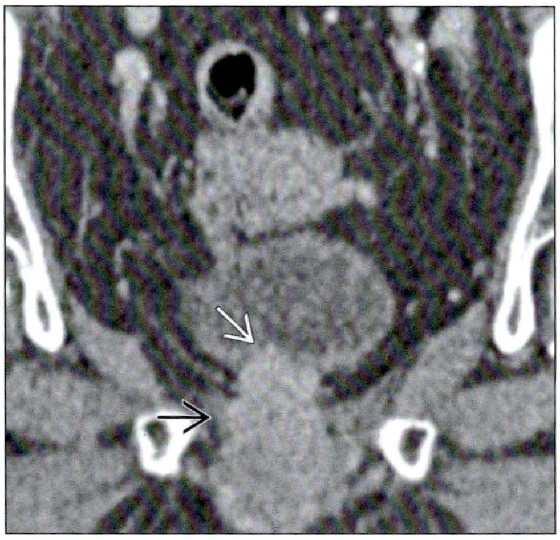

(Left) *Axial CECT shows an enhancing, ill-defined tumor replacing the urethra* ➔. ***(Right)*** *Coronal CECT in the same patient shows an enhancing, ill-defined mass replacing the urethra* ⇨ *and invading the base of the urinary bladder* ➔.

Recurrence

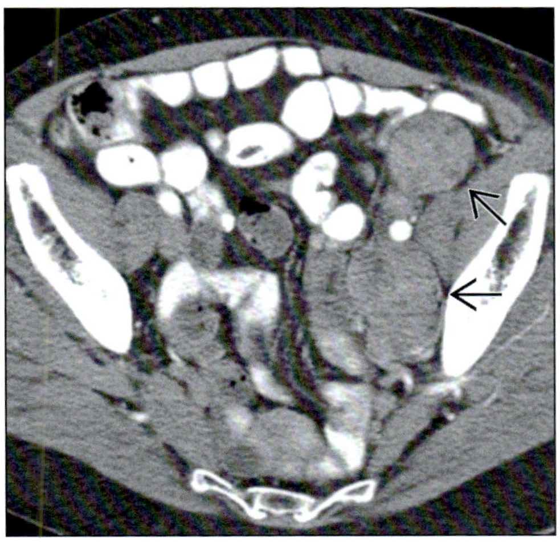

Recurrence

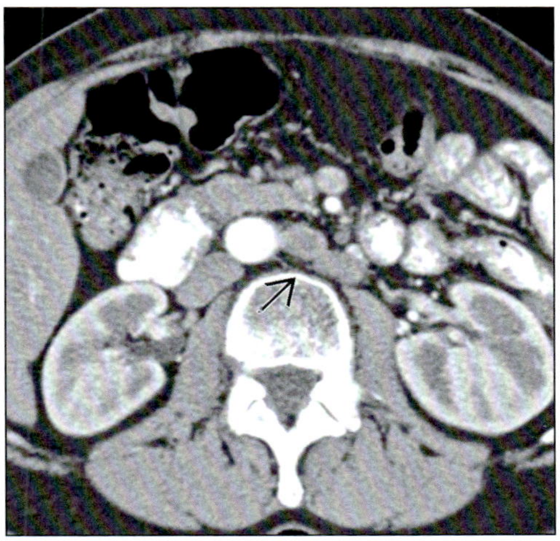

(Left) *Axial CECT in a patient with history of vulvar cancer status post left vulvectomy shows bulky left external iliac adenopathy* ⇨. ***(Right)*** *Axial CECT in the same patient shows necrotic left paraaortic adenopathy* ⇨. *Pelvic and abdominal adenopathy is usually seen with recurrence, as in this case. The prognosis is poor and usually fatal.*

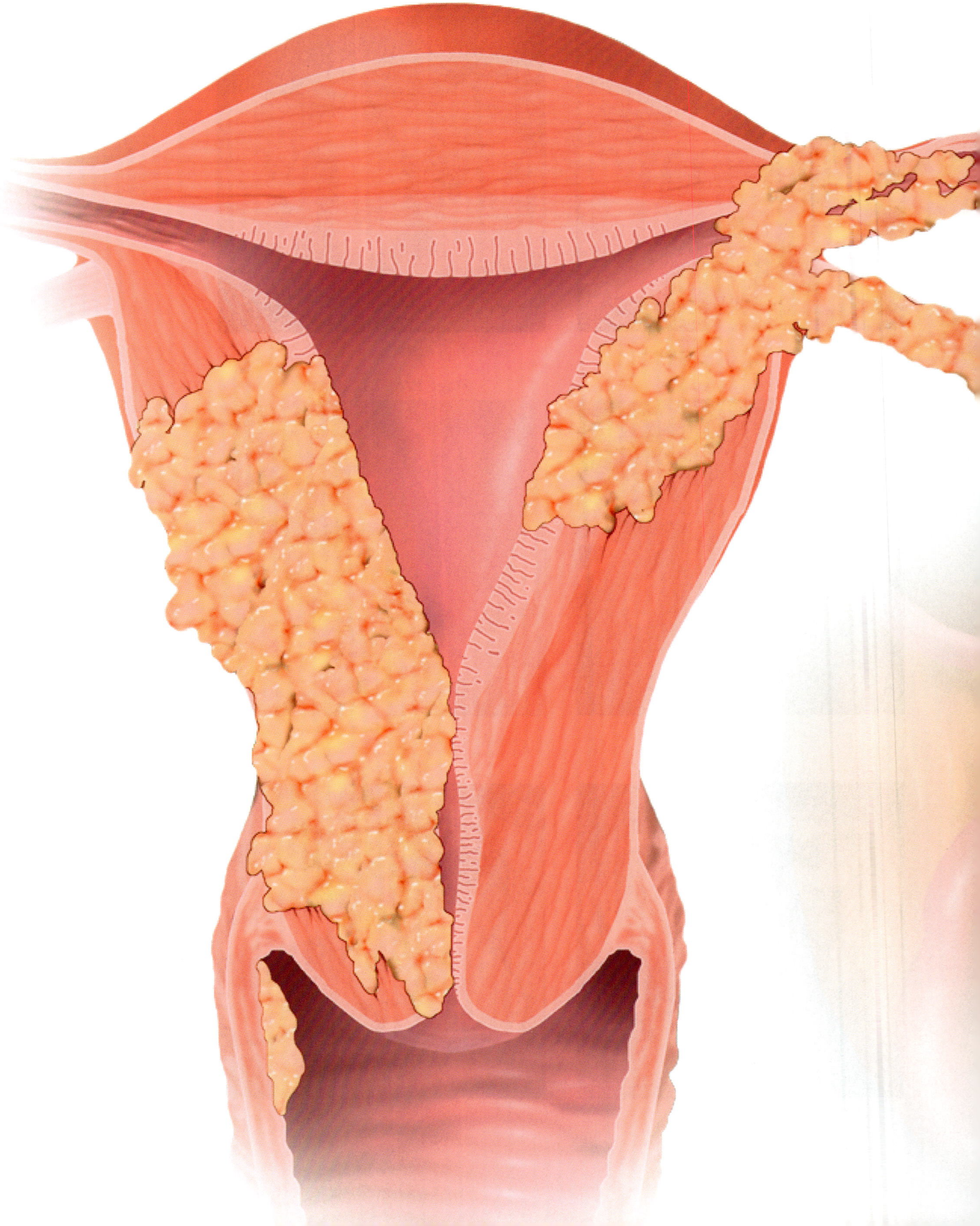

Gestational Trophoblastic Disease

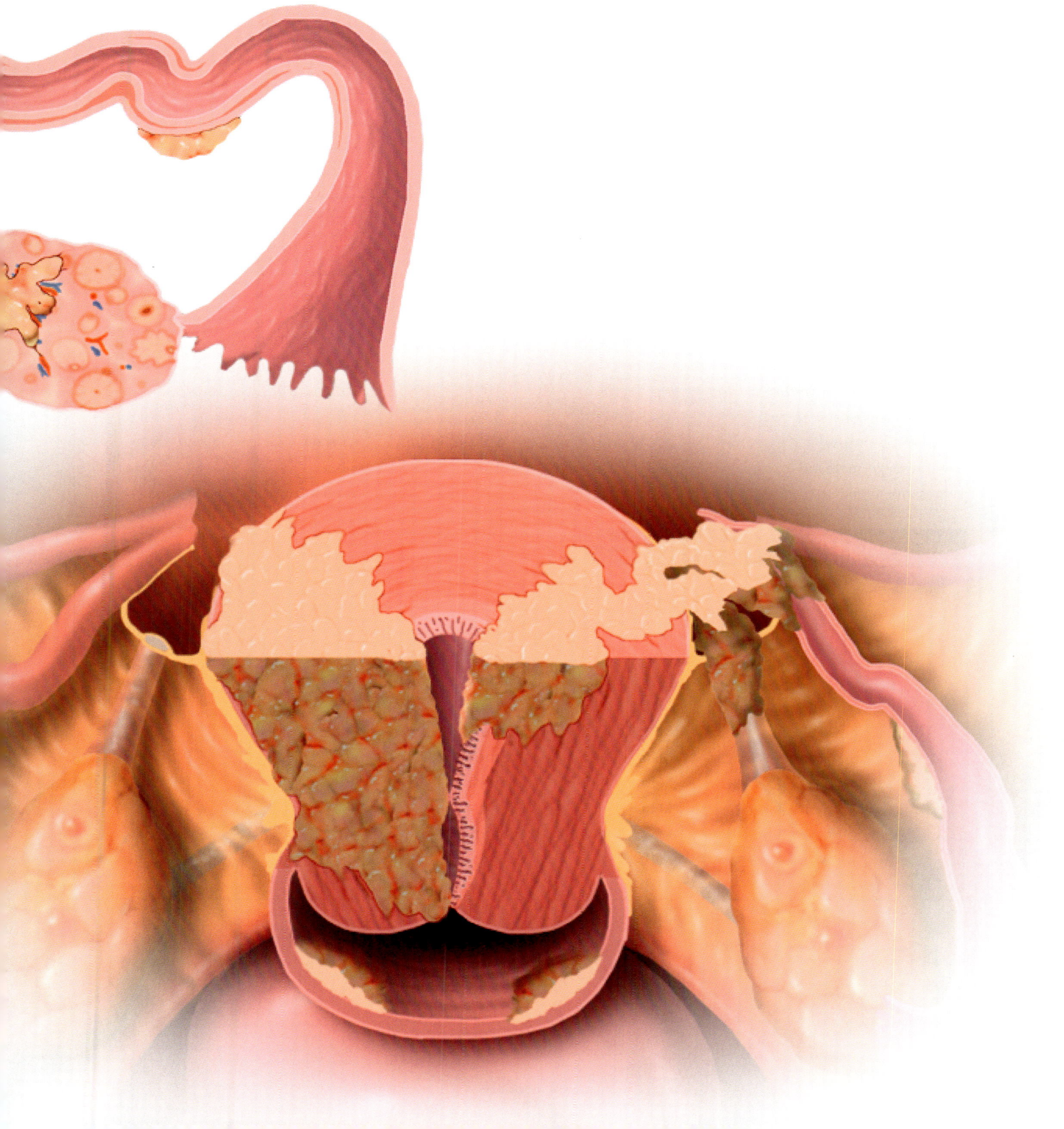

GESTATIONAL TROPHOBLASTIC DISEASE

(T) Primary Tumor

Adapted from 7th edition AJCC Staging Forms.

TNM	*FIGO*	*Definitions*
TX		Primary tumor cannot be assessed
T0		No evidence of primary tumor
T1	I	Tumor confined to uterus
T2	II	Tumor extends to other genital structures (ovary, tube, vagina, broad ligaments) by metastasis or direct extension

(M) Distant Metastasis

M0		No clinical metastasis
M1		Distant metastases
M1a	III	Lung metastasis
M1b	IV	All other distant metastasis

Prognostic Scoring Index for Gestational Trophoblastic Tumors

Risk Factors	*0*	*1*	*2*	*4*
Age	< 40 years	≥ 40 years		
Antecedent pregnancy	Mole	Abortion	Term pregnancy	
Interval months from index pregnancy	< 4	4-6	7-12	> 12
Pre-treatment serum hCG (IU/L)	$< 10^3$	10^3 to $< 10^4$	10^4 to $< 10^5$	$\geq 10^5$
Largest tumor size in cm	< 3 cm	3 - 5	> 5	
Site of metastases	Lung	Spleen, kidney	GI tract	Brain, liver
Number of metastases		1-4	5-8	> 8
Previous failed chemotherapy			Single drug	≥ 2 drugs

AJCC Stages/Prognostic Groups

Adapted from 7th edition AJCC Staging Forms.

Stage	*T*	*M*	*Risk Factors*
I	T1	M0	Unknown
IA	T1	M0	Low risk
IB	T1	M0	High risk
II	T2	M0	Unknown
IIA	T2	M0	Low risk
IIB	T2	M0	High risk
III	Any T	M1a	Unknown
IIIA	Any T	M1a	Low risk
IIIB	Any T	M1a	High risk
IV	Any T	M1b	Unknown
IVA	Any T	M1b	Low risk
IVB	Any T	M1b	High risk

GESTATIONAL TROPHOBLASTIC DISEASE

Complete Hydatidiform Mole

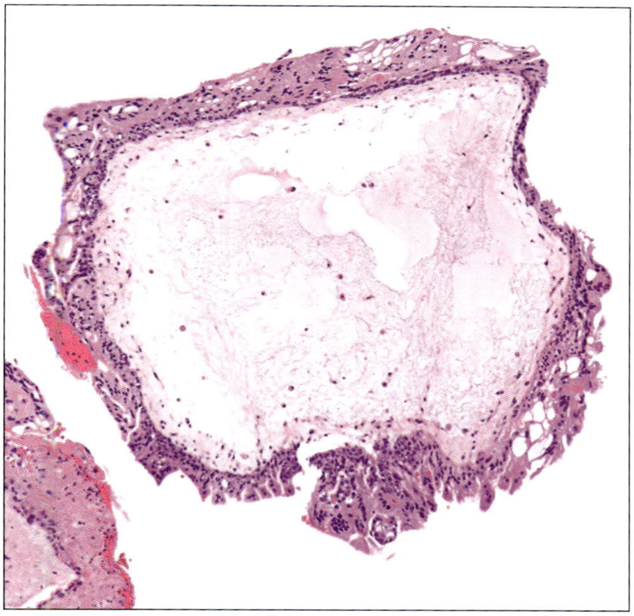

H&E stain shows 2 key features of a complete hydatidiform mole: Trophoblastic proliferation and villous edema. Note the enlarged villus that has central cistern (entirely acellular space), stromal edema, and a circumferential proliferation of trophoblasts around the surface. (Original magnification 200x.)

Partial Hydatidiform Mole

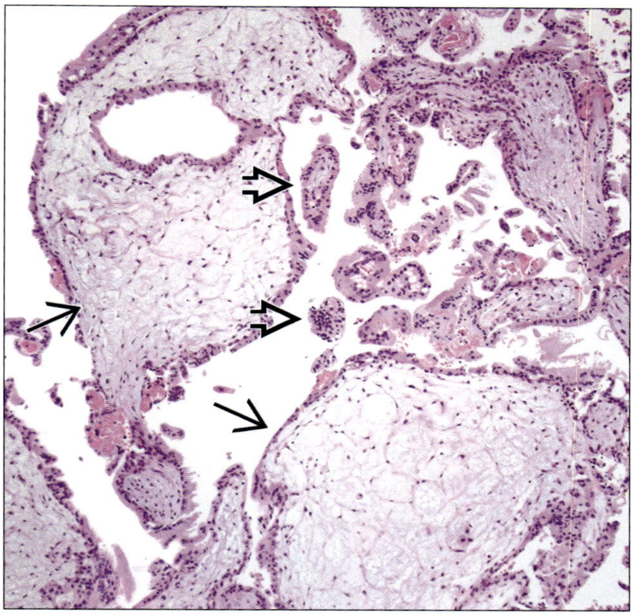

H&E stain shows a mixture of enlarged, edematous villi with cisterns ➔ and small, normal-sized villi with fibrotic stroma ⇨. The large villi have scalloped surfaces with trophoblast infolding, forming inclusions. The trophoblastic proliferation is focal and composed of haphazard tufts of trophoblasts. (Original magnification 200x.)

Choriocarcinoma

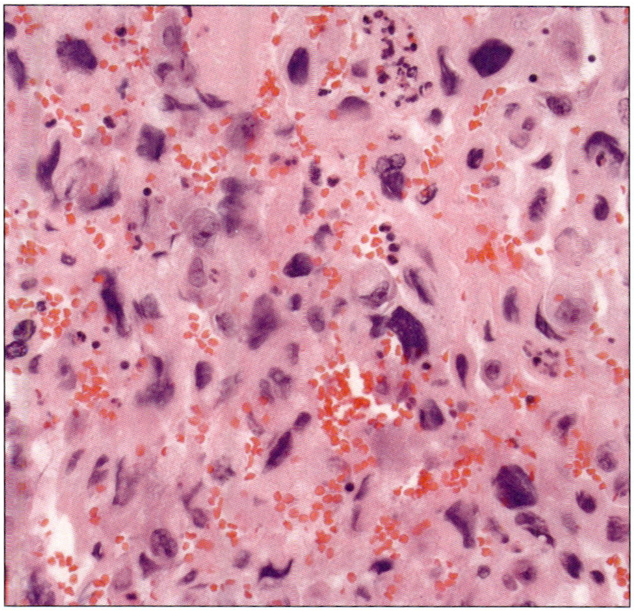

High magnification of an H&E stain shows highly atypical cytotrophoblast cells with irregular hyperchromatic nuclei mixed with syncytiotrophoblasts. (Original magnification 1000x.)

Placental Site Trophoblastic Tumor

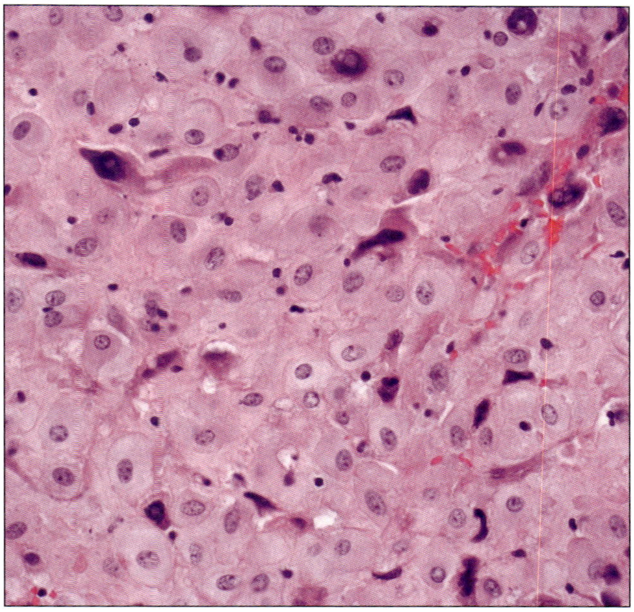

H&E stain shows sheets of intermediate trophoblasts, characterized by large polygonal cells with irregular nuclei and dense eosinophilic cytoplasm. In contrast, choriocarcinoma is composed of a mixture of cytotrophoblasts, syncytiotrophoblasts, and intermediate trophoblasts. (Original magnification 1000x.)

GESTATIONAL TROPHOBLASTIC DISEASE

T1 (FIGO I) Disease

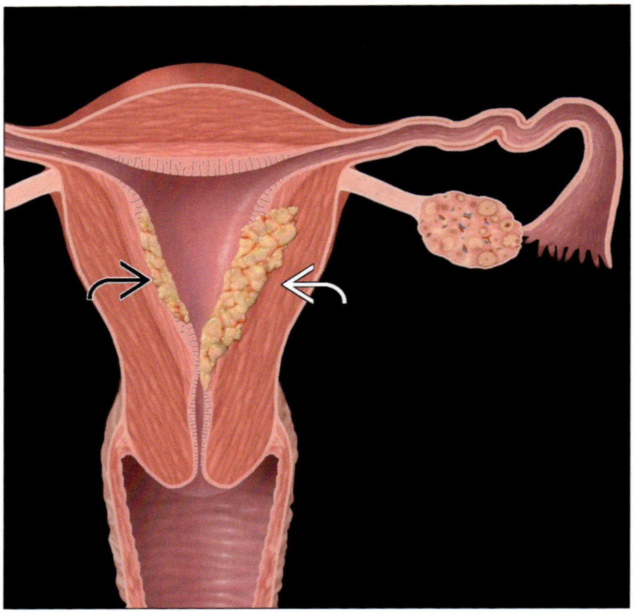

This graphic demonstrates the uterus in the coronal plane and shows gestational trophoblastic disease that is either limited to the endometrium ➚ or invades into the myometrium ➚. In T1 disease, the tumor is confined to the uterus.

T1 (FIGO I) Disease

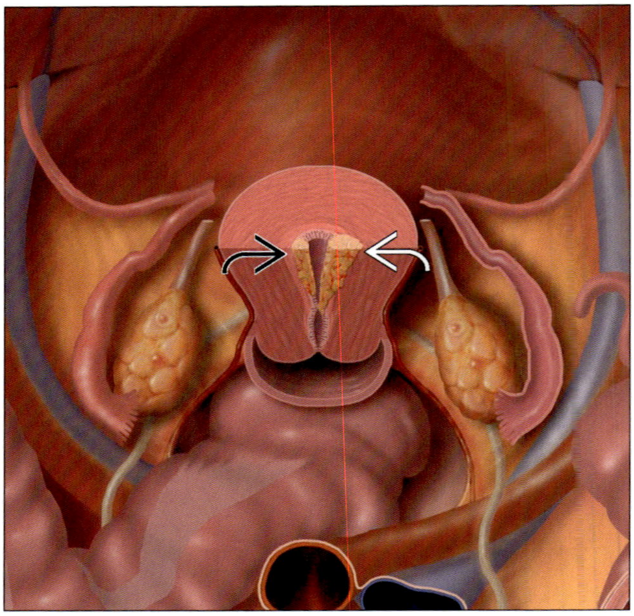

A cut section of the uterus as viewed from above demonstrates gestational trophoblastic disease that is either limited to the endometrium ➚ or invades into the myometrium ➚. In T1 disease, the tumor is confined to the uterus.

T2 (FIGO II) Disease

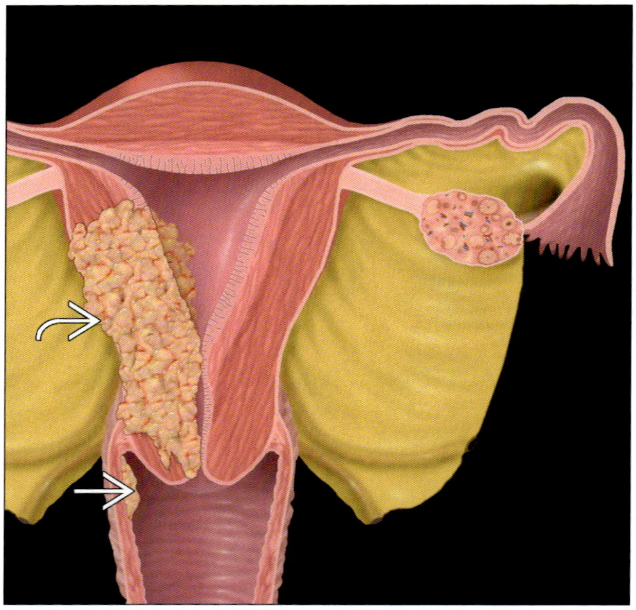

Coronal graphic illustrates gestational trophoblastic disease extending to the broad ligament ➚ and involving the vagina ➔. Either circumstance would constitute T2 disease, in which the tumor extends outside the uterus but is limited to the genital tract.

T2 (FIGO II) Disease

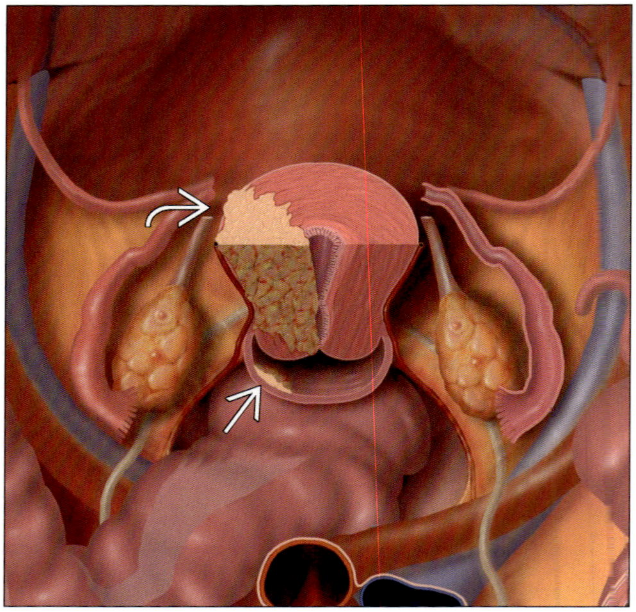

Graphic demonstrates a cut section of the uterus as viewed from above and shows tumor extending to the broad ligament ➚ and involving the vagina ➔. In T2 disease, the tumor extends outside the uterus but is limited to the genital tract.

GESTATIONAL TROPHOBLASTIC DISEASE

T2 (FIGO II) Disease

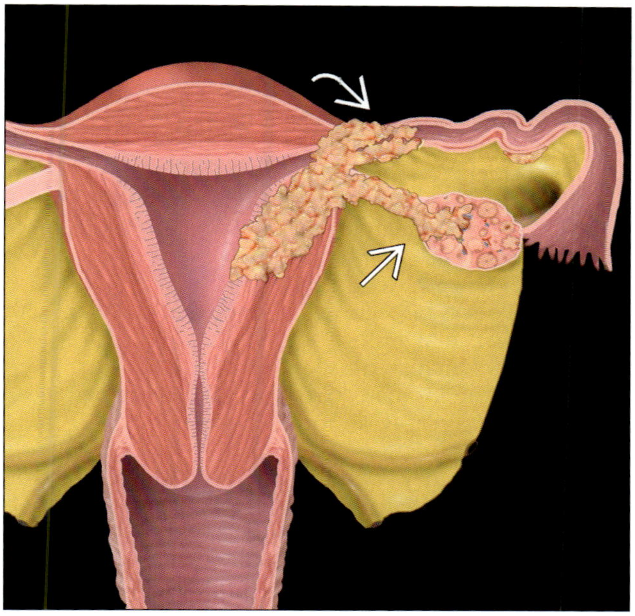

This coronal graphic shows gestational trophoblastic disease extending to the fallopian tube ➦ and involving the ovary ➔. In T2 disease the tumor extends outside the uterus but is limited to the genital tract.

T2 (FIGO II) Disease

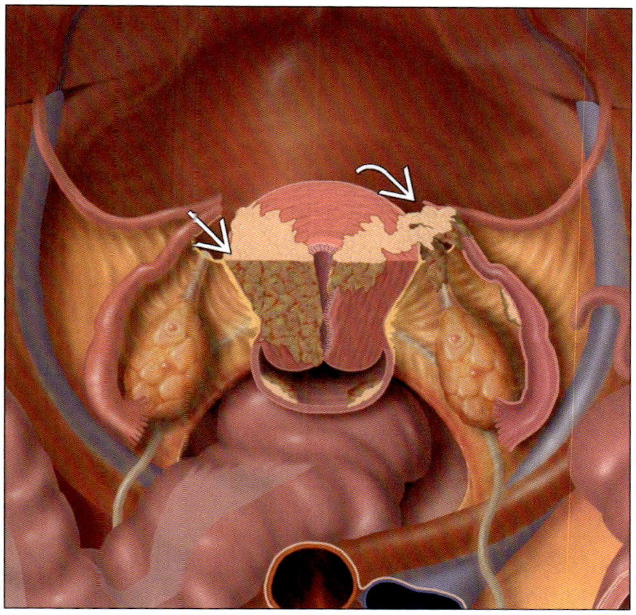

Graphic demonstrates a cut section of the uterus as viewed from above and shows gestational trophoblastic disease extending to the fallopian tube ➦ and broad ligament ➔. In T2 disease the tumor extends outside the uterus but is limited to the genital tract.

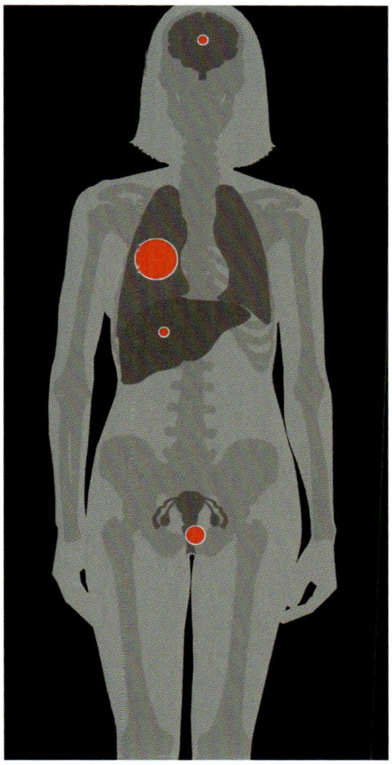

METASTASES, ORGAN FREQUENCY	
Lungs	80%
Vagina	30%
Brain	10%
Liver	10%

GESTATIONAL TROPHOBLASTIC DISEASE

OVERVIEW

General Comments

- Broad spectrum of conditions characterized by abnormal proliferation of trophoblastic tissue

Classification

- Gestational trophoblastic disease (GTD) includes
  - Hydatidiform mole
    - Complete hydatidiform mole (CHM)
    - Partial hydatidiform mole (PHM)
  - Invasive hydatidiform mole (chorioadenoma destruens) (IHM)
  - Choriocarcinoma
  - Placental-site trophoblastic tumor (PSTT)
- Gestational trophoblastic neoplasia (GTN) includes
  - Persistent hydatidiform mole
  - Invasive hydatidiform mole
  - Choriocarcinoma
  - Placental-site trophoblastic tumor

PATHOLOGY

Routes of Spread

- Complete and partial hydatidiform mole
  - By definition, benign localized tumors with malignant potential
  - Confined to uterus without myometrial invasion
- Invasive hydatidiform mole
  - CHM or PHM that invades myometrium
  - Hematogenous metastases can occur to lungs and brain
  - Vaginal metastases can occur via retrograde spread through parauterine veins
- Choriocarcinoma
  - Highly vascular with possible hematogenous spread to lungs, brain, and liver
  - Vaginal metastases are more common than in IHM
- Placental-site trophoplastic tumor
  - Tends to spread locally to uterus
  - Can involve lymph nodes, which is uncommon with other GTN

General Features

- Comments
  - Gestational trophoblastic disease encompasses heterogeneous family of lesions
    - Arise from various trophoblast subpopulations
    - Different malignant potential
- Genetics
  - CHM and IHM show diploid karyotype; completely of paternal origin in majority of patients (46,XX)
    - Single haploid sperm fertilizing ovum lacking maternal genes → duplication
    - 2 sperm fertilizing ovum lacking maternal genes
  - PHM shows triploid karyotype
    - 2 sperm fertilizing normal ovum
  - Choriocarcinoma shows many abnormal karyotypes and can follow normal pregnancy
- Etiology
  - Most important risk factor in development of GTD is previous molar pregnancy
    - Risk increases 10x in patients with previous molar pregnancy
  - Choriocarcinoma may develop after any type of pregnancy
    - 70% develop after complete mole
    - 20% after abortion or tubal pregnancy
    - 10% after term pregnancy
- Epidemiology & cancer incidence
  - GTD are uncommon (overall 1 in 1,000 pregnancies)
    - Incidence varies by geographical location
      - ~ 1/2,000 pregnancies in Europe and USA
      - ~ 1/500 pregnancies in Japan, Singapore, and Malaysia
    - Incidence varies by age
      - 2 peaks of occurrence in women (< 20 or > 40 years of age)
      - > 5x increased risk in women > 40 years
  - Choriocarcinoma is rare (1 in 20,000 pregnancies)
- Associated diseases, abnormalities
  - Theca-lutein cysts
    - Result from ovarian hyperstimulation due to high circulating levels of β-hCG
    - Often resolve 2-4 months following molar evacuation, though regression process generally takes longer than decline in β-hCG levels
    - Occur more frequently with invasive moles and choriocarcinoma than in complete moles
      - 13.8% of complete moles
      - 57.9% of invasive moles
      - 33.3% of choriocarcinoma
  - Uterine vascular malformations
    - GTD are highly vascular and associated with uterine vascular malformations
    - Vascular malformations persist in 10–15% of patients, even after complete tumor resolution following chemotherapy
    - Majority are supplied predominantly by uterine arteries
    - 1–2% of uterine vascular malformations cause vaginal or intraperitoneal hemorrhage

Gross Pathology & Surgical Features

- Complete hydatidiform mole
  - Large-for-dates uterus
  - Bulky mass, sometimes consisting of over 500 cc of bloody tissue
  - Classical bunch of grapes appearance
    - Large villi forming transparent vesicles of variable size (1-30 mm)
  - No normal placental tissue is apparent
  - Absent embryo or fetus
- Partial hydatidiform mole
  - Volume of tissue is often < 300 cc
  - Only proportion of villi are vesicular
  - Presence of embryonic or fetal tissues
    - Most spontaneously abort by 20 weeks
- Invasive hydatidiform mole
  - Pathologic diagnosis of invasive mole is rarely made because most cases are treated medically, without hysterectomy
  - All cases of invasive mole are sequelae of hydatidiform moles
  - Molar villi grow into myometrium or its blood vessels

- May extend into broad ligament and other pelvic organs
- Rarely metastatic
  - Metastasizes to lungs and brain
- Choriocarcinoma
  - May arise after normal (1/25,000) or abnormal pregnancy
  - Dark red hemorrhagic mass with shaggy irregular surface
  - Usually myometrial in location but can invade into surrounding structures
- Placental-site trophoblastic tumor
  - Rare tumor arising from placental implantation site
  - Can develop from normal pregnancy, abortion, CHM, or PHM
  - Slow growing
  - Variable in size but may present with diffuse nodular thickening of myometrium
  - Occasionally polypoid mass projecting into uterine cavity

Microscopic Pathology

- H&E
  - Complete hydatidiform mole
    - Lack of embryonic or fetal tissues
    - Cyst-like hydropic swelling of chorionic villi
    - Diffuse trophoblastic hyperplasia
    - Disintegration and loss of blood vessels in villous core
    - Diffuse & marked trophoblastic atypia at implantation site
    - Premalignant disease
      - 16% of complete moles transform into malignant GTD
  - Partial hydatidiform mole
    - Presence of embryonic or fetal tissues
    - Focal trophoblastic hyperplasia
    - Variable, usually less intense, hydropic swelling of chorionic villi
    - Focal & mild trophoblastic atypia at implantation site
    - Premalignant disease
      - 0.5% of partial moles can transform into malignant GTD
  - Invasive hydatidiform mole
    - Molar pregnancy in which molar villi grow into myometrium or its blood vessels
    - Molar villi with trophoblasts within myometrium or at extrauterine site
  - Choriocarcinoma
    - Malignant neoplasm of trophoblastic epithelium
    - Masses and sheets of trophoblastic cells without villi invading surrounding tissue and permeating vascular spaces
    - Spread to distant sites
    - Most cases present within year of antecedent pregnancy
      - However, cases described after latent periods of up to 25 years
  - Placental-site trophoblastic tumor
    - Neoplastic proliferation of intermediate trophoblasts that invade myometrium at placental site
    - Relatively poorly vascularized
    - Serum hCG only modestly elevated due to lack of syncytiotrophoblastic tissue

IMAGING FINDINGS

Detection

- Ultrasound
  - Complete hydatidiform mole
    - Early in pregnancy
      - Enlarged uterus filled with solid hyperechoic tissue
      - Only 56% of CHM shows cysts in 1st trimester
      - Gestational sac surrounding echogenic mass may be seen
      - Can be difficult to differentiate early CHM from retained products of conception following miscarriage
    - Late in pregnancy
      - Hydropic villi appear as multiple anechoic spaces 1-30 mm in diameter
      - Cysts become more numerous and visible in 2nd trimester
    - Low resistance arterial flow on Doppler interrogation (resistive index [RI] ≈ 0.55)
    - 5 sonographic features are more often seen with GTD compared to retained products of conception
      - Myometrial epicenter
      - Depth of myometrial invasion > 1/3
      - Placental venous lakes
      - Maximum mass dimension > 3.45 cm
      - Maximum endometrial thickness < 12 mm
    - Theca lutein cysts: Large ovaries with multiple anechoic cysts
  - Partial hydatidiform mole
    - Size of placenta depends on genetic profile
      - Large placenta with focal numerous cysts if extra paternal chromosome (69,XXY)
      - Small placenta if extra maternal chromosome (69,XXX)
    - Maintained overall shape of placenta
    - Gestational sac (GS) is present
    - Ratio of transverse to anteroposterior diameter of GS > 1.5
    - Abnormal fetus with multiple anomalies and growth restriction
  - Invasive hydatidiform mole
    - CHM with myometrial invasion
  - Choriocarcinoma
    - Uterine disease may be absent in patients with metastatic disease
    - Focally irregular, echogenic, heterogeneous regions within myometrium
    - Sonolucent areas surrounding echogenic foci correspond to myometrial hemorrhage
    - Highly vascular on Doppler US
  - Placental-site trophoblastic tumor
    - Heterogeneous hyperechoic mass with cystic changes within myometrium
    - Doppler US: Both hypervascular & hypovascular forms have been described
- CT
  - Limited role in detection of GTD

GESTATIONAL TROPHOBLASTIC DISEASE

- Complete and partial hydatidiform mole
  - Heterogeneously enhancing endometrial mass
  - Reticular pattern of enhancement between low-signal vesicles
- Invasive hydatidiform mole
  - Similar to hydatidiform mole with myometrial invasion
- Choriocarcinoma and PSTT
  - Myometrial mass ± endometrial component
  - Heterogeneous enhancement with prominent enhancing vessels

- MR
  - Complete hydatidiform mole
    - T1WI: Isointense to myometrium (areas of hemorrhage are hyperintense)
    - T2WI: Markedly hyperintense mass distends endometrial cavity
    - Gadolinium-enhanced T1WI: Numerous cystic areas may be seen in mass
    - Normal myometrium surrounds mass
  - Partial hydatidiform mole
    - Appears as complete hydatidiform mole
    - Abnormal fetus may be identified
  - Invasive hydatidiform mole
    - Endometrial mass with irregular interface between mass and myometrium
    - Disruption of junctional zone may be seen
    - T1WI: Isointense to myometrium with scattered foci of high signal intensity because of hemorrhage
    - T2WI: Heterogeneous mixed signal intensity with myometrial invasion
    - Gadolinium-enhanced T1WI: Vesicular structures appear as tiny low signal structures within enhanced zone of trophoblastic proliferation
  - Choriocarcinoma and PSTT
    - MR findings are not specific
    - Numerous signal voids on all sequences
    - Myometrial mass ± endometrial component
    - T1WI: Iso- or hyperintense to myometrium
    - T2WI: Slightly to markedly hyperintense to myometrium
    - Prominent blood vessels are seen in most cases
    - Arterial phase dynamic gadolinium-enhanced images: Prominent enhancing vessels

Staging

- Local staging
  - Imaging is indicated in patients with persistent trophoblastic disease
    - MR is superior to CT and US in establishing myometrial invasion in GTN
    - MR and CT can be used to evaluate for extrauterine genital involvement
      - Manifests as enhancing parametrial soft tissue mass
- Nodal staging
  - Nodal involvement is rare in GTN
    - More common with PSTT
  - Both CT and MR can be used to evaluate for regional adenopathy
  - No regional nodal designation in staging of GTN
    - Classified as metastatic M1 disease
- Metastatic disease
  - Lung involvement
    - Chest x-ray is adequate to diagnose lung metastasis and is used for counting number of lung metastases to determine risk factor score
      - Chest CT may be used as alternate
      - Use of chest CT instead of chest x-ray in staging of GTN does not alter outcome
    - Patterns of lung involvement
      - Discrete rounded densities
      - Alveolar or "snowstorm" pattern
      - Pleural effusion
      - Embolic pattern caused by pulmonary arterial occlusion
      - Arteriovenous fistulae can occur
  - Liver metastases may be diagnosed by CT or ultrasound imaging
    - Occur late
    - Poor prognosis
    - Can be hemorrhagic and enhance avidly after contrast administration
    - Hypervascular mass with aneurysmal dilatation of intraparenchymal hepatic artery on arterial phase and vascular lakes on venous phase is characteristic appearance
  - Brain metastases
    - MR is preferred for staging of brain metastases
      - CT can be used as alternative
    - Imaging features
      - Usually multiple
      - Occur at gray-white matter junction
      - Most commonly in parietal lobe
      - Surrounding edema and secondary hemorrhage
      - Cerebral metastases enhance avidly
      - Many lesions show high attenuation on unenhanced CT
      - On MR signal characteristics are variable depending on age of associated hemorrhage
    - CTA, MRA, and cerebral angiography can show arteriovenous fistulae
    - β-hCG level should be used to screen for GTN in any woman of reproductive age with brain metastasis or cerebral hemorrhage of unexplained etiology
  - Intraabdominal metastases
    - Abdominal CT scanning is preferred
  - Vaginal metastases
    - 30% of patients with metastatic GTN
    - Most commonly located suburethrally or in fornices
    - Highly vascular and may bleed vigorously if biopsied
- PET/CT
  - May identify occult disease not seen with other imaging modalities

CLINICAL ISSUES

Presentation

- Hydatidiform mole
  - 1st or 2nd trimester presentation
    - Vaginal bleeding
    - Rapid uterine enlargement
    - Large uterine size for dates (> 4 weeks larger than gestational age)

- Hyperemesis gravidarum
- Preeclampsia before 24 weeks
- Absence of fetal heart tones
- β-hCG is greater than expected for gestational age
- Expulsion of vesicles (80%)

- Gestational trophoblastic neoplasia
  - Should be considered in cases of persistent abnormal bleeding following normal pregnancy, abortion, or ectopic pregnancy
  - Persistently rising or plateauing β-hCG levels after evacuation of molar pregnancy
  - FIGO Council 2000 criteria for diagnosis of post-hydatidiform mole GTN
    - Rise in β-hCG level of ≥ 10% of 3 values recorded over 2 weeks (days 1, 7, and 14)
    - Plateau in β-hCG level (± 10%) of 4 values recorded over 3 weeks (days 1, 7, 14, and 21)
    - Persistence of detectable β-hCG level at 6 months or more after evacuation of mole
    - Histologic diagnosis of choriocarcinoma

Cancer Natural History & Prognosis

- CHM and PHM require only uterine evacuation for complete cure
- Cure rate approaches 100% for other invasive tumors with appropriate chemotherapy

Treatment Options

- Major treatment alternatives
  - Complete and partial hydatidiform mole
    - Evacuation with suction curettage
    - Hysterectomy in patients who do not want to preserve fertility
    - Serial hCG measurement weekly until undetectable for 3 weeks and then monthly for 6 months
  - Placental-site trophoblastic tumor
    - Hysterectomy (relatively chemoresistant)
  - Gestational trophoblastic neoplasia
    - Single or combination chemotherapy depending on stage and risk factors
    - Hysterectomy
  - Uterine vascular malformations
    - Treated either by uterine artery embolization or hysterectomy
- Treatment options by stage
  - GTD are effectively treated with chemotherapy, even when widely metastatic
  - Traditional staging based on anatomical tumor location is not adequate to fully categorize patients for treatment and prognosis
  - Other prognostic factors have been added to guide therapy
    - Cumulative score ≤ 6 is considered low-risk disease treatable by single agent chemotherapy
    - Cumulative score ≥ 7 is high-risk disease that requires combination chemotherapy
  - Stage I (low-risk GTN)
    - Single-agent chemotherapy with either methotrexate (MTX) or actinomycin D (ACTD)
    - Single-agent chemotherapy with sequential MTX/ACTD
    - Hysterectomy + single-agent chemotherapy if patient does not desire to retain fertility
    - Combination chemotherapy in patients who develop resistance to single-agent
    - Hysterectomy in patients who develop resistance to combination chemotherapy
  - Stage I (high-risk GTN), II, and III
    - Combination chemotherapy with EMACO (etoposide, MTX, ACTD, cyclophosphamide, and vincristine [Oncovin])
  - Stage IV
    - Combination chemotherapy
    - Whole brain irradiation for cranial metastases
    - Hysterectomy to control bleeding or sepsis
    - Surgical resection of resistant metastatic lesions

REPORTING CHECKLIST

T Staging

- Evaluate for myometrial and extrauterine involvement
  - MR is superior to CT and US

N Staging

- No regional nodal designation in staging of GTN
- Nodal metastases are rare except with PSTT
- Can affect pelvic and inguinal lymph nodes
- Nodal metastases are classified as metastatic M1 disease

M Staging

- Lung metastases are most common
  - Chest x-ray is adequate for staging
- Abdominal metastases
  - Appear as enhancing masses, usually in liver or spleen
  - CT is modality of choice
- Brain metastases
  - Heterogeneous lesions with avid enhancement
  - MR is modality of choice

SELECTED REFERENCES

1. American Joint Committee on Cancer: AJCC Cancer Staging Manual. 7th ed. New York: Springer, 2010
2. Berkowitz RS et al: Current management of gestational trophoblastic diseases. Gynecol Oncol. 112(3):654-62, 2009
3. Darby S et al: Does chest CT matter in the staging of GTN? Gynecol Oncol. 112(1):155-60, 2009
4. Allen SD et al: Radiology of gestational trophoblastic neoplasia. Clin Radiol. 61(4):301-13, 2006
5. Betel C et al: Sonographic diagnosis of gestational trophoblastic disease and comparison with retained products of conception. J Ultrasound Med. 25(8):985-93, 2006
6. Brandt KR et al: MR appearance of placental site trophoblastic tumor: a report of three cases. AJR Am J Roentgenol. 170(2):485-7, 1998
7. Green CL et al: Gestational trophoblastic disease: a spectrum of radiologic diagnosis. Radiographics. 15(6):1371-84, 1996
8. Wagner BJ et al: From the archives of the AFIP. Gestational trophoblastic disease: radiologic-pathologic correlation. Radiographics. 16(1):131-48, 1996

GESTATIONAL TROPHOBLASTIC DISEASE

(Left) *Transverse ultrasound in a patient presenting in the 1st trimester with hyperemesis shows an echogenic endometrial mass* ➔ *distending the uterine cavity. Note the lack of cystic changes, which is typical for a hydatidiform mole in the 1st trimester.* ***(Right)*** *Longitudinal duplex Doppler ultrasound in the same patient shows that the mass is highly vascular with low resistance arterial flow.*

Complete Hydatidiform Mole (Early)

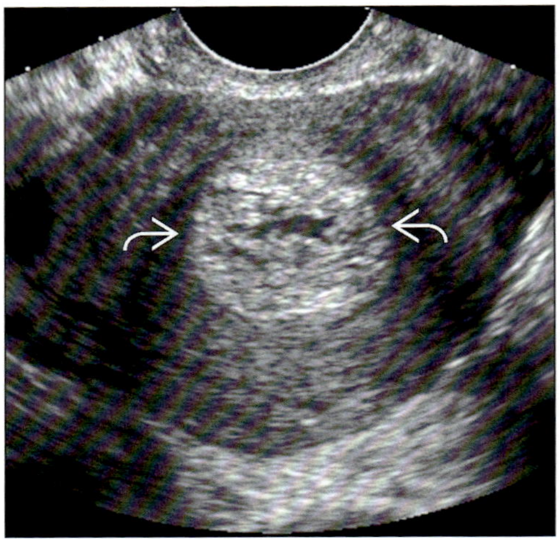

Complete Hydatidiform Mole (Early)

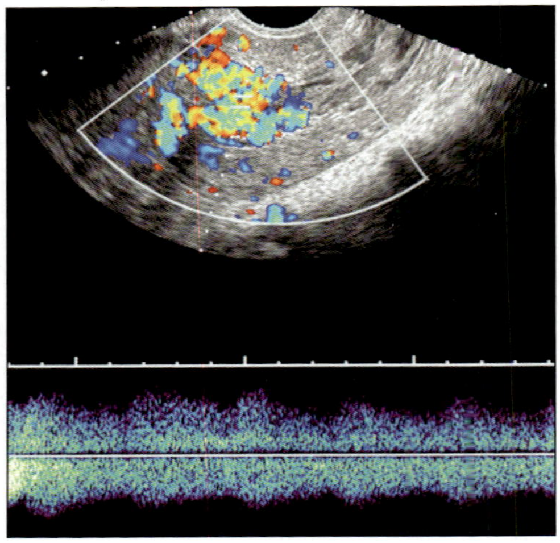

(Left) *Transverse ultrasound shows a uterine mass in a pregnant woman with marked elevation of β-hCG in the 2nd trimester. The mass is echogenic and contains multiple small cysts. The increased echogenicity of the mass is due to the presence of innumerable small cysts below the resolution of ultrasound.* ***(Right)*** *Longitudinal ultrasound in the same patient shows the uterine mass with multiple, small, cystic areas representing the hydropic villi. No fetal parts are seen.*

Complete Hydatidiform Mole (Late)

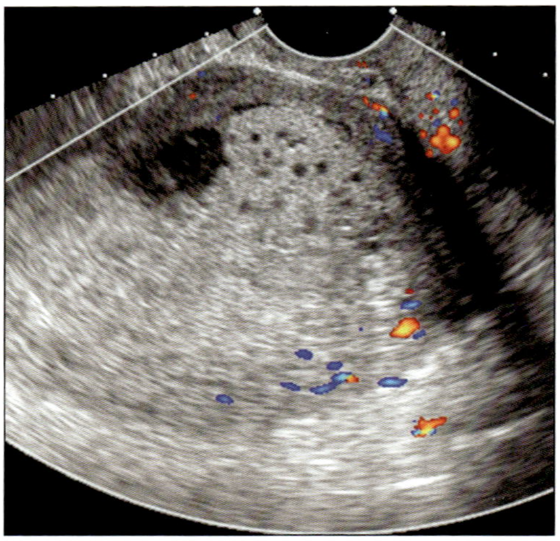

Complete Hydatidiform Mole (Late)

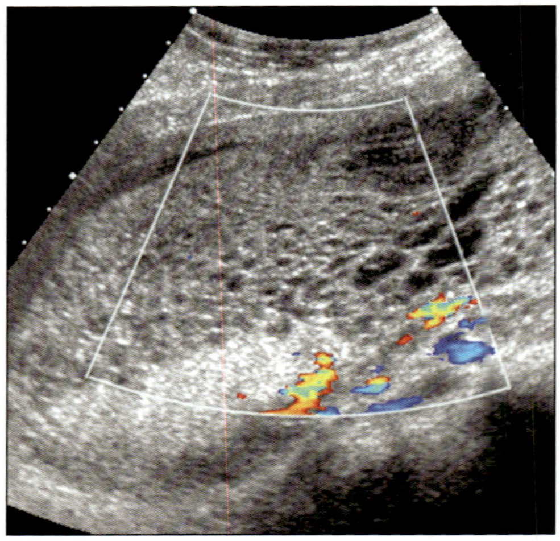

(Left) *Sagittal T2WI MR in a patient with rising β-hCG 3 weeks after an abortion shows a fundal high intensity mass* ➔ *without invasion into the myometrium. Although the appearance is nonspecific and can be seen with retained products of conception, pathology after suction and curettage confirmed the diagnosis.* ***(Right)*** *Axial T2WI MR in the same patient shows the mass* ➔ *with small signal void structures* ➔ *representing prominent vessels.*

Complete Hydatidiform Mole

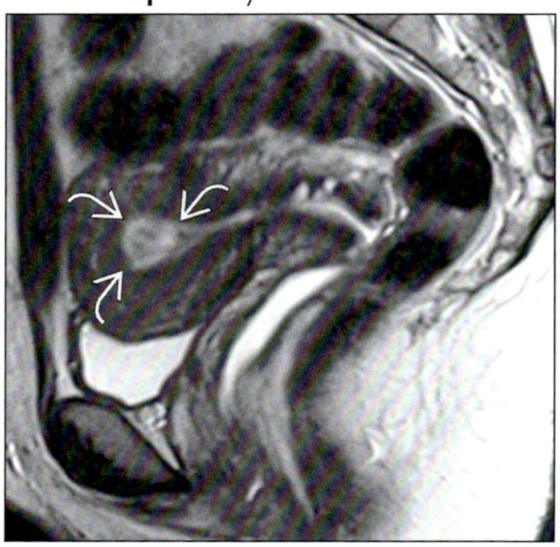

Complete Hydatidiform Mole

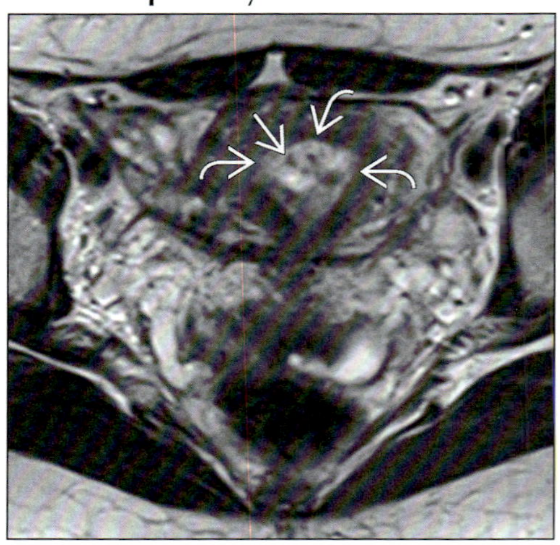

Complete Hydatidiform Mole

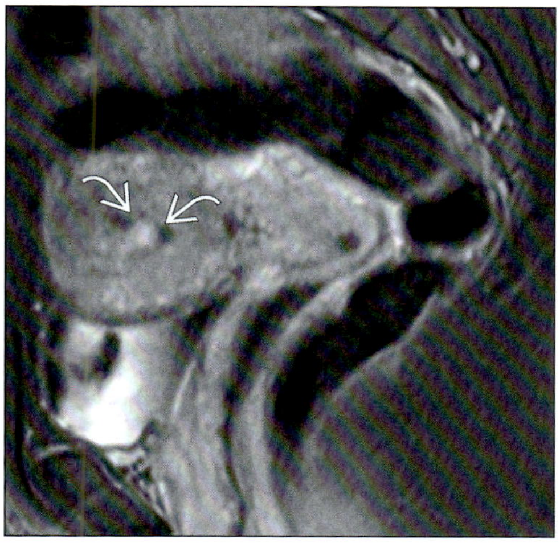

Complete Hydatidiform Mole

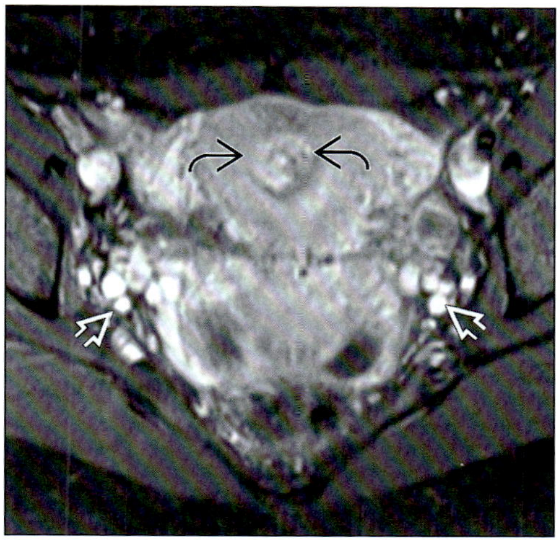

(Left) *In the same patient, sagittal T1WI C+ FS MR also shows an enhancing fundal mass ➔ without evidence of myometrial invasion.* ***(Right)*** *Axial T1WI C+ FS MR in the same patient also demonstrates the enhancing fundal mass ➔. The degree of enhancement correlates with the amount of active trophoblastic tissue and the level of β-hCG. Note the increased parametrial vascularity ➔.*

Complete Hydatidiform Mole

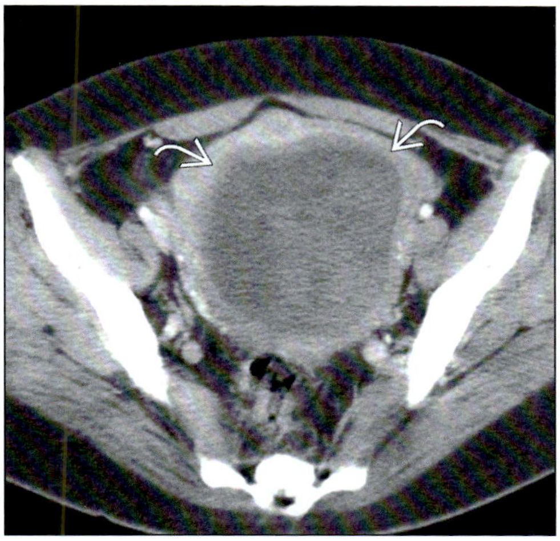

Complete Hydatidiform Mole

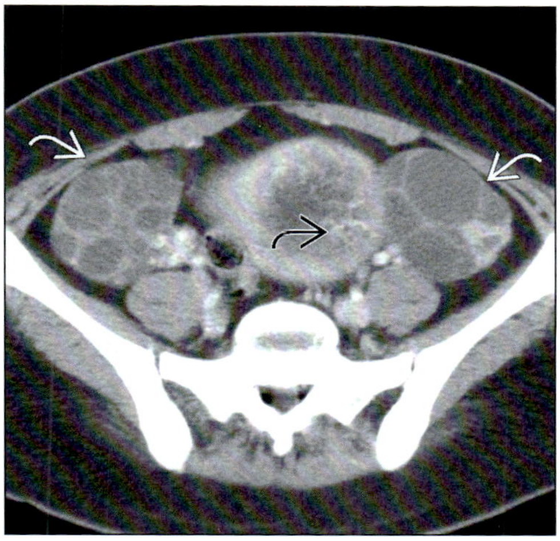

(Left) *Axial CECT at the level of the uterus shows a distended uterine cavity with mixed density soft tissue ➔ representing a molar pregnancy. There is no evidence of extrauterine involvement.* ***(Right)*** *Axial CECT in the same patient shows distended uterus with areas of increased vascularity at the periphery of the uterine mass ➔. Both ovaries are enlarged ➔ and contain multiple large cysts, which represent theca lutein cysts.*

Complete Hydatidiform Mole

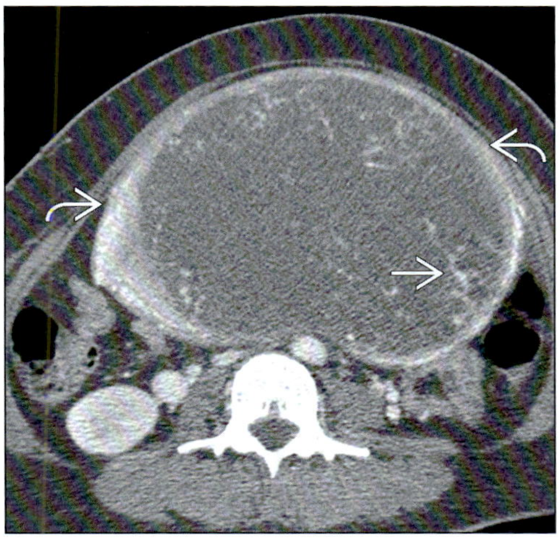

Complete Hydatidiform Mole

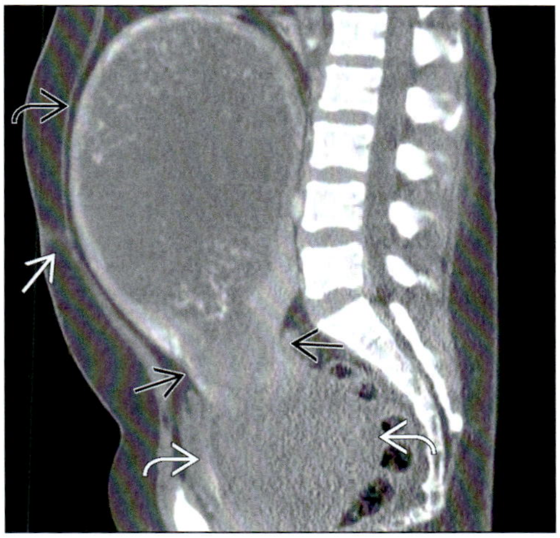

(Left) *Axial CECT shows marked enlargement of the uterus ➔. The uterus is filled with predominantly low density material representing abnormal hydropic villi with enhancing septa ➔ giving the uterine contents a reticular appearance.* ***(Right)*** *Sagittal CECT MIP image in the same patient shows marked uterine enlargement ➔ with the fundus above the umbilicus ➔. The molar pregnancy distends the cervix ➔ and fills the vagina ➔.*

GESTATIONAL TROPHOBLASTIC DISEASE

*(**Left**) Transverse transvaginal ultrasound in an early pregnancy shows a yolk sac adjacent to echogenic trophoblastic tissue. (**Right**) Transverse transabdominal ultrasound shows a large placenta with focal cystic changes. Other parts of the placenta appear normal. Fetal parts are seen. The fetus showed growth restriction and multiple anomalies. Cystic placental changes are seen in triploidy if the extra set of chromosomes is of paternal origin.*

Partial Hydatidiform Mole (Early)

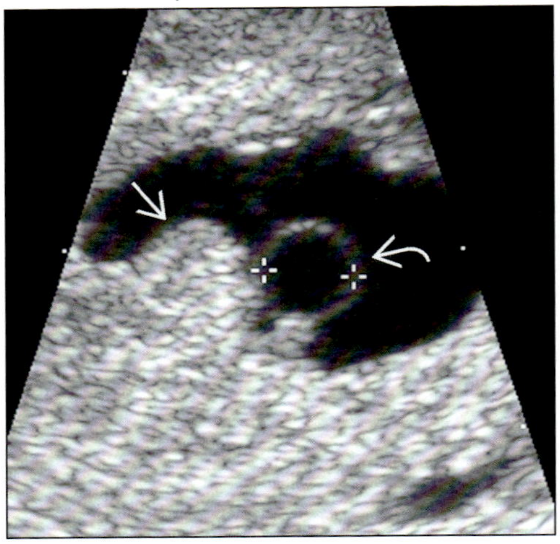

Partial Hydatidiform Mole (Late)

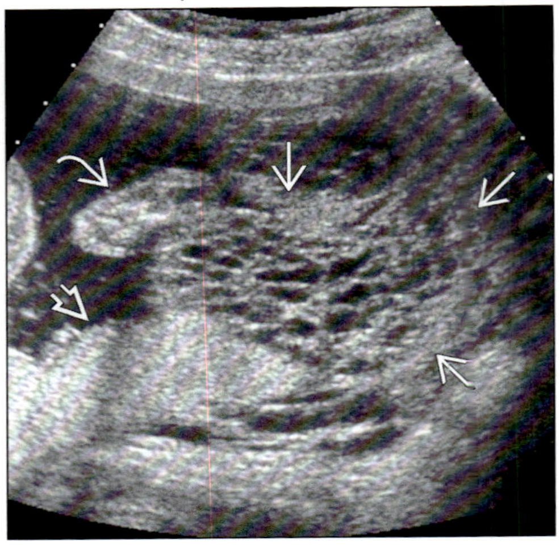

*(**Left**) Axial T2WI MR shows a high signal intensity mass, which fills the uterine cavity and appears to be limited to the endometrium. (**Right**) Sagittal T2WI MR in the same patient shows a retroverted uterus containing an abnormal high T2 signal mass that fills the uterus. Note the sharp interface between the mass and the myometrium of the posterior uterine wall, as well as the loss of endometrial-myometrial interface of the anterior wall due to tumor invasion.*

Invasive Mole

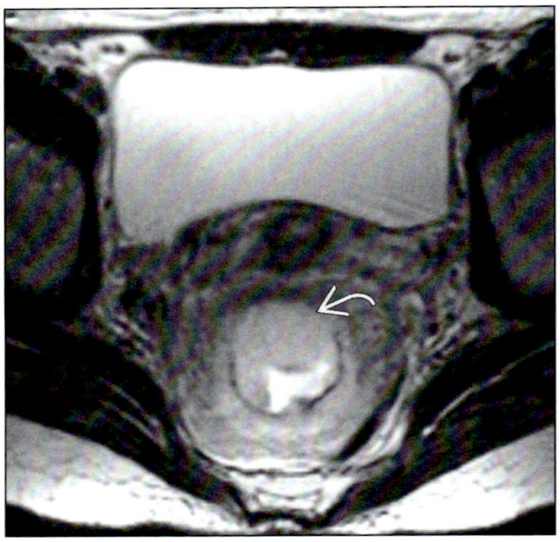

Invasive Mole

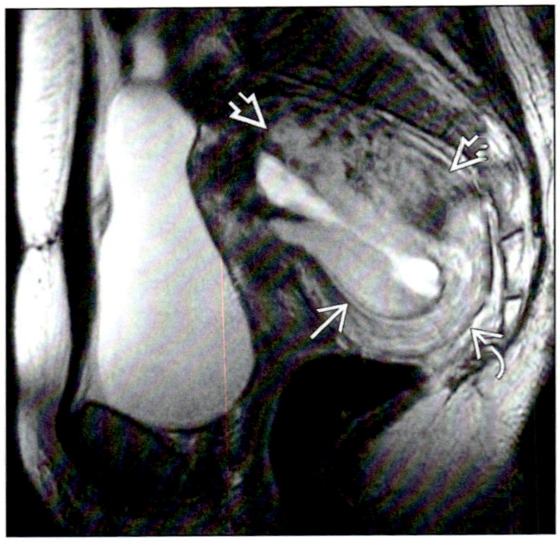

*(**Left**) Sagittal T2WI FS MR in the same patient shows an endometrial mass that is isointense to the normal myometrium. High signal intensity intraluminal blood is also seen. (**Right**) Sagittal T1WI C+ FS MR in the same patient shows the enhancing circumferential endometrial mass with focal extension into the myometrium along the anterior wall. Compare this to the well-defined endometrial-myometrial interface along the posterior wall.*

Invasive Mole

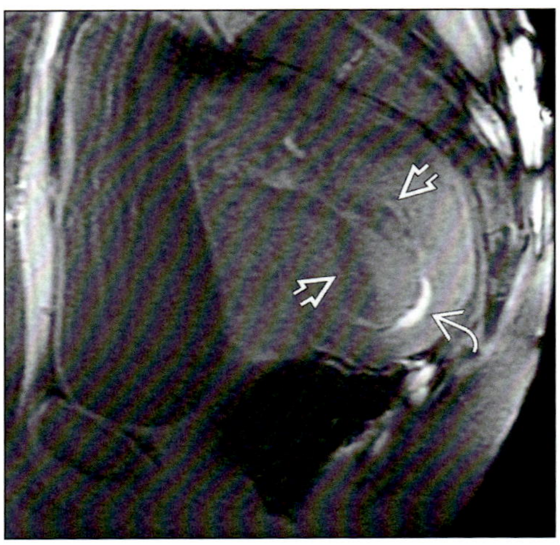

Invasive Mole

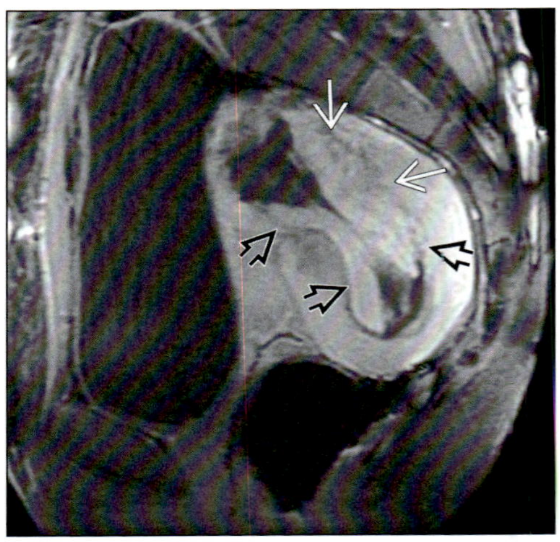

Choriocarcinoma

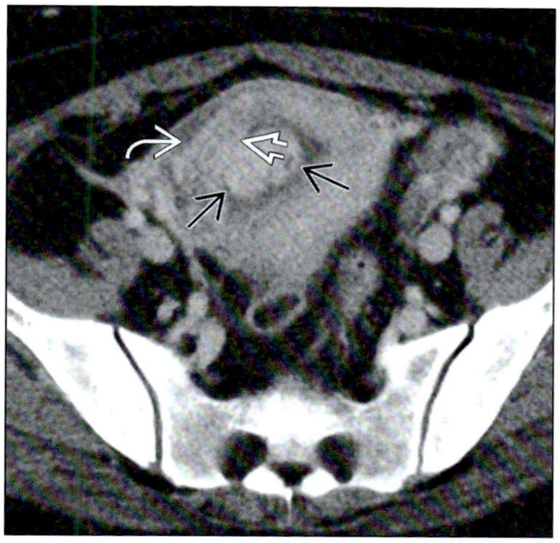

Choriocarcinoma

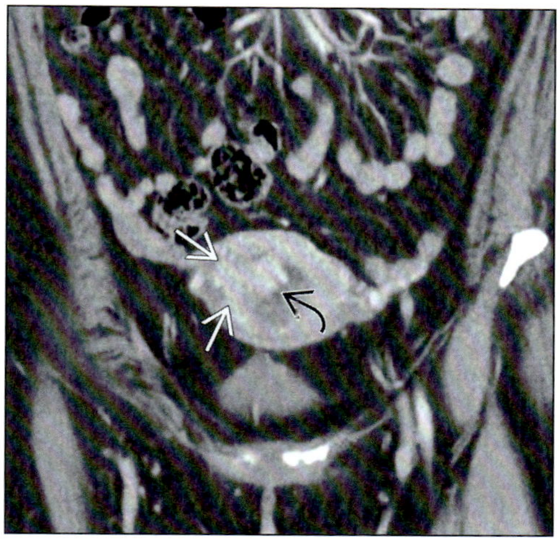

(Left) *Axial CECT in a 25-year-old woman who presented with vaginal bleeding 3 months after full-term delivery shows an enhancing, predominantly endometrial mass distending the uterine cavity with ill-defined interface with the myometrium. Note the increased vascularity within the underlying myometrium.* ***(Right)*** *Coronal CECT in the same patient shows the enhancing mass invading into the myometrium without extrauterine extension.*

Choriocarcinoma

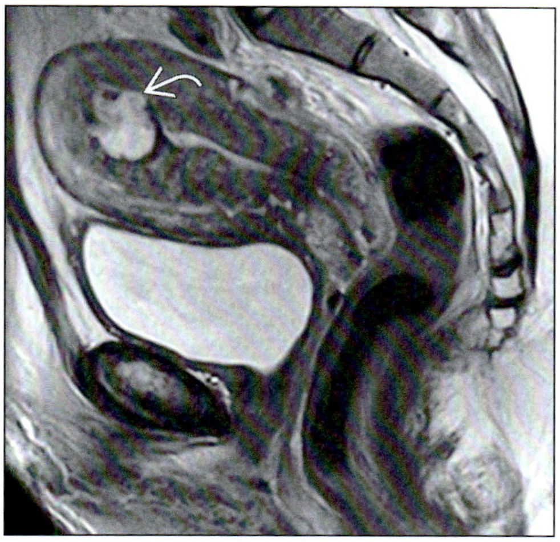

Choriocarcinoma

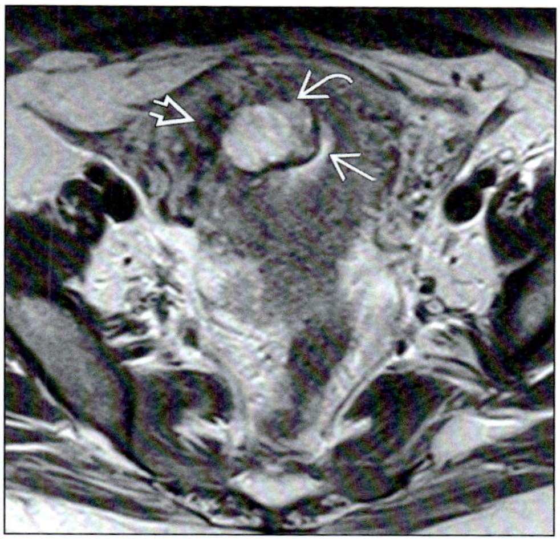

(Left) *Sagittal T2WI MR in the same patient shows a predominantly myometrial mass of high signal intensity in the region of the fundus.* ***(Right)*** *Axial T2WI MR in the same patient shows the hyperintense myometrial fundal mass indenting the endometrium. Note also the prominent vessels appearing as round and tubular signal voids within the myometrium.*

Choriocarcinoma

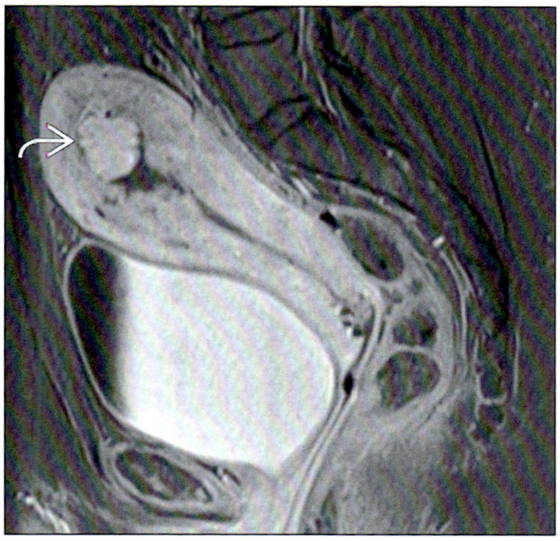

Choriocarcinoma

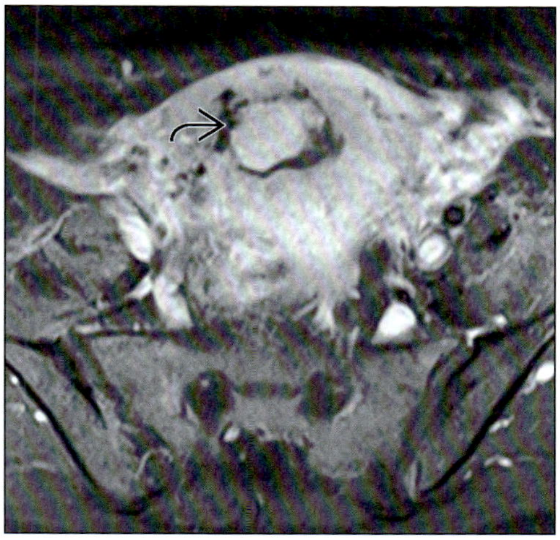

(Left) *Sagittal T1WI C+ FS MR in the same patient shows an enhancing fundal mass. The mass shows more intense enhancement compared to the adjacent myometrium, indicating its high vascularity.* ***(Right)*** *Axial T1WI C+ FS MR in the same patient shows the intense enhancement of the predominantly myometrial mass.*

GESTATIONAL TROPHOBLASTIC DISEASE

*(**Left**) Sagittal T2WI MR in a patient with elevated β-hCG 3 months after the conclusion of a normal pregnancy shows a large high signal intensity mass that appears to distend the uterine cavity with poor endometrial-myometrial interface. (**Right**) Axial T2WI MR in the same patient shows a heterogeneous high signal intensity mass filling the uterine cavity. Myometrial invasion is not clear on these images. Note the low signal intensity septae within the mass.*

Choriocarcinoma

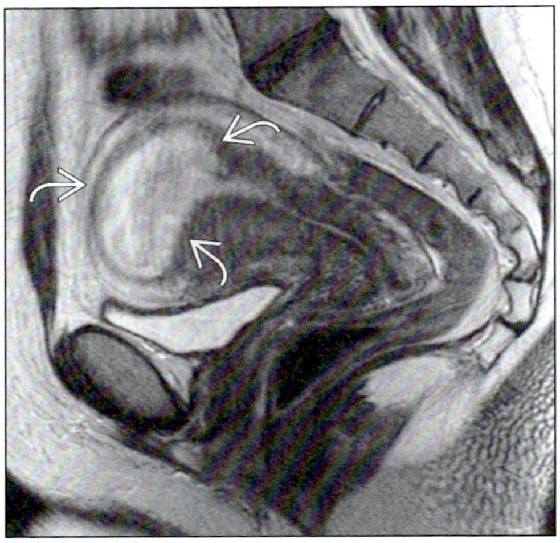

Choriocarcinoma

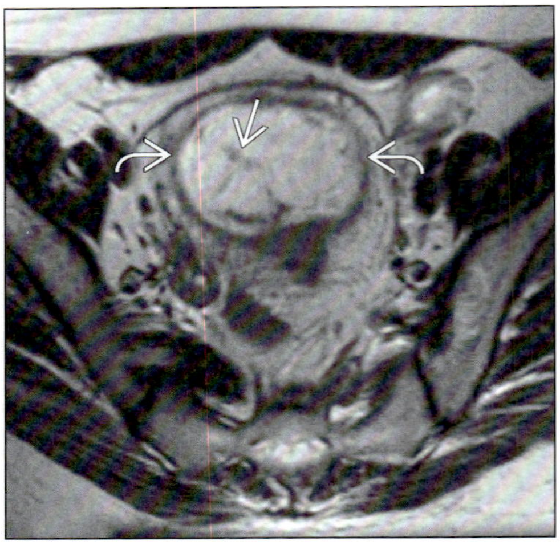

*(**Left**) Sagittal T1WI C+ FS MR in the same patient shows an enhancing fundal mass that invades the myometrium and extends to the serosal surface of the uterus. This and the previous 2 images show that the mass is actually myometrial in location with displacement of the enhancing endometrium. (**Right**) Axial T1WI C+ FS MR in the same patient again shows the enhancing, predominantly myometrial mass that displaces the enhancing endometrium.*

Choriocarcinoma

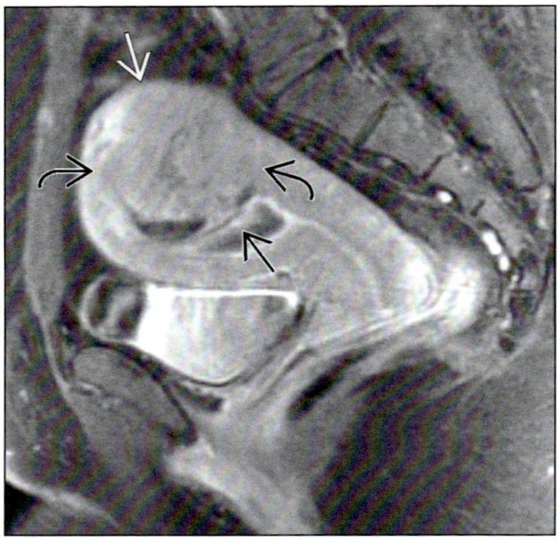

Choriocarcinoma

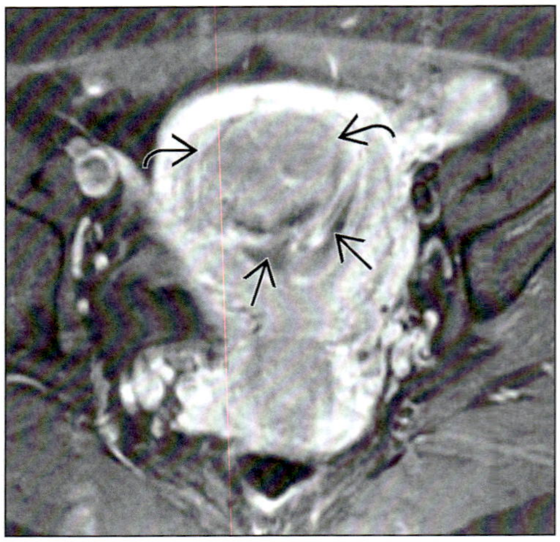

*(**Left**) Axial T2WI MR in a 34-year-old woman, who presented with persistent elevation of β-hCG 3 months after spontaneous abortion, shows a fundal mass that is predominantly of high T2 signal intensity with a central area of low signal intensity, likely due to intralesional bleeding. (**Right**) Axial T1WI C+ FS MR shows a peripherally enhancing fundal mass that reaches to the serosal surface without extrauterine extension.*

Choriocarcinoma

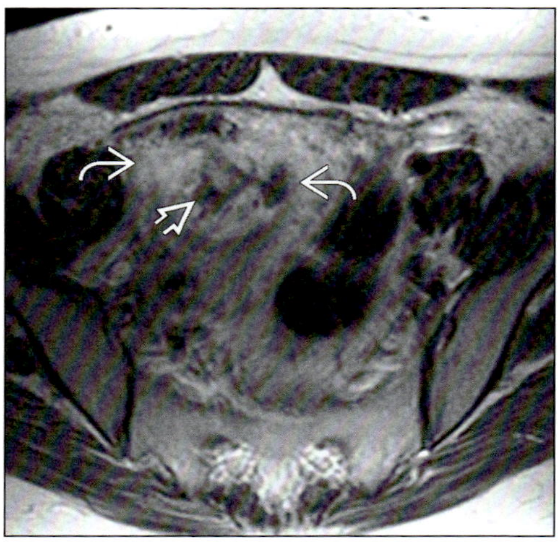

Choriocarcinoma

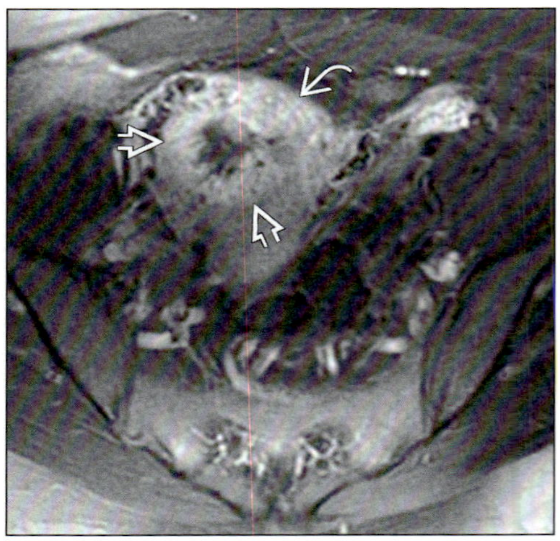

GESTATIONAL TROPHOBLASTIC DISEASE

Placental-Site Trophoblastic Tumor (T1)

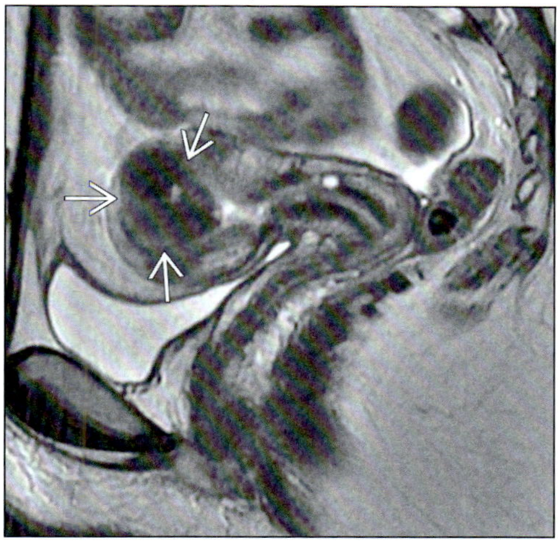

Placental-Site Trophoblastic Tumor (T1)

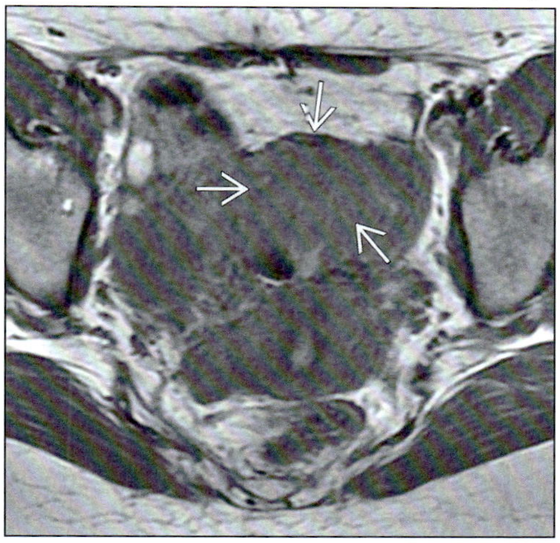

(Left) *Sagittal T2WI MR shows a fundal mass ➡ of low signal intensity relative to the myometrium with small intralesional foci of high T2 signal intensity in a 31-year-old woman who had an abortion at 7 weeks gestational age and continued to have elevated β-hCG. The mass extends to the serosal surface without penetrating the serosa.* ***(Right)*** *Axial T1WI MR in the same patient shows that the uterine mass ➡ is isointense to the myometrium on T1W images.*

Placental-Site Trophoblastic Tumor (T1)

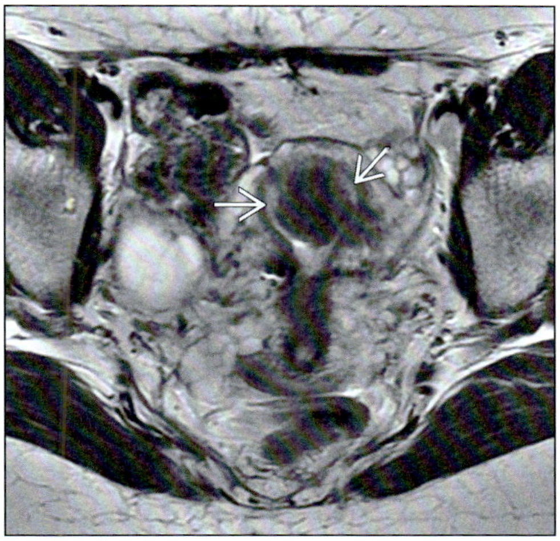

Placental-Site Trophoblastic Tumor (T1)

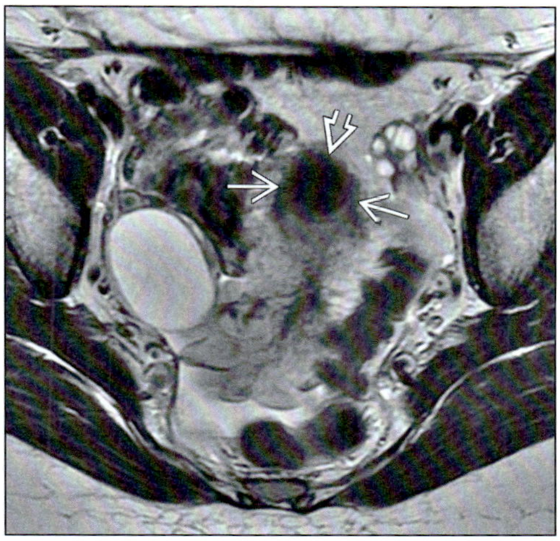

(Left) *Axial T2WI MR in the same patient shows an endometrial mass ➡ of low signal intensity relative to the myometrium.* ***(Right)*** *Axial T2WI MR in the same patient at a higher level shows the low T2 signal mass ➡ extending into the myometrium to the serosal surface ⮚ without actual serosal penetration. At hysterectomy, the mass was confined to the uterus without extension to other pelvic organs, consistent with T1 disease.*

Placental-Site Trophoblastic Tumor (T1)

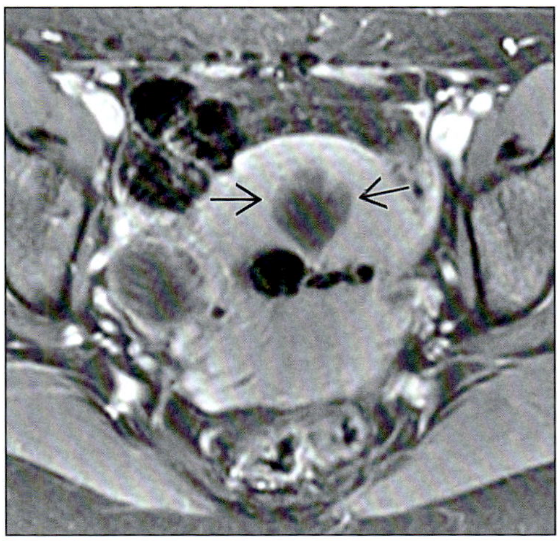

Placental-Site Trophoblastic Tumor (T1)

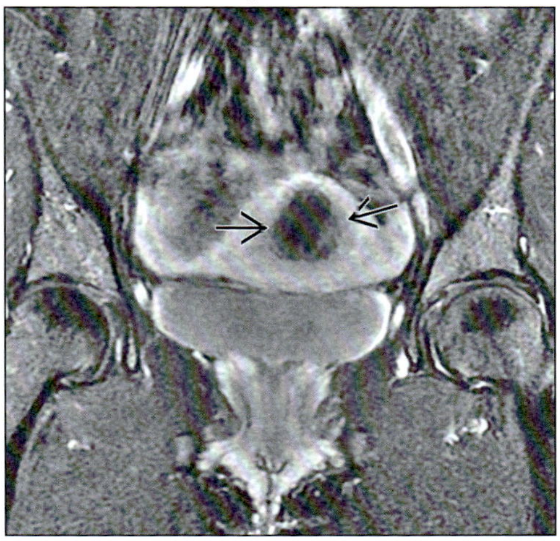

(Left) *Axial T1WI C+ FS MR in the same patient shows that the endometrial/myometrial mass ⇨ is poorly enhancing relative to the normally enhancing myometrium.* ***(Right)*** *Coronal T1WI C+ FS MR in the same patient shows the hypovascular mass ⇨ within the myometrium. Both enhancing and poorly enhancing patterns may be seen on imaging, which correspond to the hypervascular and hypovascular patterns seen on pathologic evaluation, respectively.*

GESTATIONAL TROPHOBLASTIC DISEASE

(Left) *Axial CECT in a patient who presented with modest elevation of β-hCG following a normal pregnancy shows a highly vascular mass that invades the myometrium. The uterus is filled with high-density material due to an intraluminal hemorrhage.* ***(Right)*** *Coronal CECT in the same patient shows a highly vascular myometrial mass with tumor extending into the left parametrium. Extrauterine tumor extension constitutes T2 disease.*

Placental-Site Trophoblastic Tumor (T2)

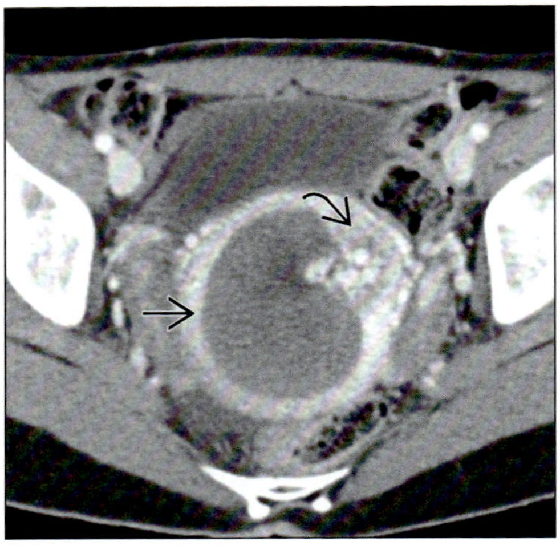

Placental-Site Trophoblastic Tumor (T2)

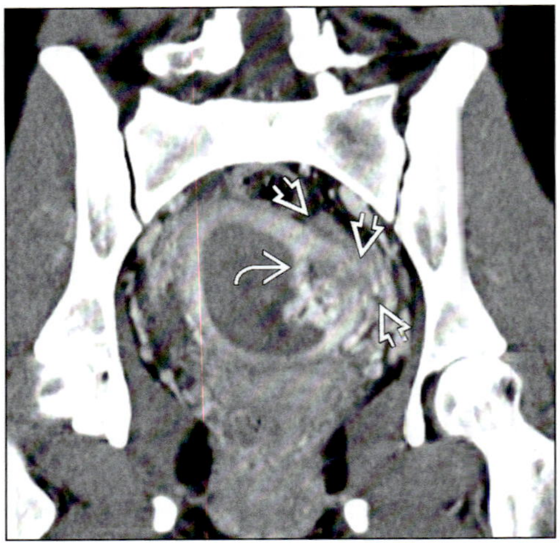

(Left) *Sagittal T2WI MR in the same patient shows an anterior wall myometrial mass of high signal intensity in a retroverted uterus. Note the multiple signal void structures within the mass due to a rich vascular supply.* ***(Right)*** *Axial T2WI MR in the same patient shows a predominantly myometrial mass of high signal intensity containing multiple signal-void-like rounded and tubular structures due to increased vascularity.*

Placental-Site Trophoblastic Tumor (T2)

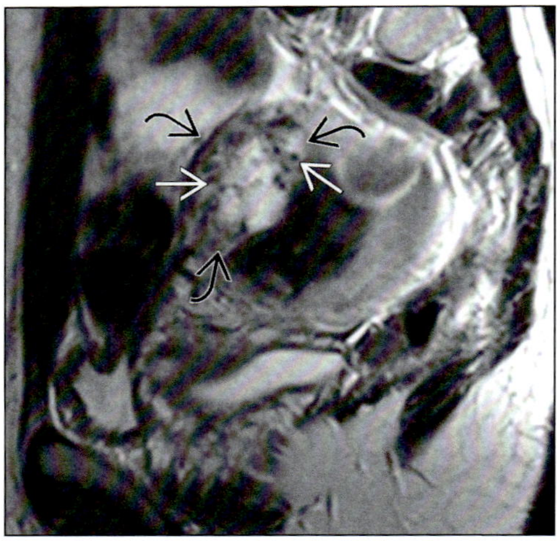

Placental-Site Trophoblastic Tumor (T2)

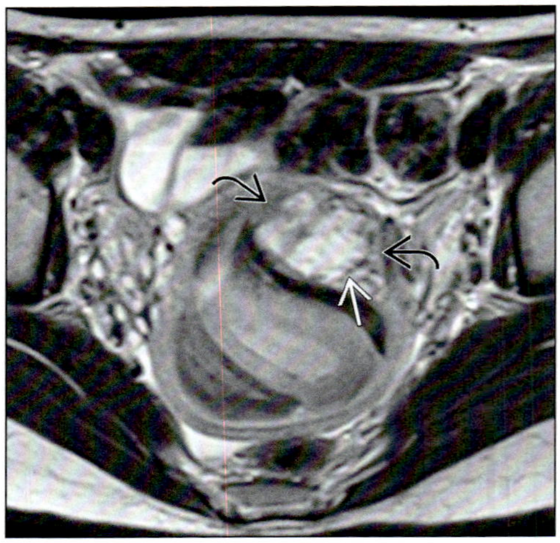

(Left) *Sagittal T1WI C+ FS MR in the same patient demonstrates the enhancing, highly vascular, myometrial mass and blood filling the uterine cavity. This case represents the highly vascular pattern of PSTT.* ***(Right)*** *Axial T1WI C+ FS MR in the same patient shows a highly vascular mass with heterogeneous enhancement. The uterine cavity is filled with high T1 signal intensity blood products. Left parametrial tumor extension is seen.*

Placental-Site Trophoblastic Tumor (T2)

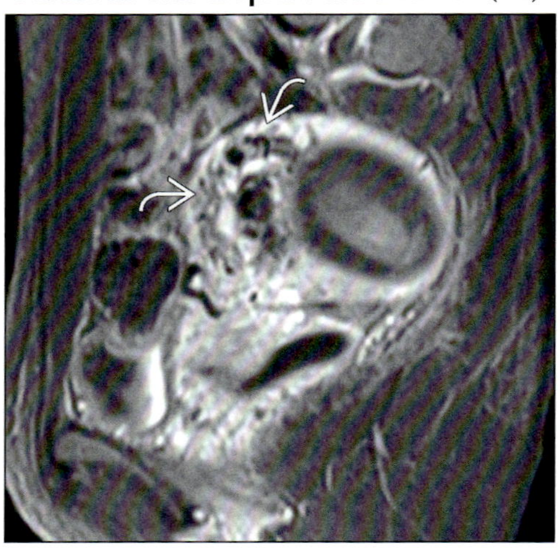

Placental-Site Trophoblastic Tumor (T2)

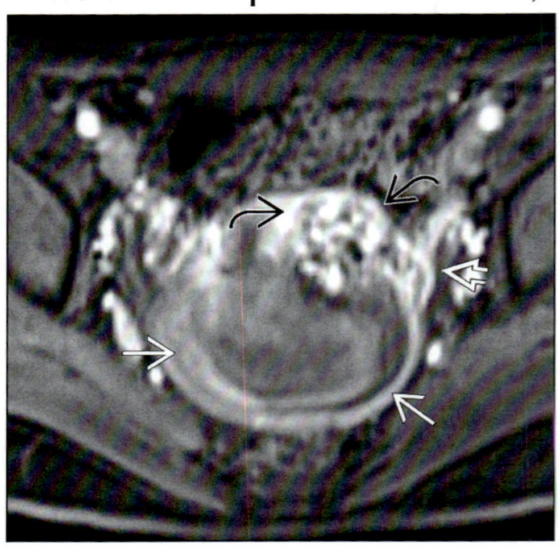

GESTATIONAL TROPHOBLASTIC DISEASE

Post-Treatment Arteriovenous Fistula

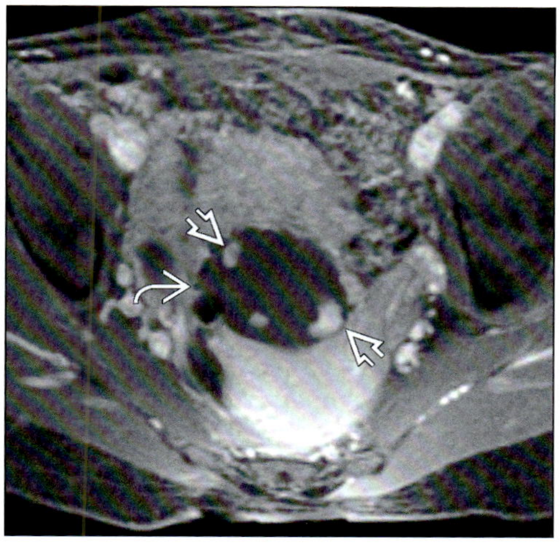

Post-Treatment Arteriovenous Fistula

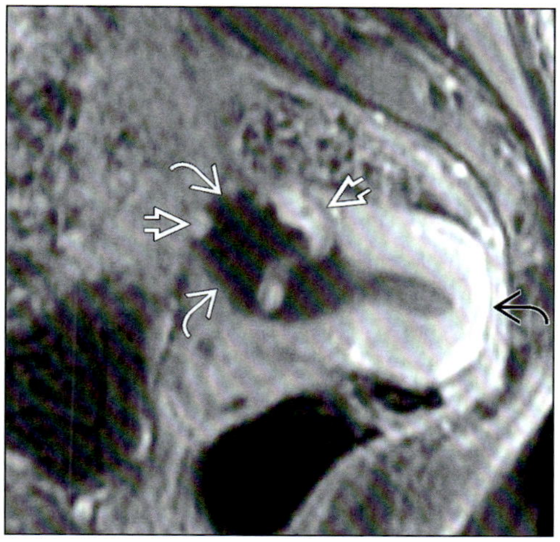

(Left) *This patient received single-agent chemotherapy for treatment of an invasive mole and presented with vaginal bleeding. This axial T1WI C+ FS MR shows a fluid-filled cavity at the site of the treated mass that contains multiple large blood vessels at its periphery.* ***(Right)*** *Sagittal T1WI C+ FS MR in the same patient shows the retroverted uterus and a large cavity with large serpiginous vessels at the periphery of the cavity.*

Metastatic Choriocarcinoma

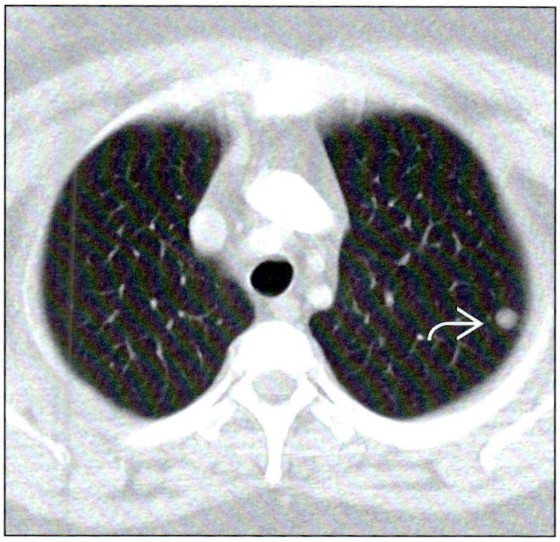

Metastatic Choriocarcinoma

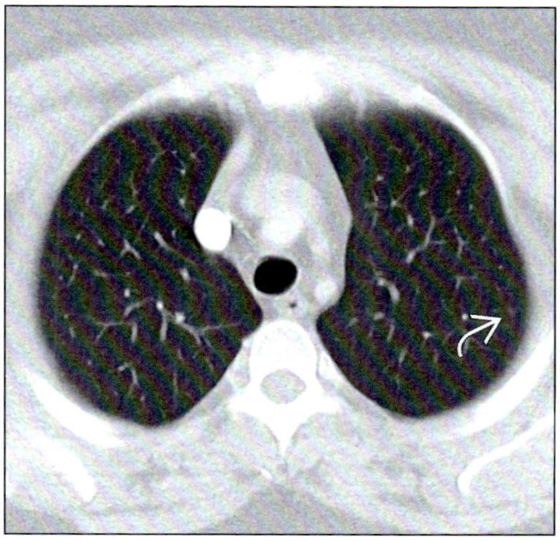

(Left) *Axial CECT in lung window shows a round, soft tissue density nodule in the left upper lobe in a patient with an invasive mole diagnosed after CHM.* ***(Right)*** *Axial CECT in lung widow in the same patient obtained 3 months later, after the patient received methotrexate, shows almost complete resolution of the nodule. Two other smaller nodules completely resolved with treatment.*

Metastatic Choriocarcinoma

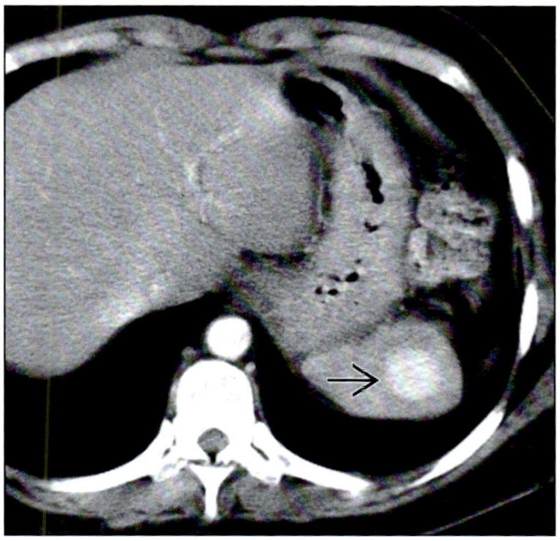

Metastatic Choriocarcinoma

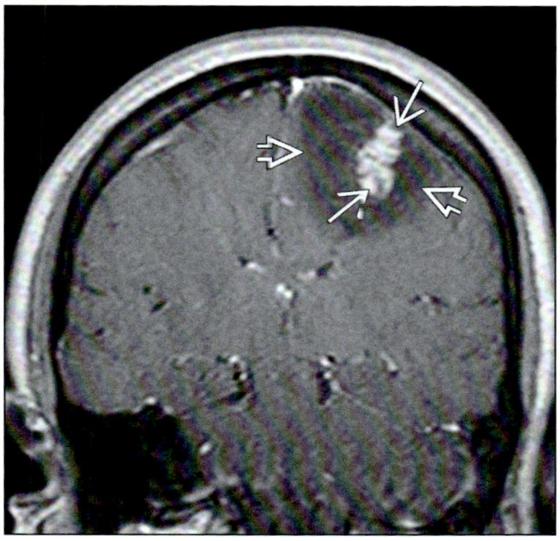

(Left) *Axial CECT in a patient with persistent elevation of β-hCG shows an intensely enhancing splenic mass. The patient also had lung metastases. It is uncommon for patients with gestational trophoblastic neoplasia to present with abdominal metastases in the absence of lung metastases.* ***(Right)*** *Coronal T1WI C+ MR shows an enhancing lesion in the left parietal region with surrounding edema.*

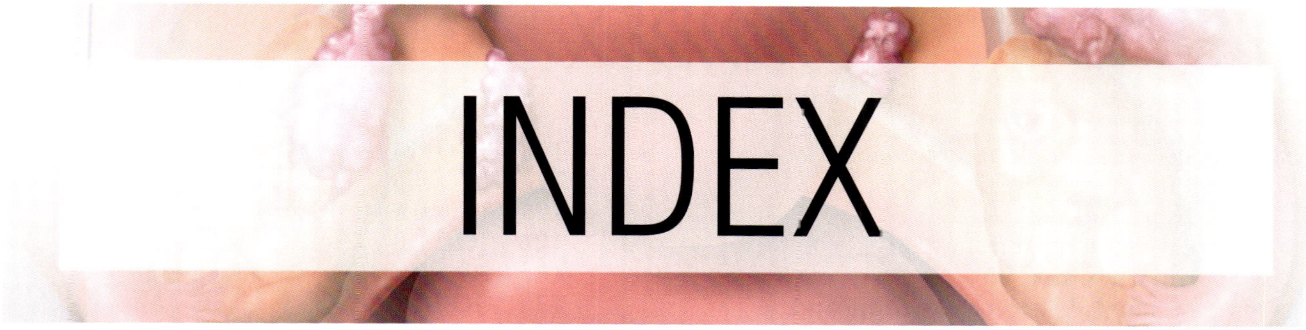

INDEX

A

C

INDEX

INDEX

L

M

O

S

T

U

V

INDEX